SURVIVAL STRONG

SURVIVAL STRONG

A GUIDE TO STREET SURVIVAL AND STRENGTH

PHIL ROSS

Copyright © 2016 by Phil Ross.

Library of Congress Control Number: 2016901545
ISBN: Hardcover   978-1-5144-5514-2
               Softcover   978-1-5144-5513-5
               eBook   978-1-5144-5512-8

All rights reserved. No part of this book may be reproduced or transmitted in any form or by any means, electronic or mechanical, including photocopying, recording, or by any information storage and retrieval system, without permission in writing from the copyright owner.

Any people depicted in stock imagery provided by Thinkstock are models, and such images are being used for illustrative purposes only.
Certain stock imagery © Thinkstock.

Print information available on the last page.

Rev. date: 02/26/2016

To order additional copies of this book, contact:
Xlibris
1-888-795-4274
www.Xlibris.com
Orders@Xlibris.com
731011

CONTENTS

Prelude xv

Acknowledgments xix

Forewords... xxi

Introduction xxvii

1. Undeniable Self-Defense Truths 1
2. Real-World Application 9
3. Mind-Set... 15
4. Physical Fitness and Strength 33
5. Weapons of the Human Body 91
6. Targets of the Human Body 101
7. Generation of Power.. 111
8. Grips and Locks 117
9. Entry and Single Techniques 135
10. Movement and Zones.. 163
11. Basic Grappling 167
12. Combinations and Series 171
13. Street Applications and Tactics 175
14. Practice and Training Routines 247
15. Dog Attacks 261

16. Unconventional Weapons...265

17. Conventional Weapons..271

18. Home Preparedness..275

19. Everyday Public Places 277

20. Mass Hysteria...281

21. Car Safety 287

22. The Importance of Training: Practice Cycle......................................291

23. Breathing and Meditation 297

Epilogue..299

Recommended Training Aids..301

It's dark, and you're alone walking down a deserted street in a strange city. You hear footsteps behind you. They are quickening. You pick up your pace, and the footsteps become faster and louder. You look over your shoulder and . . .

You are awakened from your slumber to the sound of your windows being jostled. A faint crash as the windowpane gets broken and the glass smashes to the floor. Then you hear the window hinges creak open and a pair of feet land. The intruder makes his way across the room, and you hear the door to your bedroom open and . . .

The elevator doors are about to close. An arm reaches in and props the door open, enabling six rowdy youths to enter. They look at you, laughing, and the comments begin as the circle closes around you and . . .

You are at the mall, and you have forgotten where you parked your car. Your arms laden with packages, you search in the darkness for your vehicle. Suddenly, you hear a voice break the silence. "Are you lost?" You turn around and . . .

It's date night, and you and your girl just had a great dinner, and you decide to go dancing at a local club. You're out on the dance floor, and there's a group of guys out there, and they begin to bump into you and start to grind your girlfriend. The dance floor is crowded, and there's no way for you to get out of the circle, nor can you get the attention of security. You see the fear in the eyes of your girl, and then . . .

Your car breaks down on a deserted highway. It's going to take an hour for AAA to arrive. You are traveling with your wife and two small children. You see a pickup arrives and pulls up behind you. Three large, scruffy gentlemen get out and approach your vehicle. Two of the men come to your window, and the other goes to your wife's car door. With a gap-toothed grin, the man closest to you says, "You havin' a little car trouble, er ya?" You see a crowbar in his hand and . . .

Scary scenarios, aren't they? What would you do? Read this book and find out how to be prepared for *similar* situations as they arise.

Praise for Survival Strong

I'm constantly asked by my students what books I'd recommend for self-defense, and because of my own experiences, I always have mixed feelings about putting my name behind something. Not anymore! Phil Ross's new manual, *Survival Strong*, is now *the* go-to book on defending your life and the lives of the folks you care about. This is the only book I've ever read which can genuinely give you all the bleeding-edge psychological and physical tools to take yourself to the ultimate level of personal ability. I'd be surprised if this manual is ever surpassed in its field—that's how f—ing good it is.

—**Paul "Coach" Wade**
Calisthenics guru and author of The Convict Conditioning Series

Very few people in this world practice what they preach . . . Phil Ross has been walking his talk for as long as I have known him . . . humble yet confident, this book is an illustration of what it takes to physically face the uncertainties today's world can bring to your doorstep.

—**Jason Rich**
Naval Special Warfare Operator/SEAL TEAMS 8 and 10.

Phil has been a lifelong athlete and martial artist, but has truly taken to the academic study of human movement and performance. While he's been unable to become certified in every single martial art, chase a degree in each branch of science, or proclaim to be on the cutting edge of every buzzword-generating fitness fad, what he has done is even more impressive. He's cut through the BS, the marketing, the sense-saturating hype that many fads generate. All the while, keeping an eye on fundamentals, concepts, and strategies . . . He's studied, practiced, been lectured to, lectured to others, taught a plethora of classes (martial arts, fitness, etc.), studied some more, and certainly spent time reflecting on it all . . . For this reason, I'm excited to read this book!

Phil's unique experiences have led him to become a reputable instructor for athletes of all ages and abilities. His education allows him to craft training programs for people seeking wide-ranging results, aiming for various goals . . . And knowing that, I'm quite excited for the final product; the result of time spent, experiences had, lessons learned, and, finally, crafted with a sense of perfectionism that Phil brings to every endeavor.

If there's a brain to be picked on the subject of human movement, it's Phil's. He's seen it all, and in the pages that follow, he shares his views . . . If you're looking to bypass years of attending lectures, the reading of numerous encyclopedias, and paying for dozens of personal training lessons, this book is for you.

Learn what is worth learning, and avoid some of the most common (but sometimes most subtle) mistakes that athletes and martial artists habitually make as they seek improvement.

—**Brian Ebersole**
UFC Fighter (ret., 68 professional fights), Division 1 Wrestler

I first met Phil Ross in 2012. Both he and I were cornering our fighters at a UFC event. After speaking to him for 30 minutes, I knew that he was a guy that could add value and knowledge in my life. We quickly became friends and later, training partners. Phil is a "martial arts guru" and, a pioneer in the training that the body requires to accomplish the technique and objective. Phil is methodical, detailed, and talented in his unique approach to training people. I admire him greatly and recommend this book to anyone serious about acquiring or polishing their skills to defend themselves' or loved ones.

—**Mitch Coats**
Jiu Jitsu Black Belt (2nd degree)

Phil's book Survival Strong isn't so much a manual on Self Defense as it is the love-child of a combat encyclopedia and the autobiography of a man who as actually been in just about every violent altercation you can imagine. Drawing on DECADES of training from a very wide range of experts in the field and tons of personal experience, Phil Ross takes you on a journey through self defense, and self mastery. You could easily spend the next 10 years learning and implementing the strategies and movements you'll find within. This thing is absolutely PACKED to the rafters with no fluff.

—**Max Shank**
International Presenter, Owner: Ambition Athletics,
Creator: Ultimate Athleticism

There is an old saying, "them that can, do – them that can't, teach". Phil is one of the rare few that can do and teach. Heed his advice and become a better fighter, simple as that. Phil blends decades of empirical experience in a multitude of fighting disciplines with an unquenchable and ongoing thirst for knowledge. Too many "elder" athletes become fossilized in their thinking and morph into the fundamentalist mindset that accepts no more impute and disses anyone that dares disagree from their frozen commandments. Phil, ever the fight scientist, always seeks new avenues of progress. This book is a compilation of techniques and tactics over a lifetime of immersion. This is no moldy retrospective written by a feeble retiree reminiscing about the good old day—this is an active, alive document chock full of ideas and strategies that, if implemented with the ferocity and exactitude required, will break you, the active fighter, through whatever stagnant plateau you find yourself mired in.

—**Marty Gallagher**
IPF powerlifting world champion
World champion coach

It is my pleasure and distinct honor to provide a foreword to Survival Strong, this body of work written by my friend and brother of over 25 years, Master Phil Ross. Our friendship did not consist of weekly beer runs or poker games. We trained together, mourned together, worked together and kept each other on a path that so many stray from. It is a friendship where the other person took as much interest in your well being as you did their's.

While reading Phil's book, I felt as if I were back next to my friend training, or on a detail, or just running the trails in the woods. His written words are as genuine as the man himself, and I can attest to his complete belief in himself, his philosophy, and his techniques.

Phil's views on experience, as requisite to being an authority in conflict resolution, could not be more accurately stated. I was reminded of a detail we worked together, where members of our team were checking the mouths of everyone entering, looking for hidden razors. I'm sure you can picture how different that environment was compared to the places most people frequent.

Throughout Phil's comprehensive manual, his pearls of wisdom flow as naturally from his pen as they did during our decades training together. It's always been black or white with Phil, and if he can't wrap it up in one or two sentences, it isn't worth much. No fence riding; no maybes; no middle ground; "no getting squished like grape".

Phil's mind is in tune, and perfectly suited to the science of Confrontation Resolution; a field where he is considered an expert of the highest order. With the passion of an Evangelist, he delivers his message on the conditioning required, for that one time many will never experience, but none can afford to ignore.

The Close Quarter Armed Combatives training that I provide to those who carry firearms, is a direct evolution of my training with Phil. My curriculum, which qualified me as a NEVADA P.O.S.T. Instructor, also earned me a third stripe from my friend and Instructor. It is built upon the "Cooler Heads Prevail" concept mentioned early in Phil's book, and emphasizes muscle memory training, allowing you to engage instinctively during the first 1 to 2 seconds. As Phil states multiple times, your actions must be immediate and committed. A significant body of research has been produced documenting the fact that the average person takes 1 to 2 seconds to make a decision...any decision! So, what is the aggressor doing while you are deciding? You guessed it. He is attacking. If you embrace and employ Phil's philosophy, techniques, AND train consistently and purposefully, you will maintain a cool head and prevail.

A truth that most people ignore is, those who would harm you do not live by your values. They don't freeze when witnessing something horrifying, because their lives are horrifying; and they lack the conscience to see it any other way. Survival Strong provides a comprehensive recipe for success. It clarifies for the mind; it fortifies your commitment; and it strengthens the body for the sheer physicality required.

There was never a day instructing when a pearl from Phil didn't drop into my memory to benefit my students. I never would have succeeded, as I have, if not for his constant training comments that stunned me with their clarity and applicability to the situation at hand.

Now, this body of knowledge is available for all to benefit. An informational text of this size is a demanding undertaking. I can attest that money was never a motivation. Phil's love for his fellow man and genetic sheepdog character, provided the inspiration and energy required to complete this task.

The Bible says, "To those He has given much, much is expected". In producing Survival strong, Phil has certainly lived up to that expectation.

For you my brother, "Nemo me Impune Lecesset"

—John (Bob) Pierson
B.S., NREMT - I, 3rd Degree Inst., American Eagle MMA., 3rd Degree Inst. McCoig MMA, Nevada P.O.S.T. Close Quarter Armed Combatives Inst., Edged Weapons Inst. -Valencia-Lamenco Eskrima, C.D.T. Inst.- Tom Patire, NRA Firearms and CCW Inst., Personal Protection Spec., Owner, Dir. Training - Eagle Guardian Solutions (CQDR), Author - 3 manuals on Empty Hand and Edged Weapons Defense, Senior Range Master, Dir. Martial Arts - Front Sight Firearms, North American Recipient of First Annual Project A.W.A.R.E. Award, PADI. International

> Violence is inherent in our society.
>
> You need not like it, but you better know how to deal with it.

PRELUDE

I will first tell you what I am not. I'm not a retired Navy SEAL, Marine Recon, or Green Beret. I wasn't a police officer in a high-crime area. I didn't do any hard time (although I spent a few overnights locked up but was later found not guilty). I was not part of a street gang, motorcycle club, or any organized crime. I was not an MMA (cage) fighter, although I did compete successfully in the components that comprise MMA.

You may be asking yourself, "If you weren't all of these things, then what qualifies you to write a book on self-defense?" In the 2002 movie *The Knockaround Guys*, Vin Diesel's character says, "Five hundred." He then explains to the guy he is squared up with that to be considered a tough guy; you have to have had over 500 fights. This is where my qualifications come in. If you tally up my list of conflicts/confrontations/competitions, the number far exceeds 500.

I was victorious in over 300 martial arts competitions primarily comprised of point contact but also a fair number of bare knuckle karate, kickboxing, full contact tae kwon do, submission fighting, Brazilian jujitsu, and continuous fighting. I fought in some of the toughest areas in the east: Paterson, Newark, Camden, and South Plainfield in New Jersey; Washington, DC; Baltimore, Maryland; Brooklyn and New York; Youngstown, Ohio; and Philadelphia, Pennsylvania, to name a few.

Then you must add in the over 200 street confrontations inclusive of my time as a bouncer and bodyguard.

Then factor in the additional street fights and living in a high-crime area (Prince Georges County, Maryland). This does not include the hundreds of wrestling matches and the thousands of hours spent in live combat training of various types with another human being trying to beat me.

I have been on the wrong end of knives, nunchucks, guns, clubs chains, and bottles, faced multiple attackers, and have been in some other extremely precarious situations where I had to rely upon my wits and training to extract myself. I will be the first to say that I've been extraordinarily fortunate not to have had more serious injuries or met my demise; although I did sustain one heck of a beating when I fought six guys. Not a smart move, but hey, sometimes those things happen.

I will also tell you that I'd rather be lucky than good. But I am convinced that you create your own luck, whether it be good or bad. As the great coach Vince Lombardi said, "Luck is when opportunity meets preparation." As a street fighter, bouncer, or protection specialist, you want to be prepared as possible so when the opportunity arises, luck will be on your side!

Victory favors neither the wicked nor the righteous. *Victory favors the prepared.* Fail to prepare, prepare to fail. There are endless slogans regarding being prepared for good reason. Being prepared not only has you trained for the situation and equipped with the proper tools, but it also gives you the confidence and belief in yourself to employ your skills when called upon.

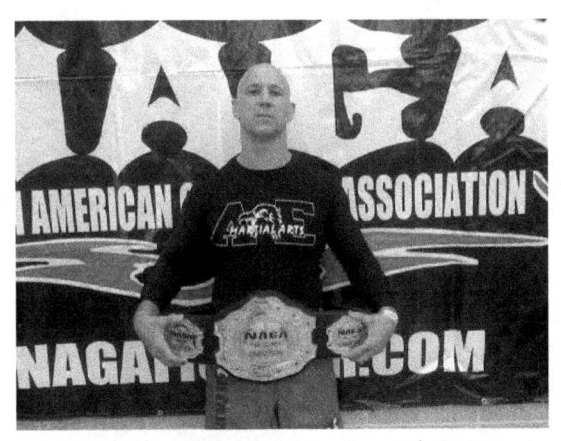

Battle at the Beach, August 8th, 2010
5 fights, undefeated and unscored upon.

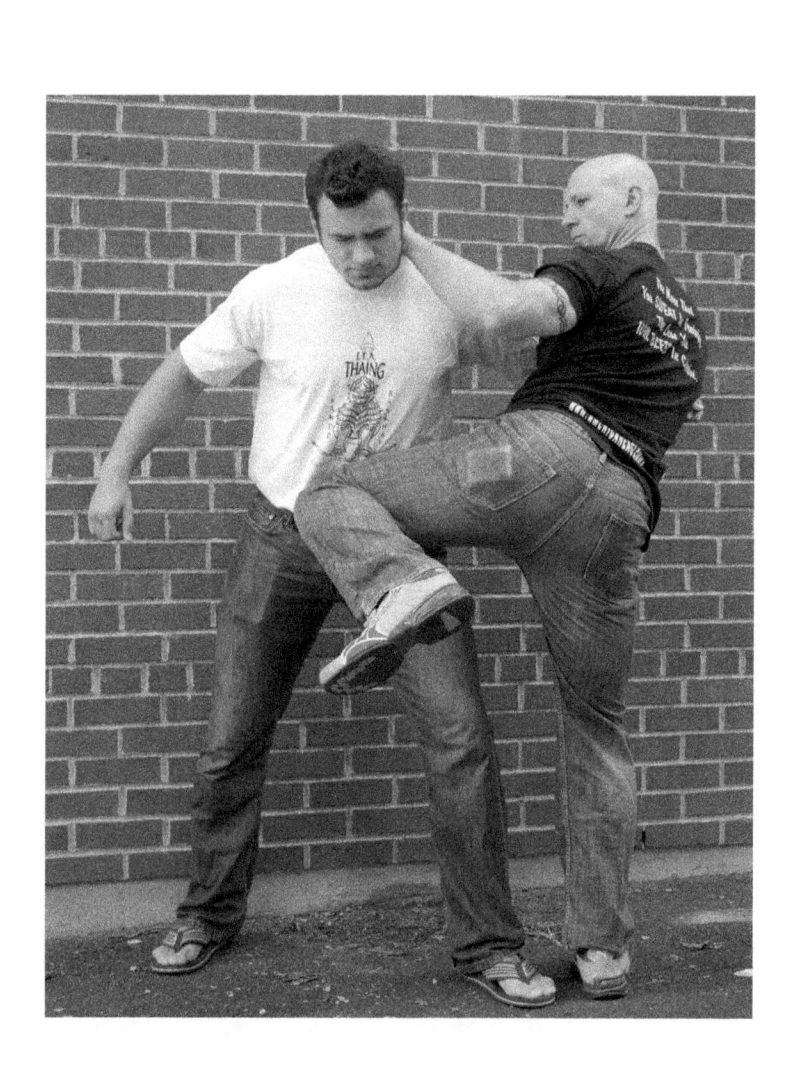

Acknowledgments

I would like to thank my parents, for providing me with a solid mental and emotional foundation that is the basis for my vision, indomitable spirit, and belief in myself.

There are many people who have had a positive influence on my life, especially regarding my training in the martial arts. I have had the great fortune of having some incredible instructors, coaches, and training partners over the years. I also have trained and worked with war veterans, police officers, security professionals, and "street guys." I would like to thank them for their knowledge, influence, and being part of my journey.

Major Influences: My grandfather Cosmo Ferro; my father, Phil Ross; Coach Rich Wittie (wrestling); Tim and Chris Catalfo (wrestling); Sensei James Martin (karate); Instructor Bill Timmie (tae kwon do); Dr. Mike Evangel (tae kwon do); Professor Jon Collins (bando); Dr. Pat Finely (arnis, Jun Fan, bando); Dr. Tony Palminteri (Japanese jujitsu), Brendan Behr (student and training partner), Steve Cirone (security, bodyguard, martial arts, defensive tactics instruction, firearms instruction); Joe Rubino (boxing, kickboxing); Frank Shamrock (MMA and submission fighting); Robert Smith (martial arts student and training partner); Tom Patire (bodyguard and security, defensive tactics, firearms instruction); Carl Cestari (defensive tactics and combato defendo); Mitch Coats (Brazilian jujitsu); Jay Hayes (Brazilian jujitsu); Percy Alston (security and martial arts and strength training partner); Brain Ebersole (MMA, grappling, former UFC fighter); John Holster (AEMMA 4th Degree black belt, student and training partner for 25 years), and John R. Pierson (student and martial arts training partner, weapons instruction, security details). There have been others along the way, but these people have had the most profound influence on me and what I've done in the street, in the mat, and in the ring.

My students who helped me with the photographs: Drew Donofrio, Scott Crisanto, Matt and Andres Burgos, Zack Fox, and my family—Amy, Nicole, Spencer, and Adrienne Ross. Thank you for taking the time to pose for and take pictures.

I'd also like to thank Max Shank, who is not only the strongest pound-for-pound person that I know but is also one of the strongest people I've ever met, period. His consultation on the bodyweight training in this book have made this system complete.

Forewords

Most books have one foreword; we have two. We are fortunate enough to have passages from two exceptional martial artists with a great deal of experience and wisdom to share. Enjoy.

Kioshi Joe Rubino
Boxing and *k*ickboxing *c*hampion

Let me begin by congratulating you on your decision to purchase and read this book. It will be a very enlightening journey resulting in your acquisition of life-changing knowledge.

Let me tell you a little bit about my background. I've been involved in the martial arts for about forty-five years. I have successfully competed as a martial artist, a boxer, and a kickboxer. I am not going to pat myself on the back by listing the trophies, awards, belts, or titles that I may have won in competition because that is just not my style. Let's just say that I was fortunate enough to have achieved a high level of success during my years of competition. I was raised in a tough section of Brooklyn where you had to learn how to fight at an early age to earn respect, or suffer the consequences. I probably had more street fights as a young kid from elementary school through high school than most people have in a lifetime. After high school, the street fights were, fortunately, far fewer, so martial arts, boxing, and kickboxing competition were what I utilized to satisfy and cultivate my warrior spirit.

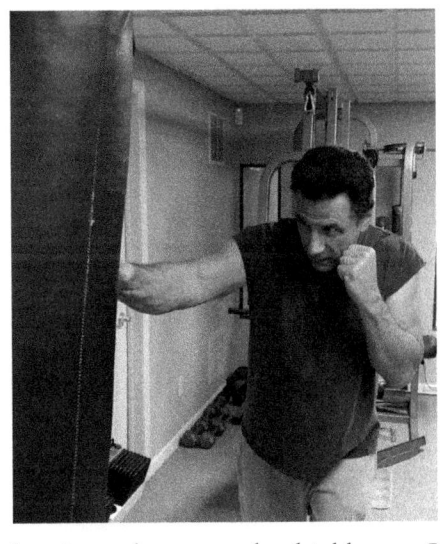

While traditional martial arts schools serve a specific purpose for many, as an instructor and coach, I am a proponent of having a school/dojo/gym/ academy that mixes effective techniques from many different martial arts into a system and training regiment that develops well-rounded fighters that are capable of successfully defending themselves in a real street fight and/or compete at a high level.

I believe that when it comes down to one-on-one competition, boxing, wrestling, kickboxing, judo, sambo, and Brazilian jujitsu are the *real* combat sports. My belief has been proven to be true as is evidenced by the real combat sports backgrounds of the most successful fighters in the MMA since its inception. MMA competition is the pinnacle of real combat competition. I wish the MMA was around when I was still young enough to compete; I would have definitely been prepared and energized to train to compete in this sport.

Those few who do decide to compete in any of the real combat sports quickly realize that mental toughness is even more important than athletic prowess and technical skills. In competition, I have won fights against some superior athletes just because of my stronger desire to win, and perhaps even more so my hatred for losing. Many coaches will speak of heart when they refer to mental toughness. To me, *heart* and *mental toughness* are synonymous and can be defined as the drive, determination, confidence, courage, and perseverance to do whatever it takes to win or be the best at your chosen sport.

To excel at any of the real combat sports, a top competitor will need to possess the following five characteristics: athletic ability, heart (mental toughness), conditioning (aerobic and anaerobic), technical skills, and discipline. That is it—it is *that* simple, or difficult, depending on your perspective. Just think about this reality: you are born with heart (or not) and athletic ability (or not), and it is your coach's/instructor's job to transfer the sport-specific technical skills to you; then you have to practice these skills over and over again perfectly until they become ingrained in your muscle memory. Now that leaves just conditioning and discipline both of which are totally under your control. Of course, your coach or instructor can help, but believe me, these two characteristics are totally within your control to acquire. *It is all on you.* Anyone who loses a real combat sport match because of poor conditioning or lack of discipline should be embarrassed and should not be competing. The difference between the champions and all other competitors is that the champions will exhibit all five of these characteristics and excel at every one.

So, to be a top-level competitor and/or to be capable of defending yourself in a tough street fight requires the body and mind to be in perfect accord as follows: the mind (drive, determination, confidence, courage, and perseverance) and the body (athleticism, conditioning, and technical skills).

The only other factor is fear, and overcoming your fears is all about mental training. There are many fears—such as fear of losing, fear of looking bad, fear of getting hurt, fear of dying, fear of failure. To help my students overcome their fears, as a coach/instructor, I taught my students to always try to "think about and visualize what you *do* want to happen, not what can happen or what you don't want to happen."

As I stated previously, I have been in the martial arts for about forty-five years, and during that time I have met and observed at least one hundred martial arts instructors, and trained with some of them as well. Of those one hundred, I will tell you that there are maybe a half dozen instructors that I would consider to be the real deal; Phil Ross is one of them.

I have known Phil for well over twenty years, and he is one of the few people that have earned my respect as a martial arts competitor and instructor. Phil has always exhibited all of the aforementioned characteristics of a champion. Phil has done what most so-called master black belt instructors have never dared to do—that is, he has put his knowledge, ability, and reputation on the line in real combat sports competition. Phil has been a well-respected competitor in wrestling, martial arts, kickboxing, sambo, and grappling. In addition, apart from his share of street fights, he has worked as a bodyguard, bouncer, and protection agent for many years. Phil is the real deal, as measured by his martial arts and real combat fighting skills, knowledge, experience, ability, and warrior spirit.

Some people have what it takes to compete at a high level in a specific sport but do not necessarily have the understanding, qualities, or ability to become great coaches or instructors. Phil epitomizes the essence of a great instructor and coach. To me, the best way to determine just how great a coach or instructor really is would simply be to observe the students who have trained with him for many years. From my own personal observation, those who have been fortunate enough to train with Phil for many years exhibit superb physical and mental conditioning and tremendous technical skills and fighting ability.

Phil is the real deal as an exemplary and complete martial arts instructor and coach.

In addition, Phil is an RKC (Russian Kettlebell Challenge) Master certified kettlebell instructor and avid exercise guru. Phil himself is the best example of what conditioning really means, for if you met Phil and observed him training, there is no way that you would be able to guess his age.

I am very fortunate to have met Phil and known him for all of these years. I have absorbed as much of his martial arts insight and knowledge that time would allow over the years, all of which has made me a better instructor and coach.

Within the pages of this masterful book on fitness and fighting, Phil has successfully conveyed to the reader many important concepts from his vast knowledge of martial arts, fitness, and real-life experiences in a captivating and concise manner.

Read, absorb, analyze, and enjoy this book, for the knowledge you will gain will benefit you for the rest of your life.

Respectfully,
Joe Rubino

Jon Collins
Assistant professor, health education and stress management

I am Professor Jonathan A. Collins, an assistant professor teaching college courses in health education and stress management for forty years. I was an NCAA Top Ten Gymnastics competitor, a professional and international kickboxer up to age thirty-five, and an elite fitness competitor up to age fifty. I have coached both men's and women's collegiate gymnastics programs, and have trained/coached national and world champion athletes/professional boxers, kickboxers, and martial artists as well.

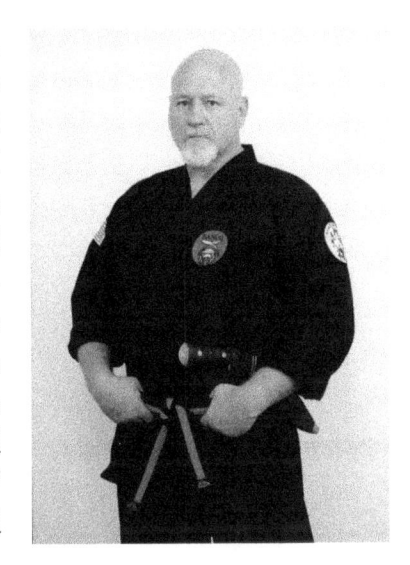

I met Mr. Ross in 1980 while he was a student/athlete at the University of Maryland. He was already an accomplished wrestler, extremely fit, and was working as a security agent to help put himself through college. Having known Phil for over thirty years, I can say that he has always demonstrated an amazing work ethic and commitment to learning, especially when it comes to being the very best he can be—in sports, in school, as a teacher, and as a person.

Over the years, I have watched Phil develop into an amazing and impressive man—as a devoted family man, teacher/trainer/coach, sports competitor, and friend. It is no wonder that his own, and the many children whom he has taught and influenced over the years, have become the courteous, attentive, respectful, successful, and health-conscious young adults that they are!

One of the things I find most relevant about Mr. Ross's perspective on training is his approach to personal responsibility and methodic progressions in learning, which he imparts in his teaching of conditioning/fitness, sports skills, and self-defense tactics. He is also one of the few instructors I've worked with who have been able to successfully make the transition and distinction between the concepts of martial sport/martial arts and realistic self-defense. He has always been a proponent of the fact that when it comes to being able to effectively defend oneself, "there is no substitute for physical conditioning and mental preparation." As a teacher myself, I especially understand and appreciate his views and philosophy toward this, and the idea that a proper self-development/defense plan involves the three components of *awareness*, *avoidance*, and *action*.

Mr. Ross explains to his student and clients that "awareness involves knowing what and where the risks are, and what your personal options/ limits/ abilities and strategies to deal with these are. Avoidance means staying away from dangerous people, dangerous places, and dangerous things!" And "action means to apply learned strategies and skills when other options are no longer viable or available." I also concur with his thought that self- defense is not fighting but, rather, getting to or escaping to a safe place . . .

Phil is an extraordinary example and role model for representation of his personal beliefs on how being healthy and fit are paramount to a person's total well-being. He not only talks the talk, but he absolutely walks the walk in his leadership and guidance down life's paths of learning, so that his charges can/ will live longer, healthier, safer, less stressful, more productive, fulfilling, and fun lives!

Much respect,
Professor Jonathan A. Collins

Introduction

The Survival Strong System is based on several principles:

How to avoid a situation
How to recognize situations
What to do when they arise
Strategic options
Situation-specific responses
The 4 ranges of combat
How to get and stay strong and fit
The importance of being in good physical condition
Conventional and unconventional weapons

The defensive tactics included in the Survival Strong System are largely based upon the SAVE Self-Defense and Fitness video series that was spawned for the program that I developed in the late 1990s. I had instructed at a multitude of seminars and workshops for members of law enforcement, security, and educational agencies as well as for the general public. I noticed that no matter how good the material was (whether it was from me or another instructor), most participants were unable to commit the movements to their immediate recall. This was primarily due to the lack of practice. In 2005, I developed the complete training system with a train-along video series. The program received several #1 ratings. In 2012, I collaborated with Max Shank, one of the top bodyweight specialists in the world as well an accomplished martial artist, to develop the Survival Strong Workshop and Certification.

The book *Survival Strong* is an in-depth depiction of the philosophy, techniques, and ideals that the system is built upon. Enjoy the journey to discovering techniques and strategies that work in real life situations. Your view on training, self-defense, martial arts, and self-protection may be changed forever!

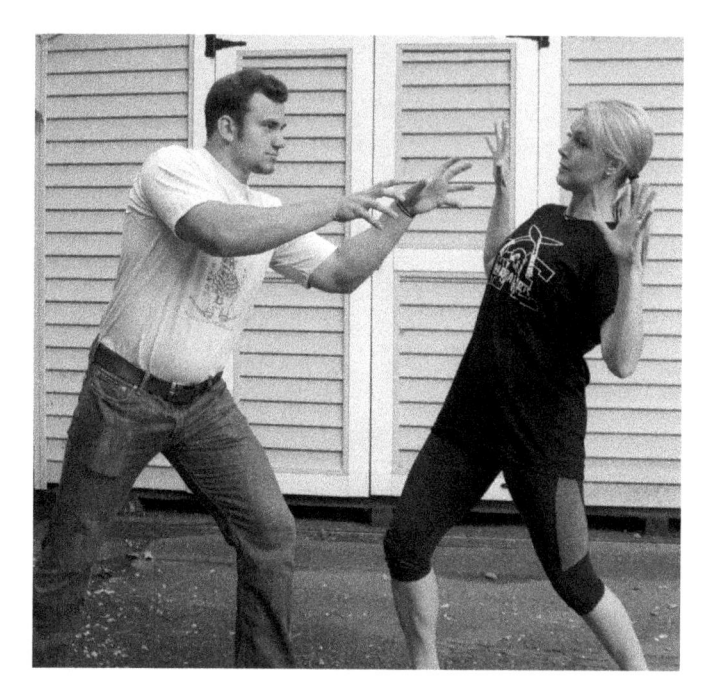

Statistics demonstrate that everyone will be a victim of a violent crime at some point in their lives. What measures have you taken to beat the odds? Are you prepared to handle the situation when violence comes knocking at your door? How will you react? Will you be able to protect yourself and your family? What will you do in the face of a home invasion? How will you handle a terrorist attack? What will you do if faced with multiple attackers?

How will you address the various weapons that you may face? What will you do if you are in faced with an execution type assault?

The most important factors are your mind-set and your training. Notice that I put mind-set first. Your mind is your best weapon. It is your mind that drives you to train and have the proper attitude to fight back. Your training must be purposeful and regular. It's not enough to think that you know what to do. I know how to hit a baseball, yet I don't play for the Yankees. You need to practice so you will be able to react without thought to the impending threat. IT, or instinctive technique, needs to be developed. There is a *kukri* (short sword) recitation in the Burmese martial art bando that states, "Repeat draws, cuts, and blocks. Repeat steps, turns, and locks, until sword frees from thought." In layman's' terms, you need to practice so you are able to simply react without hesitation and without thought. If you have to stop to think, it's too late. The time you needed has cost precious milliseconds. Maybe that's all you had. Do not permit yourself to be a statistic.

We need to employ the 3 As (Awareness, Avoidance, and Action) and SIPDE (Scan, Identify, Predict, Decide, and Execute). These two components go hand in hand. They are essential survival skills and should be practiced until they become second nature.

1
UNDENIABLE SELF-DEFENSE TRUTHS

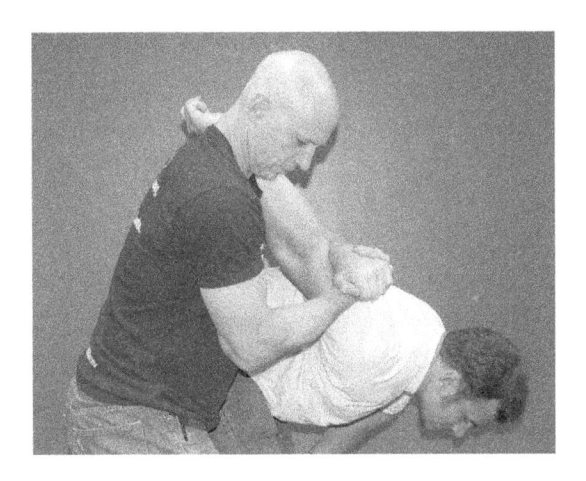

The art of learning how to defend oneself is developed through skills acquired during your defensive tactics training. It's not as simple as how to defend against a choke. There are a multitude of factors and determinants to consider during your preparation. Not only must we consider mind-set and avoidance, but we have to look at the actual types of technique application. There are different levels of threat, for lack of a better word. These are determined by distance of the offender, speed of the attack, and circumstances. None of which you have control over. You can only control how you respond to these situations. The levels or types of situations are as follows:

1. Confrontation with a verbal exchange
2. Confrontation with no verbal exchange
3. Surprise attack when you are caught off guard
4. Hostage situations
5. Intercepting an attack with a preemptive strike

All these scenarios will be addressed.

The Survival Strong Self Defense and Strength Training

The Survival Strong System of Self Defense and Strength System combines body weight and defensive tactics. The system that is practical, concise, and unmatched. Not everyone has the time, inclination, or the circumstances to join a full-blown martial arts school and train for hours and hours a week to advance in belt level. This system is devised to either be a part of an existing martial arts program or as a stand-alone means to develop great strength and defensive skills with very little or no equipment at all.

The movements and techniques espoused are designed for partner, small group, and for solitary practice. If it's inconvenient at times to train with another, many of the techniques—pad work as well as the strength and conditioning elements—may be practiced while alone. There are certain aspects of the training that do require a partner. For when training for actual combat, *there is no substitute for actual human-to-human movement.* Even though bag and pad work are strongly recommended, the variables of another human body cannot be replicated with any apparatus or in your solo training. The bag and pad work are necessary for helping you develop power in your techniques and ensure that your hands and feet are properly positioned when executing your striking techniques. Whatever your circumstance is, train often, mix your methods, and make your training part of your life.

Gross motor skills are far superior to small, intricate, and complex techniques. You will discover that many of our defensive tactics responses end up in one of a few (7 basic) positions. In a stressful situation, you are only going to be able to recall 5 to 9 strategies and/or concepts. The magic number 7 plus or minus *2* theory was developed by the Princeton University cognitive psychologist George Miller. According to Miller, the human mind can hold only 7 +/- 2 objects in their working memory. This is referred to as Miller's law and is one of the main reasons that phone numbers and social security numbers have 7 and 9 digits (less the area code, of course!) Additionally, the more components involved, the greater the chance is for something to go wrong.

There are certain principles to be aware of that must be adhered to when practicing and when in application. Anticipate the worst at all times and always maintain good physical condition. Trust no one and always assume that there is more than one attacker. Operate on the all-or-nothing principle. Either do nothing or completely incapacitate the opponent(s) to ensure your survival and escape. Always practice vigilance and look for unconventional weapons and escape routes.

Your stance is extremely important: you must be able to move quickly, comfortably, and with power, take angles and improve your position in relation to your opponent. Keep your hands up at all times; even when speaking, place your hands up (open palm) and out front and one foot slightly back in a "hidden" fighting stance. Your assailant will not feel threatened or may have no idea that you are already in a fighting stance. However, your hands are in a defend-and-counterattack position and with your one foot back, you have moved your center line out of the direct line of attack, plus, you have increased your ability to move and strike.

Maintain your balance by keeping your nose over your navel; maintain a good posture and a neutral spine. Don't use force against force, the stronger opponent will always win. The navel points in power direction; your hip position is crucial. Never have straight knees when you are facing your opponent, this leaves you immobile and vulnerable to attacks to the knees. Point your index finger in the direction that you want to take your opponent when performing small-joint locks.

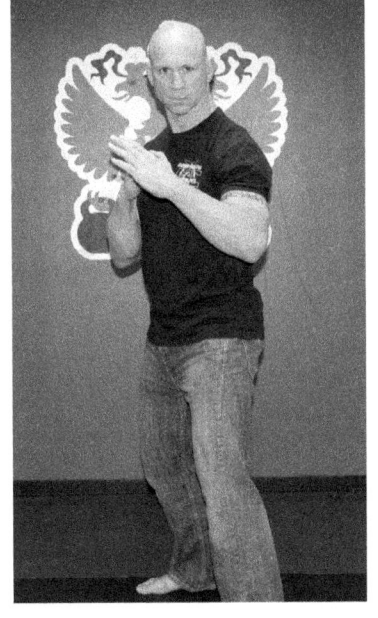

Deliver strikes to hard parts of the body with the soft part of your hand and strike the soft parts with a hard part of your body. The whole notion of yin-yang comes into play here. Dark versus light, good versus evil, and hard versus soft. It is better to strike someone with a closed fist to the abdomen rather than punch them in the head. You stand a greater chance of injuring yourself going hard to hard. Soft to soft is not as effective. Slapping an opponent with an open hand to the stomach may be annoying, but generally will not produce sufficient trauma to put them down. Now a well-placed knee to the stomach, bladder, or groin can be extremely effective.

Here are some examples: Use an open-hand strike to the face and a knee to the groin. A closed fist to the head may result in a broken hand.

Only trained, seasoned fighters stand a chance of not injuring their hands with a strike to an opponent's face or head. However, many fighters have broken their hands even while gloved in combat or training. So use the soft parts of your body to attack hard parts of your assailant and vice versa for maximum effectiveness with minimum injury to yourself.

Strike an opponent without chambering your technique, or drawing back to go forward. Doing so will significantly slow down your techniques and telegraph your strikes. It is essential to practice delivering your blows from your hips and utilize full-body tension as you lock into the technique. The incomparable Bruce Lee developed a technique called the *one-inch punch*. Starting from a completely relaxed state, move and apply full-body tension upon contact. Whether executing a one-inch, three-inch, or standard strike, employ this method for maximum power.

Distract your opponent by striking with the closest hand, foot, or knee and understand leverage to gain and maintain advantage. "Vanish" from your opponent's view by always maintaining angles and improving your ability to deliver strikes to exposed and vulnerable areas. Always keep your eyes on the lower center of your opponent's chest during initial contact. Learn basic limb dynamics and their reflexive movements. It is important to know how the body reacts to being hit and what the resulting movement will be after you deliver a blow.

Most vital and semivital target areas are located centerline. It is crucial to keep yours unavailable as much as possible and focus your strikes on your opponents. Thus, knowing and working your angles is critical. Your attacks and counterattacks should always attempt to end with a significant strike to these areas. This will increase the incident of success.

Keep the back of your hand facing your opponent (your palm facing you). This will position the back of your hand between you and a possible sharp-edged weapon. The back of your forearms are more resilient than the front. Arteries are located on the inside section of your arms (as well as the inside of your legs). Always assume that your opponent is armed even if you don't see a weapon. If he brandishes a weapon, assume he has another.

There have been many incidences of a victim disarming an assailant only to be attacked by the opponent with a secondary weapon.

When practicing disarms, *never* hand the weapon back to your training partner. This will create the improper muscle memory. Remember, "Perfect practice makes perfect." There have been many occurrences of trained martial artists disarming an assailant only to hand the weapon back to them! Don't be *that guy*! To expand on this notion even more, don't help your partner up once you've taken them down.

1. No one is going to help you up in the street, so you better practice how to get up on your own, in a defensive posture.
2. You don't want to knock a perpetrator down and then help them up because you have trained yourself to be "nice" to your training partner. Let them and you get up on your own accord, and you'll be doing both of you a favor.

Take advantage of the *element of surprise*. In every confrontation, there is one opportunity to make a decisive move. If you are smaller, appear weaker, or are unarmed, your perpetrator may not expect you to launch an attack. Use their notion of superiority to your advantage. Do your best to mentally disarm them and then take advantage of the opening.

Use the "all or nothing" principle. You either "go or you don't go." *Never* do anything halfway or hold back at all. If you are faced with an imminent threat, go all out and completely finish your assailant. You hit and hit as hard as you possibly can until you no longer see movement, or until you have rendered the opponent helpless enough for you to secure your escape. Your survival and the survival of your loved ones are dependent upon your ability to act and react swiftly and furiously.

Why do you need to be in shape? The average street confrontation lasts a mere ten seconds. Yes, most street confrontations do last only seconds, but there is a condition that occurs during stressful situations called an *adrenaline dump*. This occurs when the body goes into fight, flight, or freeze mode. The better the condition you are in, the better your body processes the stress, and the better you are able to control your breathing.

Additionally, what if you are tired after a long day of work or travel? What if you are a little sick? What if the fight does last more than a few seconds and you need to contend with multiple attackers?

Also consider that you are quicker and stronger if you are in good physical condition. Did you consider that you may go into cardiac arrest if you are overweight and become stressed? If you don't want to be in condition, this book is not for you. Either hire bodyguards or get a gun and a big dog and never leave your house.

Phil Ross:

The American Eagle Mixed Martial Arts and Defensive Tactics system was developed from a unique blend of both martial arts training and real-world experience. The Burmese martial arts of Bando, Combat Jujitsu, Korean

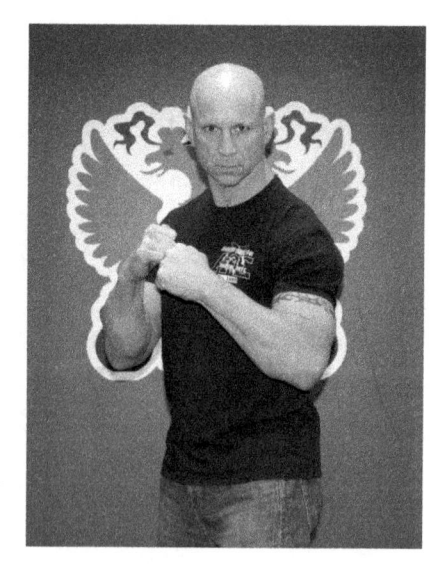

Tae Kwon Do, Filipino Arnis, Jun Fan, Muay Thai, Western Boxing and Wrestling, Submission Fighting, and Shotokan Karate. In addition to the formal martial arts, I was an executive protection agent for over ten years, as well as a bouncer in Washington, DC; New York City; and various establishments in New Jersey for more than twenty years. The real-life experience that I have had has contributed significantly to the realistic application of techniques and tried and true theories set forth. I successfully competed on the national level in wrestling, karate, tae kwon do, submission fighting, free fighting, and continuous point fighting on the national level from 1979 through 2010. Including wrestling, I was victorious in approximately 500 physical contests in the aforementioned disciplines. These numbers do not include the physical confrontations incurred during my employment as a bouncer or bodyguard.

In order to effectively teach a defensive tactics program, you have to have had significant experience in either the street, the ring, or on the mat. I have all three. The street, or real-life, experience is to be gained from the military, police, bouncer, bodyguard, incarceration, or other such situations where your life is threatened or potential bodily harm may come to you where there are no rules and anything can happen. The ring would include any of the full contact sports that involve striking. This includes, but is not limited to, boxing, kickboxing. Muay Thai, full contact (or knockdown) karate, mixed martial arts (or cage fighting), or any other type of competition where a knockout is permitted. The last area is the mat. This would include wrestling, judo, Brazilian jujitsu, Pankration, catch wrestling, and, of course, mixed martial arts. Also included on this list is any full contact grappling competition where the controlling, submitting, or manipulating of another individual is required for victory. If you are a black belt in a Kata based system or practice self-defense maneuvers learned from a DVD or a YouTube video, you are not qualified to develop, provide advice or otherwise present a defensive tactics system. You must have trained, competed, or been faced with situations where bodily harm could have come to you and you have a measure of experience being hit, taken down, or you submitted. I'm not saying that you have to be a UFC champion or a Navy SEAL to be able to teach, but you have to have had some real-world experience.

2
REAL-WORLD APPLICATION

When considering self-defense and actual application, there's nothing like hearing it from those who have "walked the walk." Many people "talk the talk," but what have they really done? I have trained and worked with both of these professionals in the field. We have seen each other in action on a multitude of occasions, both in the ring and out. Percy Alston and I were training partners for years and bounced at several bars together. We competed on the same karate team in college. Steve Cirone and I trained together on many occasions and worked a fair amount of security as well as bodyguard assignments. We also worked together as instructors for teaching defensive tactics to law enforcement agents on many occasions.

Enjoy.

Percy Alston
Retired Prince George's County police officer
Instructor (criminal law and narcotics), Public Safety and Security Institute
Municipal Police Academy, Prince Georges Community College

I have known Phil for more than thirty years. When we first met, we were bouncers at a local bar near the University of Maryland. We also trained together at the University of Maryland bando club. I had also trained in various styles of martial arts, as did Phil. I believe that we were doing what is now called mixed martial arts. As bouncers, we fought/engaged with people on a nightly basis.

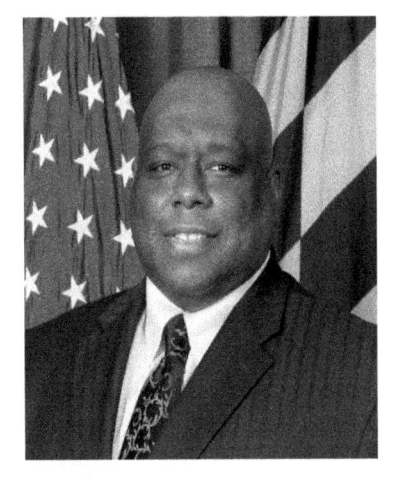

These fights were rough and sloppy. In the early 1980s, they were also more honorable. Most of the fights were one-on-one, and weapons weren't utilized. This is just what you would expect in a college bar. While working, we never lost a fight. During this time, we both competed in numerous karate tournaments. I did well, but I wasn't the best point fighter. I relied heavily on my power. Phil was more successful in the tournaments because of his speed and agility.

In 1984, I became a Prince George's County police officer. PG County is a jurisdiction that borders Washington DC and Northern Virginia. While it is considered somewhat affluent, there are many pockets that are laced with poverty and riddled with violent crime. Early on and for most of my career, I worked as a narcotics investigator in an undercover capacity. My philosophy about fighting changed from bouncing and competitive fighting to fighting for life or death. Dealing with murderers, robbers, and drug dealers, I knew that losing a fight might cost me my life. While I was a police officer, Phil and I continued to train together until he moved back to New Jersey. Phil started a martial arts gym. I gravitated to and competed in powerlifting. When we had a chance to get together, he would show me new holds, throws, and techniques that I was able to apply throughout my career. Even though these techniques weren't taught or approved by my department, I was going to do whatever it took to stay alive. I know that my martial arts training honed my ability to perceive a threat. I was able to use wrist locks, chokes, and strategic strikes in order to achieve pain compliance while arresting the bad guys.

Unfortunately, I have seen a lot of police officers receive unwanted scrutiny and criticism because they lost control and used too much force or struck someone too many times while attempting to effect an arrest. Image, appearance, and body language definitely play a part in how people size you up. If you project an image of strength and confidence, a potential adversary will take pause before deciding to confront you. On the other hand, if you look weak and vulnerable, you will appear as the perfect victim. Of course, I believe my greatest skill was/is my ability to avoid or talk my way out of or through violent encounters. All of this comes from maturity and experience.

As a law enforcement officer I observe people meander through life as what I call "sheeple". These people who always follow are not prepared for life's challenges. They present themselves as victims. Unfortunately, in our society, there are wolves or predatory criminals who are looking for the sheeple. In 2014, this is a fact of life. While Phil and I will never prey on the weak, when the wolves see us, they will turn and run or be repelled.

Steve Cirone
Black belt, security expert, VIP bodyguard, army veteran

My name is Steve Cirone. Born (1961) and raised in Hudson County, New Jersey. Across the river from New York City. I have three tough brothers. Growing up wasn't easy. Fighting with my brothers every day until we were bloody was normal. Also, I survived many street battles. I've been shot in the knee, stabbed in the arm, hit in the face with bottles, hit in the head with a two-by-four, had my nose broken six times, spent several weekends in jail, and much more. Also, the enormous number of devastating tragedies that I have endured throughout my life hardened me even more. I've been a bouncer, a bodyguard, and a boxer since 1978. A street fighter most of my life. I also worked as a corrections officer. I earned a black belt in a street combative style of martial arts, taught to me by a great instructor (Tom Patire).

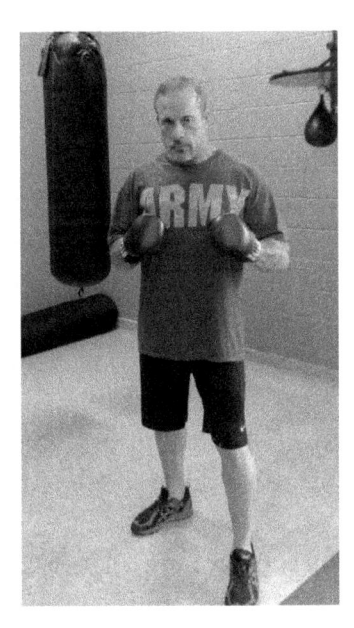

I was inducted into the International Black Belt Hall of Fame in 1999. I'm a US Army veteran. I'm an instructor of martial arts, boxing, kickboxing, fitness, and defensive tactics for police and bodyguards. I have many other certifications. I'm also deeply involved with MMA cage fighting. My résumé goes on and on. I'm a highly seasoned and experienced veteran of protecting people, crowd control, AND defusing volatile situations and confrontation. I'm about to share some real-life situations that I've experienced and how my martial arts training and street knowledge came into play.

First, I'd like to say something about Phil Ross. I've known Phil Ross for a very long time. He is like my brother. We have worked as bodyguards together, as bouncers together, as instructors together, fought back-to-back, and protected people together many times. I trust him with my life. Phil's credentials speak for themselves. I vouch for him 100 percent.

I've been involved in thousands of dangerous, hands-on, life-on-the-line, take-care-of-business situations. Let me share a few with you.

Several years back, I was hired to work as a bodyguard protecting a news crew and a news reporter in a rough area of New York City. The neighborhood was volatile and on the verge of a riot because one of the locals was killed by a cop. I was standing by the news van with the reporter and news crew. The reporter was sitting in the van with the side doors open. A man approached the news van. I stopped the man by identifying myself and telling him to step back please. He said, "I want to talk to the reporter." I once again said, "Step back, please." The reporter said, "I'll talk to him."

The man stepped closer to the van and started talking to the reporter. I positioned myself to protect the reported if needed. The man put his hand in his pocket. He started to pull a knife out of his pocket. I immediately reacted. I took the man down using a martial arts / bodyguard technique, as I disarmed him. I held him down using another technique. As I was neutralizing him on the ground, I looked across the street and noticed that the locals were looking at me and yelling at me with anger, as if I was hurting one of their own. The authorities were informed; they arrived and took the man away. I didn't think of the danger I was in. I was just doing my job. What I did came naturally, thanks to my training.

The next experience I'd like to share with you took place in a nightclub at the Jersey shore, where I was the head bouncer at the time. The place was rocking as fifteen hundred people were drinking and dancing and having a wild time. The beer muscles were flexing. A fight broke out on the dance floor. Fists were flying. I signaled my crew of bouncers. I was first to arrive. I stepped in to break up the fight. The other bouncers soon arrived to help. We had to get rough with some of the participants. We got the fight under control. Ten or so had to be escorted out of the club.

As my bouncers escorted the last few out, I was watching the bouncers' backs when suddenly, a choke hold was applied to my neck from the rear. The choke was very tight. I said, "What are you doing?" The man choking me said, "I'm a marine. You threw my friend out, this is what I know how to do." At that point, I made sure I was able to breathe, and I put my body in the position it needed to be in to defend myself. I then said to him, "You better let go." He said, "F**k you." At that point, I went into action. I used a martial arts technique to get myself out of the choke hold, and in one motion, I reversed his arm, dislocated his shoulder out of the socket, and took him down to the ground. Then I picked him up and ran him through the club and out the front door, all the while controlling his arm with a chicken wing technique and passed him off to the authorities.

My mind-set when handling a volatile situation or any situation is unique. Defusing situations and putting people in their place and standing up for what's right and trying to keep order and never backing down is who I am, and it comes naturally to me. Thank you for letting me share with you some of my life experience.

There was another time: Phil Ross and I were working security together at a 600-person private party, which turned into two rival gangs starting a riot, which Phil and I were in the middle of, trying to defuse it. That was fun. That story is for another time.

3
MIND-SET

There are certain defining moments in everyone's life, and this one propelled my street-fighting prowess. Prior, there were quite a few less severe confrontations, but this one served to have a significant impact on me, my abilities, and my mind-set when it came to defending myself. I must warn you, it's fairly graphic, and what transpired may upset you in some way. If you don't like what I did and how I defended myself, too bad. I responded to an attack by an older, larger, and more experienced assailant. I did what I felt I had to do to win and deter any further potential retaliation. There will be others reading this who may not think the incident is a big deal. I'm OK with that as well. Bear in mind that I was only seventeen years old at the time.

That being said, this is one of the incidents that I can relay without any potential of legal ramifications. One, I was only seventeen, and the assailants were above the age of majority. Two, I'm writing this book thirty-four years after the fact. So I am quite certain that the statute of limitations has long expired. Three, there was a time that the perpetrator relinquished his opportunity to press charges because he was not only involved with an assault with a minor, but he was also trespassing.

It was June 1980. I believe that it was Friday night for two reasons. I know that I graduated on a Thursday night, and the Friday night was June 20 (or at least Google Calendar shows it as the date). We were celebrating my high school graduation and were hosting a big shindig with a band and family and friends in attendance. Please note that I had quite a few friends from other towns, being a wrestler; many of us formed friendships with the area athletes. That being said, there were quite a few tough young kids at my house.

15

Three uninvited guests showed up, and a couple of my friends that I had assigned to the bouncing duties denied them entrance and subsequently threw them out. They got into their car and drove off, almost hitting me and two other guests, one of them a female (my date). I yelled at them, and they turned their vehicle around. One kid decided to throw an M-80 at me.[1] I leapt out of the way as the explosion resounded through the air. They sped off.

Little did they know that I lived on a circular court, one way in and one way out. They were traveling the long way out. I directed my friends to cut them off with their car. They sped to the intersection and blocked the road. The party emptied behind me as we ran to the corner and engulfed their car.

The driver had his window open, so I reached in, grabbed him by the throat with one hand, and pummeled his face with my other, very willing fist. The kid in the back seat got out, and one of my friends grabbed him and tossed him across the hood of the car. Another one of my friends jumped on the vehicle's hood and started to stomp up and down on it.

Before I ran to the other side of the car, I first stopped to punch dents into the car's trunk. The only guy who had not gotten hit yet was the one who threw the firecracker. I asked him, "You like throwing firecrackers?" He received the same treatment as the driver, only worse. We left the three bloodied and battered and headed back to the party high-fiving each other and espousing our accolades for administering immediate retribution. Only, it wasn't over yet.

The displaced partiers decided to recruit some muscle and attempt to exact their own revenge. They were to be met with a surprise.

Five guys showed up to my party as it was winding down. I think it was close to midnight. (I call this the A**hole Hour.[2]) They were older than my

---

[1] An M-80 is a powerful firecracker. It has the power of a 1/4 stick of dynamite.

[2] The A**hole Hour occurs after midnight. Nothing good ever happens after midnight. People are drunk or high, their emotions are reeling, and they are

friends and me. Some of them had been out of high school for a few years already, others more recently.

Set the stage in your mind now. There were approximately twenty-five or thirty people left at the party. Mostly close friends and family. We were on my front lawn. My dad was out front and speaking with one of the parents. My father was a former marine and an ex-All Metropolitan High School Football player. He played guard on offense and nose tackle on defense.[3] He did have a fairly short fuse, to say the least.

The ringleader (let's call him Will Saylor) approached me at the same time my dad directed one of the other uninvited "guests" to get off our property. The knucklehead said, "F**k you!" My dad cracked him in the chest with a forearm shiver, and as the guy was off balance, charged him again with the same blow, knocking him into the street. As the recruited muscle was sitting on his ass looking up at the world, my dad said, "Now you're off my property."

Now, the ringleader was about 6'1" or 6'2," 185 pounds or so. He had a rap sheet as long as your arm. He was thrown out of the high school for detonating explosives and had apparently done some time. He had the reputation of being the best street fighter in town, and I knew a couple of rough kids that he had beaten up. At the time, I was about 5'9" and tipping the scales at 170 pounds.

Immediately, after the confrontation with my dad occurred, I walked up to Will Saylor, put my hand on his shoulder, and said, "Get you and your girlfriends the hell out of my party and off of my property, now! Or I'll break your neck!"[4] Saylor promptly replied with "Get your f**king hands

---

looking for trouble under the cloak of darkness. Having worked in bars for many years, I've noted that most fights, issues, and DUIs occur after midnight. To avoid issues, go home before midnight.

[3] In football, those positions are considered interior linemen. My dad, at only 5'8", was a pretty tough customer.

[4] OK, there are really two footnotes here. 1) He wasn't there with girls; I was simply trying to insult him. 2) "I'll break your neck," was my tag line at that time. I'd

off of me" and swatted my hand away. With that, I punched him with a devastating overhand right that landed squarely between his eyes. Blood spurted out of his head and traveled over twenty-feet feet.[5] One of my friends dad's was picking him up, and he still, to this day claims that I owe him a shirt from the blood that he got on it! I told him, "It's not my blood. Get the new shirt from Saylor," I said with a chuckle.

After the well-placed right hand, Saylor fell backward and into his group of friends. They propped him up, and he staggered forward. I shot in on a double leg takedown.[6] At this point, I'd achieved a full-mount position with me sitting on his chest. Now the real damage began. I started raining down punches on him, smashing blow after blow into my barely moving target. I was in a frenzy. The "whirr" was in my head. I was consumed with bloodlust. I wanted to inflict more pain. I saw his throat. So I sank my teeth right into his neck and tried to tear his flesh off.

Luckily for Mr. Saylor, my friends pulled me off. They have seen me in confrontations before and knew that I wouldn't stop on my own accord. His limp, bleeding body lay on the ground. What was left of his friends picked him up and took him to the hospital.

A week or so later, I was with my cousin uptown. We saw Saylor and a few friends. He saw us. As Saylor was standing on the corner with his friends, I instructed my cousin to drive past them slowly. As I gripped my lead-filled pipe[7] in my hand, my cousin stopped the car at the corner where Saylor and his buddies were standing. He had stitches on his face and neck. Both of his

---

say this when I was about to engage in fisticuffs.

[5] The odds of winning a fight are dramatically increased by landing the first good blow. This is usually the first shot before people are moving around too much.

[6] A double-leg takedown is a very effective means to get someone to the ground. You lower your level, lunge forward, and grab your opponent's legs. Lift him off of the ground and drive him backward. You'll learn more about this move in the grappling section of this book.

[7] I used to have a copper pipe filled with lead and capped on both ends with brass fittings. It was my "backup" in case I was caught alone facing more than one opponent.

eyes were black from me breaking his nose. I looked at him and said, "Hey kid, how's your nose?" He said nothing, and we slowly pulled away. On the surface, you may think that what we did and what I said was the wrong thing, but establishing that I wasn't afraid actually squashed any thoughts that he may have had for retaliation.

Now don't get the impression that I think that this is the best course of action. At the time, it was the only one that I felt I could take. Plus, I was young and wanted to impose my will on anyone that challenged me. "Experts" falsely state that insecure people have to fight to prove themselves. Well, I think that is 100 percent incorrect. Insecure people bully others and pick on weaker victims. They are insecure and suffer from other issues. I tend to agree with the other studies that demonstrate people with high levels of confidence and opinions of themselves like the confrontations to prove that they are right.

I have since modified my outlook on fighting. I know what I can do and what I have done. A true warrior tries his best to avoid confrontation for he knows the ramifications of his actions. I know that if I get into a conflagrative situation, the results will not be good. So I tend to avoid them and go home before midnight! I will only get into a physical confrontation if I feel the safety of one of my loved ones or mine is in jeopardy. Actually, I must digress: if I see a person in need, I know that I'll jump in. It's my nature. So is the manner that I fight.

Always keep these words in mind: *Cooler heads prevail.*

Whether you are dealing with a road rage incident, a person screaming and threatening you, or a knife at your throat, *keep your cool*. This enables you to take advantage of your opportunities and make your move when the occasion presents itself. If you are still alive and have not allowed yourself to be tied up or taken from point A to point B, you will have an opportunity. If you lose your cool, you may miss your chance. Do your best to keep your cool and look for your chance to make a move. Remember that cooler heads prevail, in any situation.

If you can escape, do so. I'm not going to teach you how to run. There are a great deal of highly qualified track coaches, YouTube videos and books on running available. We're here to show you the options to your tactical defensive responses. As stated previously, your mind-set is paramount. You must adopt the "all or nothing" principle. Let us assume that you have exhausted all avoidance techniques, your verbal contact, and you have no choice but to get physical. Please note that there generally is very little time between the verbal and physical confrontations. You have to be a hundred percent committed to the execution of the technique. Do *not* hold back! You have to be mentally prepared to hit as hard and as often as you are able until the conflict is over and the assailant rendered unable to retaliate.

The target areas for your strikes are extremely important. For instance, if a 100-pound woman were to hit a 200-pound man in the chest, she may use every ounce of her power yet not yield any result, except an angered perpetrator. Yet if she pokes him in the eye, knees him in the groin, and delivers a kick to his shin, she will most likely gain a favorable reaction, allowing her time to escape. Everyone has eyes and throats. Everyone also has groins; however, groin strikes and grabs are more effective on males. It's your job to attack the vital and semivital target areas. Proper positioning and the attack on secondary targets may be necessary before reaching the primary targets. As a general rule, primary targets are located on the center line of a person. The major primary targets are the eyes, nose, throat, solar plexus, and the groin.

Applying a proper strike to these areas generally results in at least a momentary incapacitation of the assailant. Levying strikes to these areas also buys you time to either escape or deliver additional blows to areas of the head, knees, and spine to further render your assailant incapable of causing you harm. You must create a situation that gives you time to escape without allowing immediate assailant retaliation. Destruction of your assailant's limbs or the administration of a knockout blow is the best method to ensure your successful escape. Secondary targets would consist of the back of the head, temple, ears, back of the neck, floating ribs, kidneys, liver, elbows, wrists, inside the thighs (femoral artery), outside of the thighs (peroneal nerve), shin, talus, and the top of the foot.

Be mentally prepared to unleash hell when attacked. The life you save may be your own or, more importantly, that of a loved one's. Your mindset and your willingness to do whatever is necessary to win. Remember, there is no cheating in a street fight. Fair fights do not exist. You have to be prepared to do whatever it takes to emerge victorious.

How can you toughen yourself and develop the mind-set that enables you to fight, push yourself, believe in yourself, and be triumphant? You have to challenge yourself. Throughout this book, you will witness training that will challenge you physically and mentally. Here's a challenge that I came across and used to strengthen my resolve. I have heard that this test was used by certain Native American tribes and also by some Special Forces. I cannot attest to either, for I am not from any of the aforementioned groups.

I decided to test myself.

The challenge: Take a cup of water and drink the contents, but do *not* swallow. Hold the water in your mouth. Place the cup on the ground and go for a two-mile run. When you return, spit the water back into the cup. Seems simple enough, right? Try it. You can only breathe through your nose, and the temptation to swallow the water is great. I've attempted and accomplished this challenge only a few times in my life. I figured the Indian Braves only had to do it once as a rite of passage.

Apparel

What are you wearing?

You may be asking, "Why is that important?" If you can't move, you can't fight, and that's the bottom line. Go through your wardrobe and start from the ground up. If you can afford to be driven in a limo and have bodyguards, you don't need to concern yourself with apparel. Most of us don't enjoy that luxury, though.

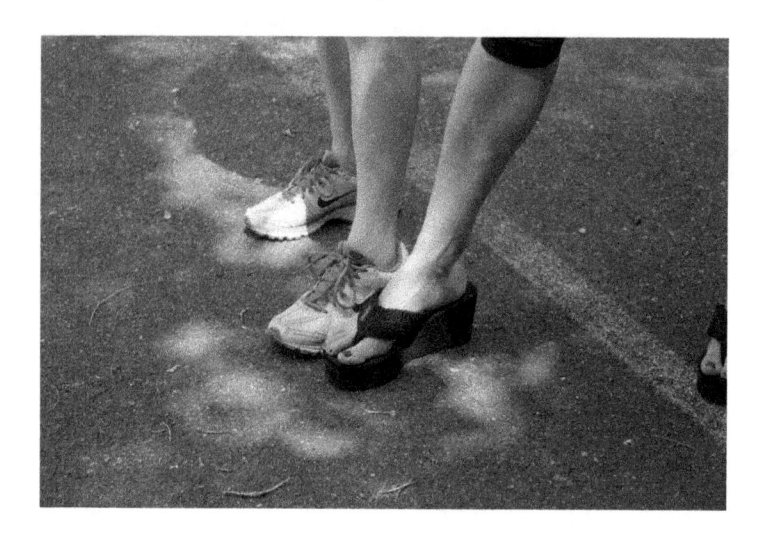

Shoes: Proper on the left, improper on the right.

First, you must begin with your shoes. I recall the response from a female executive at a S.A.V.E. corporate Workshop that I conducted. When I was speaking about footwear, this fashion plate executive exclaimed that she wasn't going to give up wearing her $350 Prada shoes. Her comment got a chuckle from the participants. My reply was, "If you ever have to run, you'll not be able to do so wearing those things." Guess what happened? Nine-eleven. She was in Tower 2 and had to run for her life.

She was forced to kick off her shoes and take off, subsequently cutting her feet on the fallen debris and shards of glass from the falling towers. Her concern for her expensive footwear went out the window. Isn't it strange how priorities change when one is faced with the reality of life and death?

I will tell you that I got a phone call from her shortly thereafter, and she asked me to come in for another workshop and to make some recommendations on "fashionable, yet practical footwear." Thank God that she escaped, but had she stepped on something large and sharp, twisted an ankle, or injured her knee, she may not not have gotten away with only minor cuts and bruises.

Examine your footwear. You need to be able to run, kick, and climb with it. If you can't, know the chances that you are taking.

Skirts, Pants, etc.

A tight skirt or skintight pants do not permit much freedom of movement. Therefore, your ability to run, jump, kick, or stretch are significantly impaired. Your pants or skirt should allow you freedom of movement.

I will not even address those who wear their pants with their underwear exposed. These guys should simply get a knock in the head and sent home. It's laughable. First of all, no one wants to see your underwear. Secondly, I will not entertain "prison-inspired style." Look at the other constraints. How are you going to run, or even move, with your pants hanging off you like that? Plain silly.

Belt

Are you wearing a belt? A belt can be used as a great unconventional weapon, especially if it's a sturdy leather one with a sizable buckle. Wrap the belt around your hand and leave a length of six to eight inches free. Wield the buckle end in a figure 8 motion and keep it between you and your opponent. The leather wrapped around your hand also serves as protection for your knuckles and adds stability to your hand. A belt can also serve as an implement to choke an assailant or as a rope substitute.

Ties and Jackets

The time of year and the weather where you live will dictate your attire. Freedom of movement is hindered if you are wearing a tight jacket. You must be able to throw a punch and move without restrictions of your clothing. If you work as a bouncer and are required to wear a tie, use a clip-on. A standard necktie is a great handle for your adversary to grab a hold of and yank you around by or choke you with. If this does happen, be certain to move with him and deliver a strike to the side of the head, from the side of the hand that is gripping the tie. He will be unable to block your strike with that hand while gripping your necktie.

I learned this from experience as a nineteen-year-old bouncer.

Luckily for me, I was comfortable at close range. When my necktie got grabbed, I went right into the guy. I was also fortunate that the rest of the bouncers were right there taking care of the others as I grappled with my attacker. I started wearing clip-ons after that incident. The additional upsides are you don't have to spend much time tying a Windsor knot, and clip-ons are generally cheaper as well. Two bonus points, and you are also protecting yourself!

Your Adversary's Attire

What is your adversary wearing? Does he have a heavy jacket on? What is he wearing on his lower extremities? How about his footwear?

You want to consider one aspect: in almost any weather conditions, people tend to not have much clothing on their lower bodies. Generally, there is only a thin layer of cloth between you and the vital and semivital target areas. Your initial strikes should be directed to the shins, groin, pubic bone, peroneal nerve, Iliotibial band (IT band), and femoral arteries of the lower body. The upper body attacks should be focused on the areas around the throat and above including the carotid arteries, eyes, ears, temple, nose, and mandibular process. These areas are generally exposed and readily accessible.

THE 3 A's: AWARENESS, AVOIDANCE AND ACTION

Awareness

Be aware of your surroundings. Where are the escape routes? What are the potential hazards in the room or area? Who is in the vicinity? Where are the friendlies and foes? Who just walked in the movie theater or the restaurant? Who is looking at my child? Why is that guy hovering around the playground? What is that knapsack doing on the floor of the train? Why are there three guys standing in the unlit doorway of that building? Where did I park my car? Who is on the plane, bus, or train? Do I have a weapon? What weapons in the environment are available to me? How am I dressed? This applies a great deal to women. As previously addressed, many women sacrifice mobility for fashion's sake. You should be able to kick, run, and jump in your attire. Know the limitations of your dress and plan accordingly. Know who is in your area and know your escape routes.

Employ the thousand-yard stare when walking in populated areas. You look almost through the other people as you pass them. Be aware of them, but direct eye contact is not recommended; though neither is shying or looking away.

Maintain a neutral disposition and a level head as you scan the area. You should be cognizant of who is in your sight path yet appear unaffected by their presence.

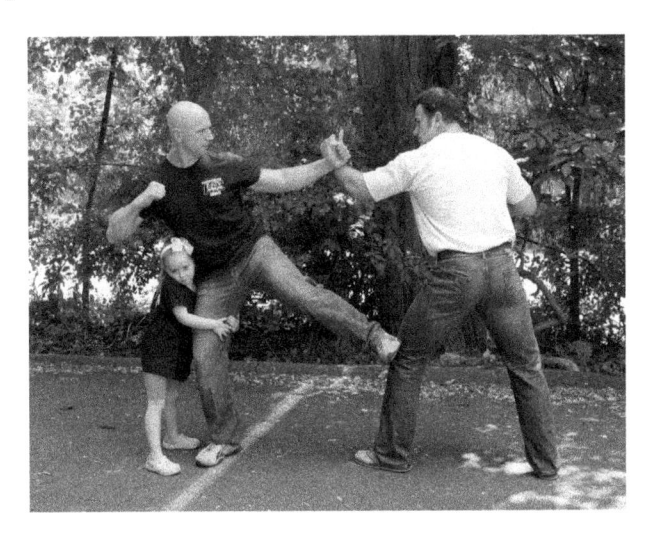

Who are you with? What is your responsibility to them? If you are alone, your immediate responsibility is to yourself. If you have travel companions, what is your responsibility to them? What are the physical limitations and capabilities of your travel companions? My responsibility is different if I am with my wife and children than if I am with my friends, training partners, or fellow instructors. Have a game plan in place. My wife and children know that if the proverbial stuff ever hits the fan to take off and quickly get to a safe haven. I'll stay and deal with the imminent threat. I'd rather deal with the assailants alone than have my mind occupied by the safety of my family. Set a designated meet-up place selected prior to traveling. This is also a helpful strategy if you get separated.

Be alert. Period. If you are walking down the street or in a parking lot and you're texting away or bopping to the music pumping into your ears through a set of headphones, how can you be attuned to your environment if you are disengaged? Do yourself a favor: pay attention to what is going on around you.

Avoidance

Most situations are avoidable. Do not unnecessarily put yourself in harm's way. Perpetrators are predatory, opportunistic creatures that seek the most gain with the least amount of effort. Does the lion attack the strongest and fastest wildebeest, or does it seek out the weak, slow, old, or young target? Obviously, the lion will take the path of least resistance and the ticket to the easiest meal. Don't allow yourself be an easy meal ticket. Avoid potentially harmful situations. It takes only one incident to end or dramatically change your life.

Know where you parked your vehicle. Make sure that it's in a lighted, highly visible area. Know where you are traveling to. Leave ample time to travel; being rushed will cause you to make mistakes. Check your routes prior to your departure. Use your GPS device and have a map and/or a printed route with you as well. Avoid bad or unfamiliar neighborhoods. *Do not get drunk or high.* Illegal narcotics should *never* be used. They should not even be a consideration in the self-preservation equation. Don't take a drink from a stranger. If you need to drink, take it from a bottle that you saw get opened or that you opened yourself. Keep your hand over the top of the beverage at all times. Don't put your drink down and come back to it. Avoid illegal parties or secret get-togethers. Listen to the little voice in your head and pay attention to your instincts. If you train long enough and focus on your awareness, your survival instincts will develop. If you feel strange or uneasy with an impending situation, *don't* do it! There is most likely a good reason that you are feeling apprehensive. Don't wear excessive or obvious jewelry. Attempt to blend. Be sure that your cell phone has a full charge and that you have a backup plan. Expect the worst and hope for the best.

When traveling abroad, if you aren't accompanied by a partner who knows the area or if you are not meeting with someone, hire a referenced guide. There are generally bilingual retired or off-duty police officers available in many countries. It's a worthwhile investment. Make certain that you budget for it and have your guide validated by a known and trusted source.

Action

Here's where the rubber hits the road! You've taken all the precautions possible. You've done everything by the book, yet there he is, sticking a gun in your face and demanding your wallet. What to do when the inevitable occurs? Look for your opening and make a concise, precise, relentless, all-or-nothing action. We have taken into consideration all the aforementioned variables: if you can run, do so; but if you are coming to your car with your baby in a stroller, you won't be able to get away. You'll have to fight or comply. I cannot and will not preach to you what your personal priorities are. Some people are willing to give up their house, their car, and their possessions. Some won't hand over a dime. I'm not here to tell you who is right or wrong. Just know that whatever your position is regarding your choice, you must be comfortable living with it the rest of your life. You don't want to put yourself in a position of would've, could've, or should've. Focus on a much smaller word—*did*. What *did* you do to prevent loss, injury, or death? Be comfortable with your mind-set before a situation occurs. Hindsight is always 20/20 vision. Predict the outcome and minimize the loss. There will always be a potential of loss or harm in an altercation. Oftentimes it's unavoidable, so do your best to keep the losses at a minimum.

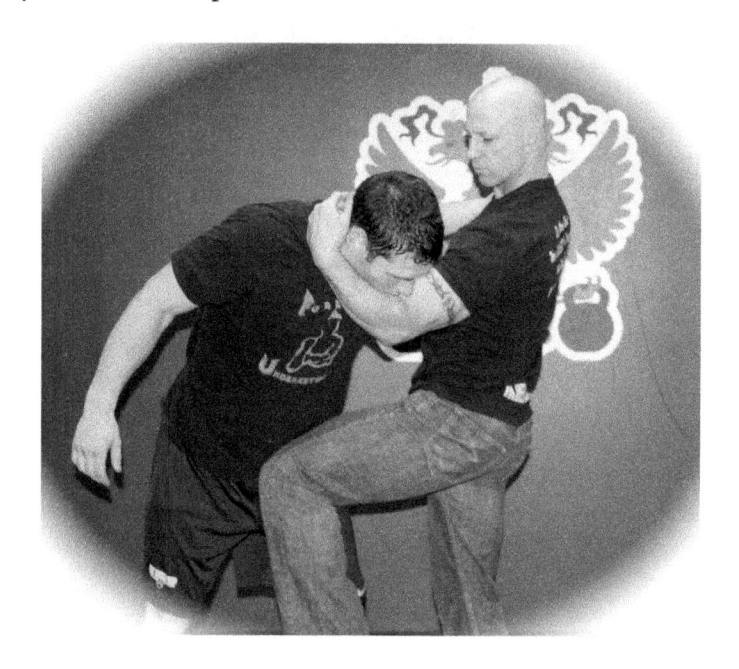

SIPDE: Scan, Identify, Predict, Decide, and Execute

Scan

Use your ears and ears to scan the area. As with Awareness, scan your surroundings and look for potential threats and escape routes. Register who is in the area and take notice of potentially dangerous people.

Identify

Identify potentially hazardous situations and persons. Recognize the threat(s). Pay attention to how the person(s) is postured. What are they wearing? Where are they positioned? Is there a road blocked off? Why are those guys hanging around the street corner? Why is there a burning tire in the middle of the road?

Predict

Predict what may occur. Given the assessment of your surroundings, the people, the escape routes, limitations, and other variables, what could happen? These assessments need to be made expeditiously. Time is of the essence. Your safety depends upon you making the right predictions.

Decide

Make a decision of what to do. Do you call 911, run, turn around and take a different route, employ verbal contact to determine threat level, attack first, nothing? The last option of nothing is what occurs in most instances, but if your senses tell you that something is awry, it most likely is. Whatever action you decide to undertake, make it decisive and complete. Don't half-do something. The end result is usually not good. Just like Mr. Miyagi said in *The Karate Kid*: "Walk on road, hmm? Walk left side, safe. Walk right side, safe. Walk middle, sooner or later, get squish just like grape. "Here, karate, same thing. Either you karate do "yes" or karate do "no." You karate do "guess so", squish like grape."[8] Sound advice, same holds true here.

Unfortunately, you have very little time to make your decision. Things happen fast—*very fast*. You cannot hesitate with whatever course of action you decide to take. Additionally, you must be totally committed.

Execute

Act upon your decision and do so in a concise, precise manner. Some course of action will have to be taken. If you are going to flee, do so and make it quick. Leave the area and be sure that you are headed to a safe haven. You may avoid an actual physical confrontation by your

---

[8] *The Karate Kid* (1984) was responsible for a huge upswing in martial arts training in the 1980s. The movie starred Ralph Macchio and Pat Morita. Neither were trained in karate.

posturing and verbal response to a potential threat. If you are going to get physical, follow through with full power and intent.

An example: I was in Philadelphia for the weekend. It was late, and I was very hungry. I decided to walk down the street and go to an all-night diner. Maybe not the best choice I could have made, but hunger took over. It was approximately 2:30 a.m. as I returned to my hotel room. As I rounded the corner, I noticed two other gentlemen across the street. No cars, no other people—just me and the two other guys. I had about a block and a half to walk until I reached my hotel as one of the guys crossed the street toward me.

OK, now, here's where the process went into action. First, I noticed them and decided that I was going to take my chances and head toward my hotel. I was too far from the diner, and there were no immediate safe havens. I know that once he crossed the street a confrontation was imminent. I had made my decision and planned to execute.

As he approached, he asked to "borrow" some money from me. Please note that I did not allow him to get closer than ten feet from me when I aggressively responded with "Stop right there. I'm in no mood for you or any of your bull--t! Tell your story walking!" The guy stopped dead in his tracks, turned around, and walked back across the street. Had he continued toward me, the first strike would have been a firmly planted low kick followed by axehands, elbows, and knees. However, he most likely listened to *his* inner voice and decided to wait for an easier victim.

The whole time, I viewed his body language and posture and watched his hands to see if he was going to pull a weapon. I also kept an eye on his partner across the street. When he left, I did not turn my back on him until he was a reasonable distance away from me. I was also aware of the position his partner had taken. He never advanced.

Fight, Flight, or Freeze

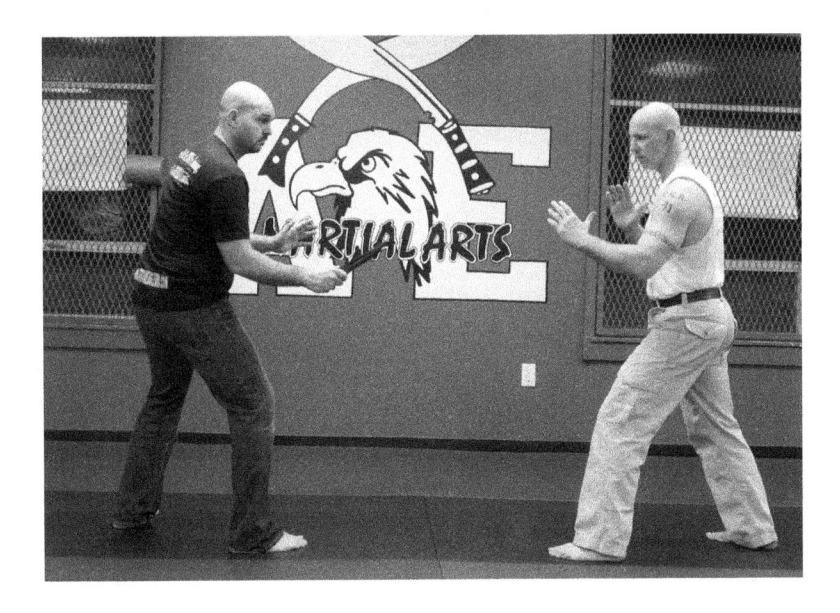

We have all heard of the fight-or-flight syndrome, but more often than not, most people freeze. Fight—you defend yourself. Flight—you run for the hills. However, there has not been much attention dedicated to the freeze segment. Most people have never even been hit, much less attacked. The moment their assailant lays their hands on them or smacks them, they freeze up like a deer in the headlights and get bludgeoned. The perpetrators are counting on this.

When the proverbial s—— hits the fan, you have to be prepared. There will be an incredible adrenaline dump, and your arms and legs will feel very heavy. Things may go in slow motion, and you will experience tunnel vision and what I call the "whirr" in your head. This whirring sound occurs right before and during a physical confrontation. This physiological reaction is a result of the infusion of adrenaline, your increased blood pressure, and the psychological stress that the mind undergoes when faced with extreme conditions. The key is to be able to maintain a clear head and allow your body to respond properly.

Following your physical training, learning what it feels like to get hit and the mental preparation involved will get you prepared. However, until you have been in an actual situation, you will not know how you react. Please also bear in mind that your reaction may differ from situation to situation, depending upon the circumstances.

In addition to the training contained here, you should also work out with kettlebells. One of the best training methods to help the body handle an adrenaline dump is to employ breathing ladders. This type of training has been successfully used by firefighters, police officers, and other military and paramilitary organizations to aid in reducing the effects of the adrenaline dump.

You need to train and become mentally and physically conditioned to instinctively respond. Thought and emotion have no place here. Concise response and action are required. This ability is acquired through consistent, meaningful training. There are no secrets.

4
PHYSICAL FITNESS AND STRENGTH

To defeat evil, good must be very strong!

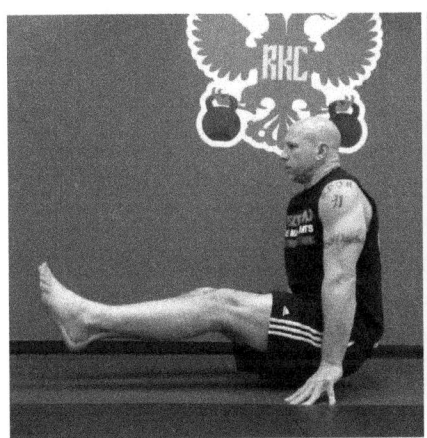

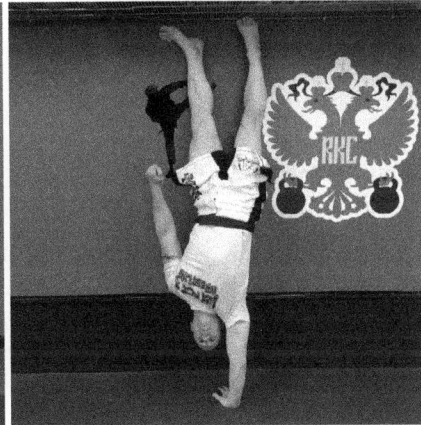

COMPLETE PHYSICALITY

There are certain minimum physical requirements you will need for proper application of most fighting techniques. You will need flexibility and strength in your hips, shoulders, and spine. It's up to you to forge your body in order to both withstand a blow and deliver one with maximum effect. If you are conditioned, your chances of survival are dramatically increased.

POWER DEVELOPMENT

The development of the upper and lower body explosive power and general strength is essential to effective striking and throwing. The stronger you are, the easier it will be to impose your will upon another and defend yourself from attack.

KETTLEBELLS, SANDBAGS, AND WEIGHT TRAINING

These are excellent methods for developing additional strength. There are many publications dedicated to these training methods. The focus of this book is based on what you are able to do with your our body, a partner or very little equipment. However, if you are using external resistance apparatus, I recommend training three to four times a week. Your workout should be an hour or less. Anything more and you are training for something other than fighting and may actually hinder your performance.

BASIC STRENGTH

In this section, our primary focus will be on bodyweight, simple suspension, and man-to-man strength-developing drills. There are other fantastic methods of strength development: kettlebells, free weights, sandbags, etc. However, there are a multitude of resources available regarding these methods of developing your strength. The advice contained in this book caters to the minimalist. The calisthenics listed below are some of my favorites for power development and conditioning. There are many others that you may incorporate in your training regimen.

Upper body strength is developed through pushing and pulling. By employing a wide variety of push-ups, pull-ups, dips, and handstands, we can develop great strength and durable tendons.

Importance: Someone may try to twist or control your limbs. If they are soft and deconditioned, you will most likely sustain an injury and not be able to free yourself from your assailant's grip. Your striking effectiveness will also increase with your strength.

Lower body strength is also developed through pushing and pulling. We use various squats and dead lifts to create lower body strength.

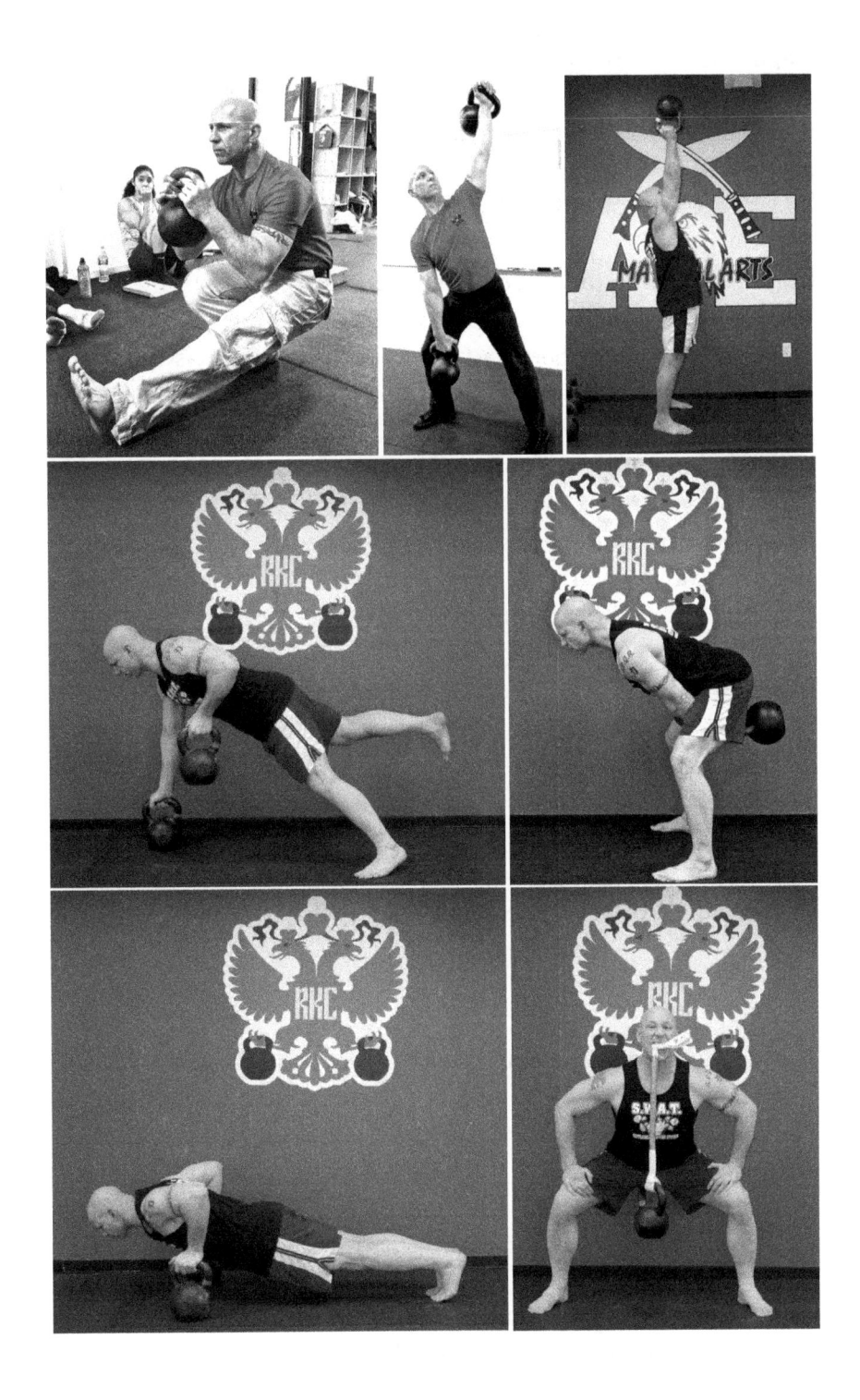

Importance: This strength will enable us to deliver powerful kicks more explosively. Our driving power comes from our lower body as well. Pushing someone off of you, standing back up after being knocked down is all aided by leg strength. Leg strength and conditioning will lessen the effects of leg attacks.

Rotational, core, and abdominal strength is accomplished through a variety of planks, bridges, and abdominal strengthening movements. These are the most important, yet frequently ignored, sets of exercises.

Importance: Development of a strong core will enable you to sustain a blow and minimize or even eliminate the damage to internal organs.

Neck strength involves wrestlers' bridge, 4-way neck dynamic tension, and static wall tension work. It is essential to have a strong neck. Most people do not work their neck muscles.

Importance: You never know when someone is going to grab you by the neck or when something will fall on you. You need to be able to withstand a beat-down. A strong neck will minimize the effect of referral shock to your brain.

Rotational and Core Strength

PLANKS

The plank is an exercise that virtually anyone can do, even if you are deconditioned or are suffering from some type of physical handicap. This exercise also serves as a means for you to develop the notion of full-body tension. This skill will help you in both delivering and absorbing blows. In all planks, tuck your hips, tighten your butt, and adopt a slightly concave position as opposed to maintaining the neutral spine.

RKC plank: Place your elbows and toes on the floor with your body straight. Start by tightening your abs, butt, and lats, and then move to apply full tension throughout the rest of your body. Your fists should be clenched and located under you face. Practice "breathing behind the shield" by bringing your breath in through your nose, down to the bottom of your lungs and exiting your mouth while keeping your abdominals taut. Vary your times holding this position, but a 30-second full-tension hold is a good place to begin your planking.

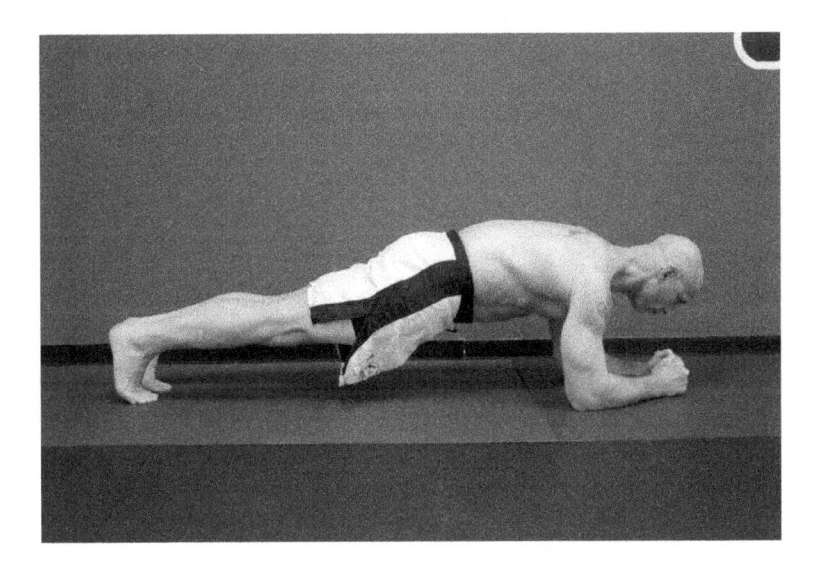

Out and back plank: Start in the RKC plank position. Walk your elbows out as far as you able while maintaining the integrity of your core. Hold for 10 seconds and then bring your elbows back to the original position for another 10 seconds. Repeat this sequence for three reps in each position as a starting point.

Power plank: How many of you like to hold a plank for 3 minutes? Neither do I. The power plank allows you to maximize your effort for a condensed amount of time. Assume the RKC plank position, and then visualize yourself bringing your elbows to toes and having them meet two feet underground. Apply full-body tension, which is no easy task, for 15 seconds. Applying full body tension for 15 seconds takes a great deal of focus, concentration, and practice. The results are fantastic, though!

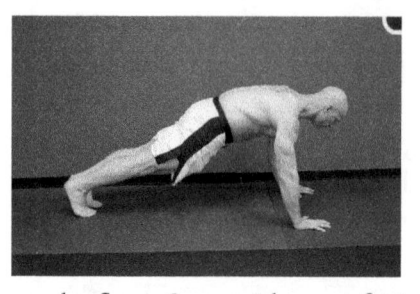

Tall plank: This is essentially the top of your push-up. Drive the heels of your palms into the ground as you grip the floor. Tighten your abs and assume the concave position. Draw your kneecaps up and into your quads as you plant your toes on the floor. Start with sets of 30 seconds.

Side plank (and tall side plank): Begin this movement on your side with your elbow on the ground lined up with your shoulder and your feet either one over the other or slightly crossed. Your hips should be perpendicular with the floor and the ceiling. Maintain this position throughout the movement. The slight crossing of the feet is a good starting position for beginners. As with all planks, apply tension to your body. From this position, drop your hip to the floor and then raise it up as high as you are able. For the tall version, post your palm on the floor as opposed to your elbow.

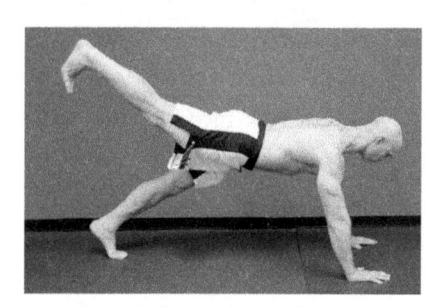

One leg plank: Assume the tall plank position and raise one foot off of the ground. Lift you leg as high as you able with keeping your hips and shoulders in the same plane and parallel with the floor. Repeat the movement on the other side. Hold the position for a duration that allows you to achieve multiple sets. Start with 10 seconds each side and increase both the time and the sets as you become stronger.

Angled plank (up and down): If you are just beginning, you may want to start your planks with your hands elevated either on a low table, bench, or chair. Once you become more advanced, switch the position so that your feet are raised. This will add difficulty to the technique.

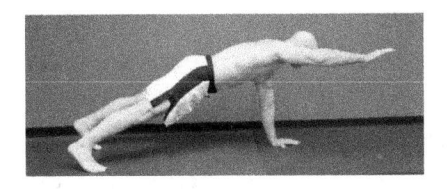

One arm plank: Assume the tall plank position and raise one arm off the ground. Bring the hand so that it is even with your shoulders. You may bring your hand up to the side or out in front. Make certain that your hips and shoulders are parallel with the floor throughout this exercise.

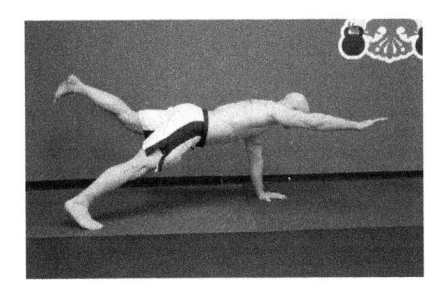

One-arm/one-leg plank (trans verse): This exercise is to be done as the one-arm plank, except that you bring the adjacent leg off the ground at the same time as your arm. So if you raise up your right hand, you elevate you left leg and vice versa.

BRIDGING

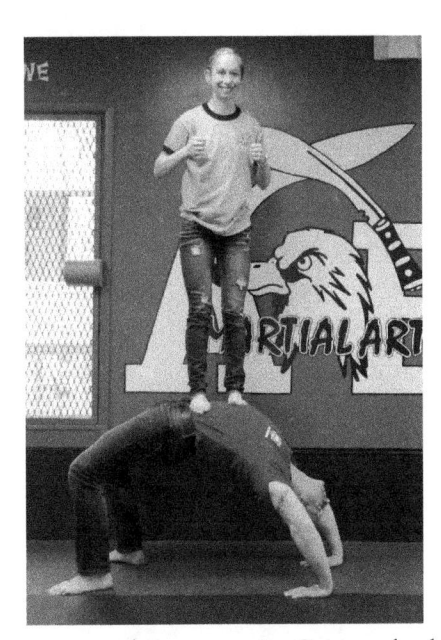

The exercise that provides the bridge between your lower and upper body. The spinal erectors are critical to real strength development and core stability. How many times have you seen a huge guy completely incapacitated because he threw out his back? I will almost guarantee that he spends quite a bit more time doing bench press as opposed to working on his bridge. Don't be that guy. Listed below are some of my favorite variations.

Whatever bridges you practice, there are several ways to train. One method is to perform a multitude of repetitions. It is important, though, to make certain to pause at the top and the bottom of the movement. This holds true for many of the other exercises.

Flat bridge: Lie flat on your back and place your arms out to the side at approximately a 45-degree angle from your sides. Have your knees bent and as close together as possible with your feet flat on the floor. If need be, place a foam roller, a small or large ball or another object between your knees to help you create tension. Perform 10 repetitions. Time under tension is essential, with 5- to 30-second holds at the peak of the movement recommended. When you become more flexible, "walk" your shoulders toward your heels and grab your ankles with your hand to help elevate your bridge even more.

Runner's bridge: Lie flat on your back in the same initial position as in the flat bridge. Dorsiflex both feet, not just the one on the leg that you are raising, but both feet. Contract your glutes and push your hips high toward the ceiling and drive your knee toward your chest while pushing through the floor with the adjacent heel.

Maintain this position for 2 to 5 seconds. Repeat the movement for 5 to 10 repetitions and then change sides.

Straight leg bridge: Sit on the floor with your legs straight out in front of you. Sit up tall and have your hands on the floor next to your hips with your fingers facing forward. Squeeze your legs together; they will want to come apart. So you'll need to contract your inner thighs and control the motion from your hips all the way down to your metatarsals. Maintain a neutral spine as you drive your hips toward the ceiling. Your head, shoulders, hips, and legs should be in a straight line at the top of the movement. Perform 20 to 40 repetitions. Vary the duration of the hold time. This bridge will tax your triceps muscles quite a bit as well.

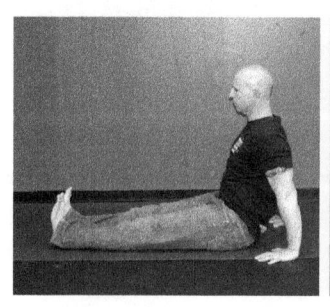

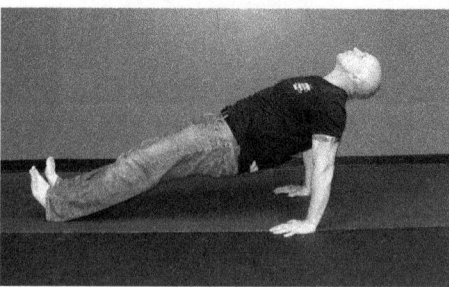

Tabletop bridge: Lie flat on your back and bring your feet close to your buttocks. Keep your knees bent and sit up. Place your hands a little behind your hips with your fingers facing your toes. Maintaining a neutral spine, bring your hips up as high as you are able by contracting your buttocks and tightening your core. Done properly, your body will form a table with your legs and arms at 90-degree angles. Hold for 2, 5, or 10 seconds, and then drop your bottom to the ground, touch quickly, and come back up. Do 5 to 10 repetitions.

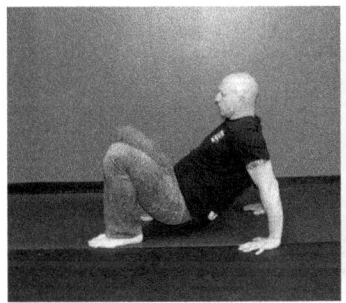

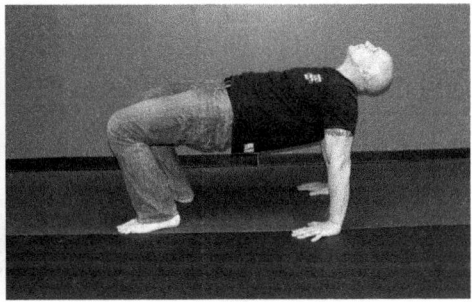

Thoracic bridges: Begin with your hands and feet on the ground, knees flexed so that your feet are almost in line with your hips but slightly behind. If we were going to the right, post on your left hand, swing your left leg through to the opposite side as you post on your left arm being certain to keep your shoulder packed.[9] Reach across your body with your right arm and drive your hips toward the ceiling. Your hips should be in a horizontal position to the floor as you drive them toward the ceiling and your shoulders should be vertical. Repeat this process on the other side for 3 to 5 repetitions in both directions.

---

[9] Shoulder packing is often described as the act of engaging your lats while pulling the shoulder joint back and down, thus elongating the neck and "packing the shoulder." This movement is the antithesis of "shrugging" your shoulders.

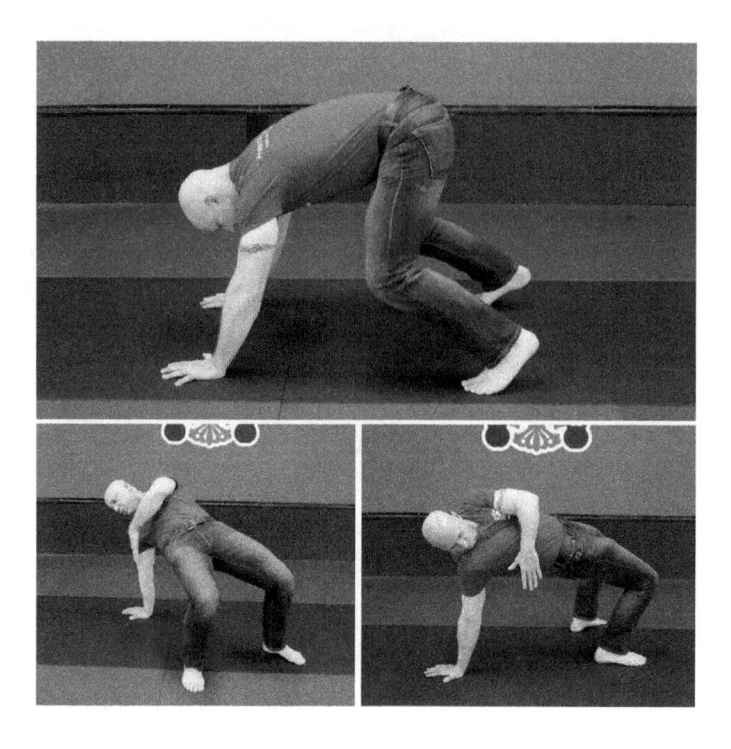

Full back bridge: Lie flat on your back and bend your knees so that your heels are as close to your buttocks as possible. Invert your hands so that your palms are on the ground with your fingers pointing toward you and on either side of your neck. Your elbows should be pointed directly at the ceiling. Feel free to make adjustments and creep your hands and feet closer together as you drive your hips upward. To maximize the effectiveness of this bridge, as well as the others, contract your posterior chain and squeeze your rhomboids together as your hips are raised. Perform 10 to 20 repetitions with 2- to 10-second holds.

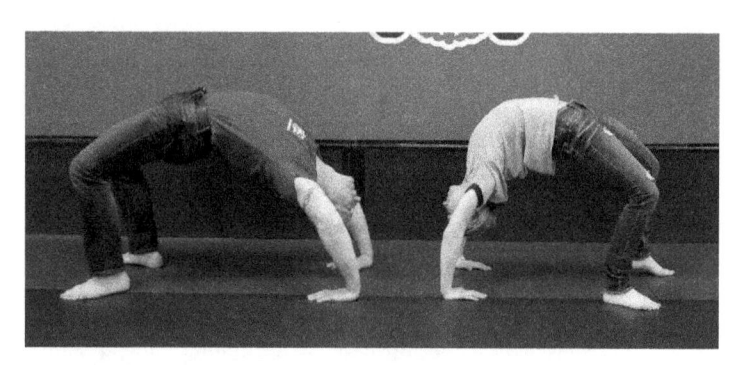

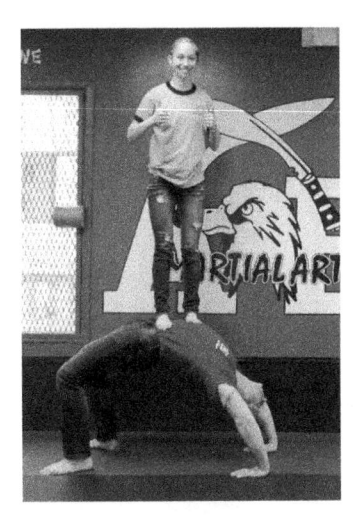

Bridge pops: Lie on the ground and bend your knees enough to allow your feet to be flat on the ground. Drive your hips upward very quickly as you punch across your body and upward. For example, as you thrust your hips upward, punch your right hand up and across to the left side of your body and past your head. Arch your body and turn your head to the same side (left in this case) that your arm is going to. Drop your hips and violently pop them up again. Alternate sides while training. This movement is crucial when someone is on top of you and you are trying to create space to move.

A basic premise to remember: When you are on top of someone, you want to minimize space to increase your control and pressure. When you are on the bottom, you need to create space to enable you to escape. When practicing bridges for strength, keep your heels planted firmly in the floor. When practicing for application and height, go up onto the balls of your feet.

Neck bridges: This is a favorite of wrestlers, football players, and other collision and combat athletes. Neck strength is essential to every collision and combat sport. If your neck is weak, you will not last long. Lie on your back as if you were going to do a bridge pop or a flat bridge, except you drive up to your head so that your heels and your head are on the ground. Once you have developed significant strength with this movement, venture onto the balls of your feet.

Next, roll from the crown of your head to your forehead in a back-and-forth motion. You should also incorporate lateral movement and "rolling" motions. Place your hands together and in line with your shoulders as you rock back and forth, side to side and in small circles. Even though your neck is part of your upper body, I consider this exercise a complete, posterior body movement linking both upper and lower sections of the body together.

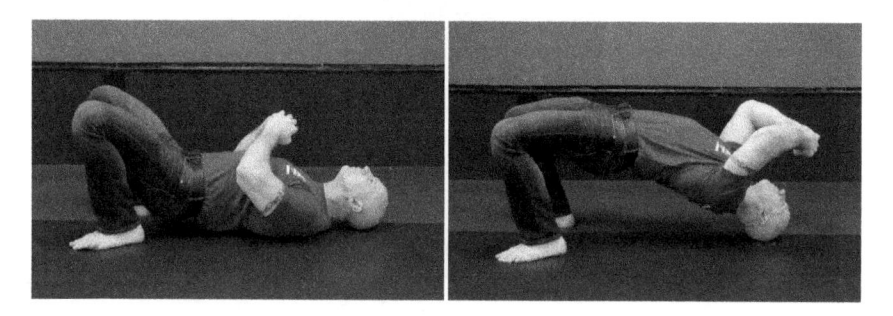

Physio ball rolling: "Sit" on a physio ball with your low back on the ball and your feet on the ground. Place your hands out front with your arms slightly bent. Then begin to roll yourself around on the ball while trying to maintain contact and not fall off. Roll around on the ball, back and forth, up and down. This is a free-form exercise. This drill is a great deal of fun and helps you develop balance. I include this movement after my bridgework. I generally do this one for time—30 seconds to a minute at a time.

ABDOMINALS

The outward visibility of "the abs" is often used as the barometer of fitness, conditioning and strength. The appearance of abdominals is not nearly as important as their strength. The fact that they can be seen is more of a function of diet. Whether your abs are visible or not, they need to be strong.

Leg thrusts: Lie flat on your back so that your lumbar (low) and thoracic (mid) back remain pinned to the ground. It's important to keep your cervical spine (neck) off the floor for most all abdominal exercises. You accomplish this by contracting your abs, not simply lifting your neck and keeping your hips "bolted" to the ground. There should be no space between your low back and the floor. *Never* put your hands underneath your low back to fill the gap with the floor. Your hands should either be on your stomach, or your fingers should be interlocked and behind your head. Bring your knees up as high as you are able toward your chest, then "thrust" your feet forward with your toes dorsiflexed.[10] Your feet should be approximately 6 to 8 inches from the ground. Perform 20 to 50 repetitions per set.

Concave abs (3 positions): Secure your lumbar region (low back) against the floor. For the beginner version, apply full tension as you force your knees into your elbows. When performing the intermediate level, extend your legs all the way out while keeping the tension in your upper body and driving the elbows toward your feet. For the advanced position, extend both your feet and hands all the way out. Be certain to keep your hips down and have no space between the floor and your back. You may have to raise the level of your feet and hands to maintain this position. There are many ways to use this method to train your abs. You can hold a specific position for 10 to 30 seconds. You may move from one position to another, holding the positions for 10 to 30 seconds before moving on. More advanced students may hold the positions for 60 seconds or longer.

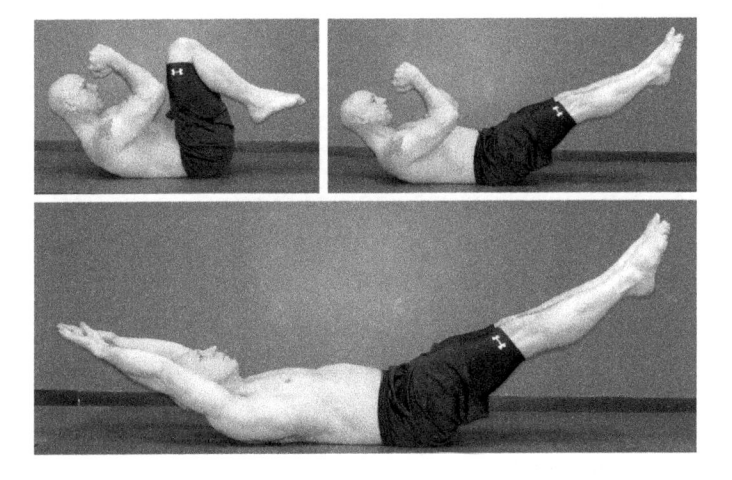

---

[10] Dorsiflexed: Toes are curled back toward the shins.

Butterfly crunches: Start in the butterfly stretch position with the bottoms of your feet together and tucked in as close as possible to your butt. Then assume the supine position as with the prior movement, except keep the bottoms of your feet together and as close to your butt as possible. Interlock your fingers and place your hands behind your head with your elbows out to the side and pressed backward as far as comfortable. Contract your abs and pull your upper body off of the ground so that only your lumbar spine[11] is on the mat while keeping your knees as far apart as possible. On the way down, your head should not touch the floor. There should be tension in your abs for the duration of the set. Perform 20 to 30 repetitions per set. Increase the reps as you become stronger.

Butt-ups and buttinators: As with most abdominal exercises, start with cervical spine off of the mat as previously explained. Hold that position and bring your knees up to your chest and then lift your butt upward. For the buttinator, bring your knees side to and up as opposed to simply raising your hips toward the ceiling. Try to keep your heels as close to your butt as possible through the movement. Your knees should be bent the whole time.

WOD (wheel of death): This great little tool can be picked up for $10 to $15. This apparatus has been a mainstay in gyms for eons—the ab wheel. We are going to review how to use this equipment properly. Start with your knees together and the wheel in both hands and directly in front of you. Grasp the handles of the wheel and try to "snap" the handle as you fire your lats, abs, shoulders, and arms. Maintain the concave, or hollow, position[12] as you roll the wheel out in front. Only go out as far as you are able with being able to return to the start position with a smooth motion while maintaining the hollow position. It is recommended that you place a pencil or weight at the far end of your reach to ensure that you don't overextend yourself. Each forward-and-

---

[11] Lumbar spine: The lower five vertebra of your spine. Often referred to as the low back.
[12] Hollow position: Used by gymnasts to brace their bodies. This is one of the few times that I will recommend that you *not* have a neutral spine. Keep a slight curve or rounding of your back by tucking your hips and head while under full tension.

back motion needs to be done under tension and take anywhere from 5 to 10 seconds. Start with 5 to reps each set. When you become more advanced, you can start on your feet.

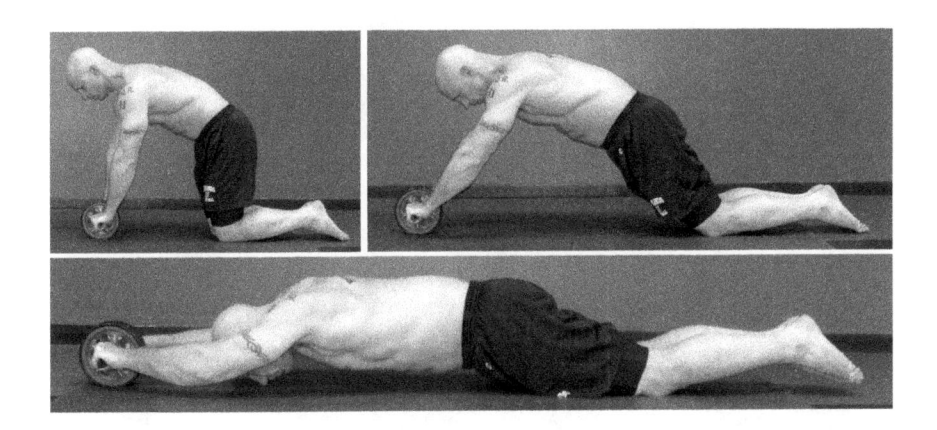

Hanging abs: The hanging abdominal exercise is most likely the best bang for your buck. There are many variations with significant difficulty ratings; however, they all begin the same way. Grasp the bar firmly, with either a thumbless (hook grip) or full grip.[13] Pack your shoulders, engage your lats and shorten your abs by lowering your ribs and drawing your hips up. Do this while maintaining a straight spine. Plantar flex (point your toes) and straighten your knees. Apply tension throughout your body and keep your elbows locked. Now you are ready to train! Here are a few of my favorites.

Knee-ups and L-sit: Hanging from a bar that doesn't allow your feet to touch the ground, assume the hanging ab starting position and bring your knees up as high as you are able. I like to raise them to at least

---

[13] Bar grips: There are several bar grips that you may use when lifting weights or gripping an overhead bar for various movements.
Full grip: Grasp the bar with your fingers on one side and your thumb on the other. Create a circle with your hand.
Hook grip: Thumbs and fingers are located on the same side of the object that you are gripping. This grip is used to reduce elbow strain and to grasp something that you can't get your hands around.
Under/over grip: Your hands face in opposite directions, both palms facing each other. Typically used for performing deadlifts. This is a very strong grip for pulling.

mid-chest level. For the L-sit version, simply extend your legs so that your profile will exhibit an *L*. Lower your legs slowly and perform 10 to 20 repetitions per set.

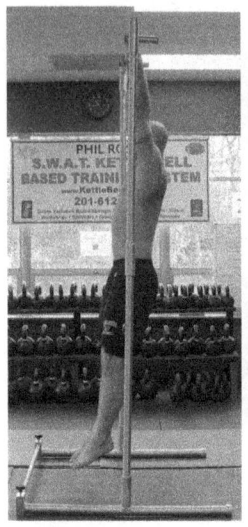

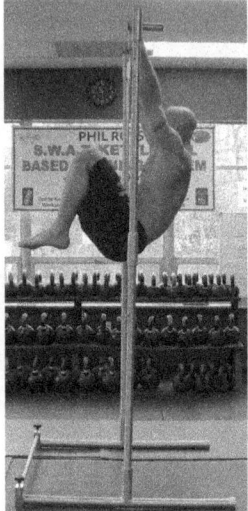

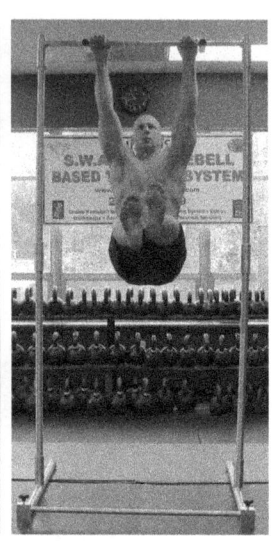

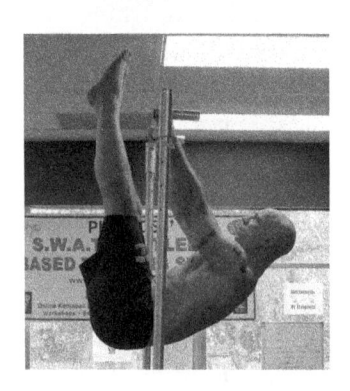

Jackknives: From the starting position, raise your feet up to the bar. Be sure to keep your knees and elbows locked. Minimize the sway by maintaining full body-tension. Sets of 5 to 10 repetitions are recommended.

Side crunch: Focusing on the obliques and serratus, lie flat on your back and slide your upper body to one side. Have the hand of the side that you slide to behind your head and your legs folded over so your knees are facing the opposite direction. Place the free hand on your knees. Keeping your shoulders in the same plane as the ceiling, contract your side abdominals and raise your upper body to the ceiling. Be certain not to twist. This is a very small but effective movement. Generally, 25 repetitions each side per set are recommended.

Ab crawl: This movement is a great deal of fun but requires some rhythm and coordination. Lie flat on your back, keeping your feet, hands, and elbows off the ground. Your elbows and knees will be close to each other, and your hands will be in line with your face. You will now pick a direction and progress laterally by shifting from having your low back on the ground to having your upper back on the ground, utilizing a rocking motion as you toggle between your upper and lower body. Make sure that you go in the opposite direction as well and do not let your feet or elbows touch the ground. Start with 10 repetitions each direction.

Leg drops: Lie flat on your back with your upper body (cervical spine) off the mat. Accomplish this by contracting your abs. Position your arms either behind your head or on your stomach. Start with your legs at a 90-degree angle from the floor, then squeeze them together, keeping your knees straight and toes pointed. Drop your feet down as far as you are able while keeping your lumbar spine pinned to the ground. Bring your feet up to 70 to 75 degrees and then drop them down to the aforementioned level again. Perform 15 to 25 repetitions each set.

Alphabet abs: Begin as you were in the leg drop exercise. With your feet, "draw" in the air the letters of the alphabet. Capital letters, no cheating with lowercase or script! Needless to say, there are 26 repetitions. Sing the Alphabet Song if needed.

SQUATS

There is no single lower body exercise more important than the squat. Strength, cardio, and balance can all be developed and enhanced with this exercise and the variations.

Standard squat: Stand with your feet approximately shoulder-width apart. Place your hands out front to act as a counterbalance. Actively pull yourself down into the squat. Your feet should be at an angle no more than 15 degrees. Your shins, knees, and hips should all be aligned. Do not allow your knees to protrude beyond your toes. Your spine neutral, ribs down, and your abdominal region taut, grip the floor with your toes and keep your heels planted. Eyes need to be level with the horizon.

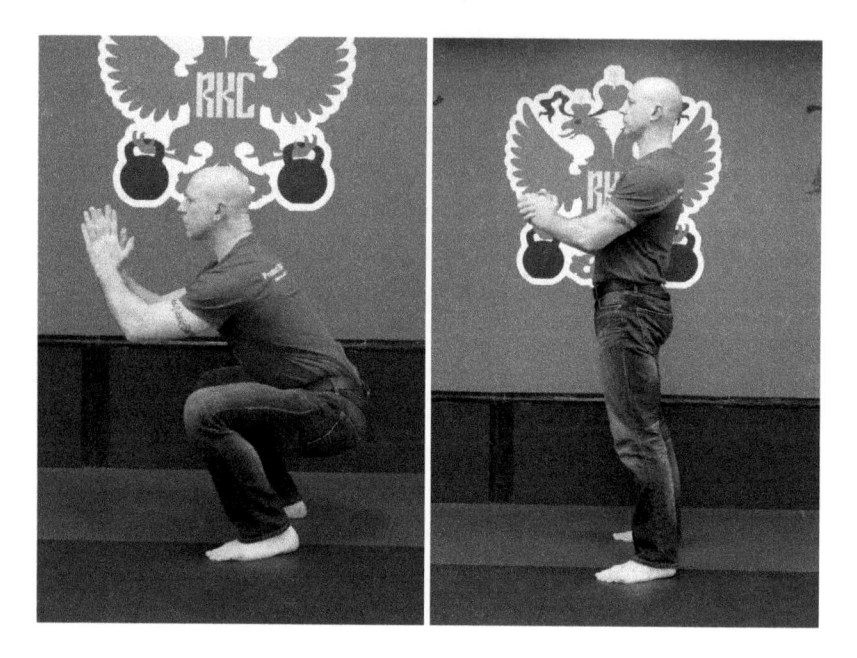

Skewed squats: An incredible squat to help you develop the strength and balance necessary for performing the pistol, or one-legged squat. Adopt as narrow of a stance as you possibly are able to maintain while keeping your balance. Plant one foot firmly on the floor and position the other foot next to the base foot so that the ball of the foot is on the ground and in line with the base foot's heel. Most of your weight should be on the base foot. The more weight you can place on it, the better. The stabilizing foot should almost appear as if you are wearing an imaginary high heel with calf flexed.

Actively pull yourself down below parallel. With practice, you will be able to get substantially below parallel and significantly improve your strength throughout the full range of motion. Sets of 10 repetitions each side is a good starting point.

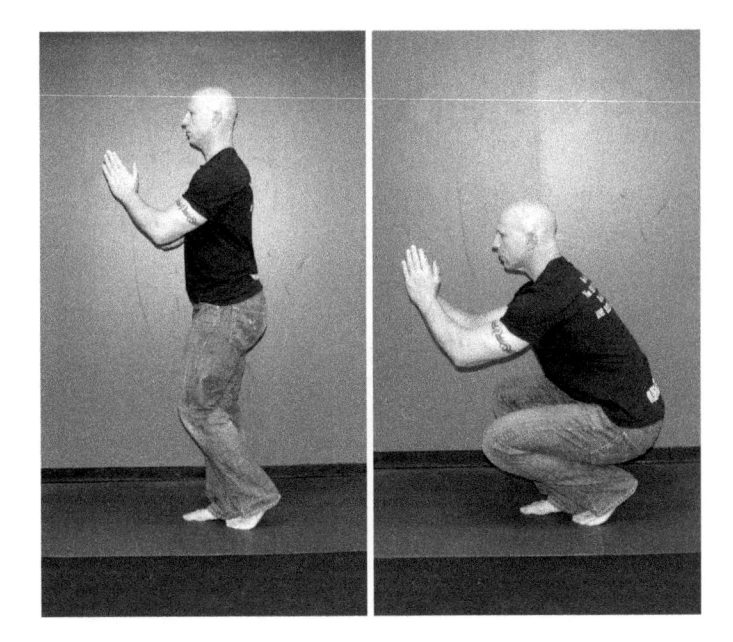

Pistols (single-leg squats): The most difficult and beneficial leg exercise. Period. The training enroute a butt to heel Pistol develops balance, trunk stability and incredible leg strength. There are weight lifters that can full squat 600 pounds, yet they collapse and fall over when attempting the Pistol.

Root your foot into the floor and extend the other leg with your foot dorsi-flexed. Pull yourself downward as you tighten your abs and put power through the heel of the extended leg. You'll want to have the crease of your hip pass below your knee joint as you maintain the full tension into the bottom of the movement. It also helps to create tension and balance when you extend your arms forward. For more advanced versions, raise your arms above your head.

Begin your training with one to three repetitions.

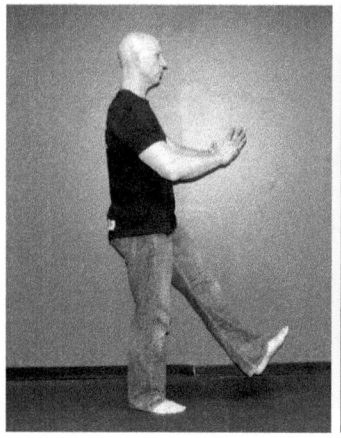

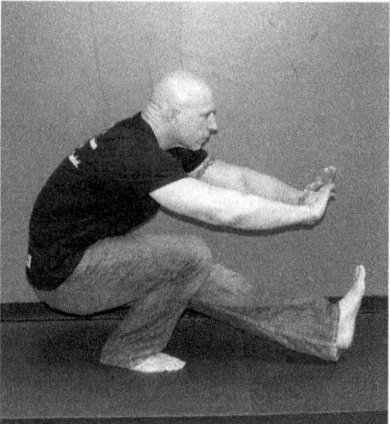

Hindu squats: This is a fantastic movement for muscular endurance. Begin with your feet relatively close together. The closer, the better, provided that you are able to keep your feet, knees, and hips collinear.

We want to use motion and get into a rhythm for this exercise. Dip down as low as you are able to, bringing your arms down and to the sides. Explode up and move your arms in a swooping motion in front of your body so that your hands are above your head when you are at the top of the movement and in line with your feet at the bottom. Exhale on the way up and inhale on the downward. This is a great endurance builder. Perform 25 to 50 repetitions per set.

Lunges: Stand tall with your feet together and your hands at your sides and on your hips. Bring one leg up and step forward placing your foot out in front only as far as you are able to go without losing your balance. Go deep enough so that the knee of your back leg almost touches the floor. Now return to your original standing by pushing the foot of the extended leg. You may do your repetitions on one leg and then the other or alternate. You may also do a backward lunge by stepping backward instead of forward. You may also lunge backward and forward on the same leg to mix things up a bit. Do 15 to 25 repetitions each leg per set.

Split squats: These are great for developing the leg power and coordination for lunging inward with a strike or for shooting a takedown.

Stand completely upright with your hands on your hips. Step one foot forward planting the foot firmly on the ground. Drop the knee of the other leg almost to the floor and be on the ball of the foot of the back leg. Be certain to keep your back straight, your spine neutral, and your abdominals and trunk tight, applying tension and stability to your movement. Perform 20 to 25 repetitions per leg, per set.

Airborne lunges: This may be the best single leg movement to perform. If not, it's a close second to the pistol. Begin standing tall with your feet together. Drop one leg back and guide your knee to touch the floor slightly behind and next to the heel of your planted foot. Do not allow the top of the back foot touch the ground as you go up and down. If you are unable to perform these, put your back foot up onto a raised platform like a step, or even a large book. Start with sets of 3 to 5 repetitions.

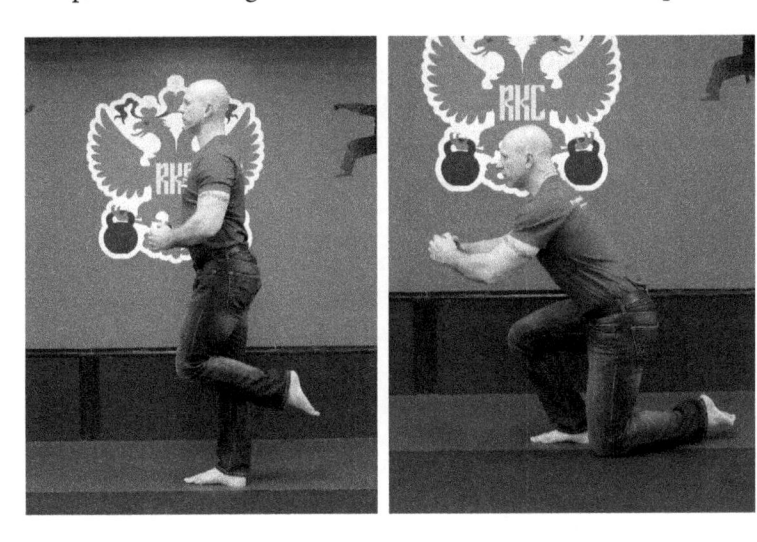

Single-leg deadlifts, unweighted: This movement is great for developing balance, flexibility and the posterior chain. As with most of the lower body exercises, start with your feet together. Maintain a neutral spine and bend forward at the hip while lifting one foot off the floor while letting it go behind you. Slightly bend the knee of the base leg, adopting a "soft" knee. Keep your shoulders and hips square to each other and the floor as you bring you upper body closer to the floor. If you can achieve parallel, great! If not, get as close as you are able while maintain the integrity of the technique. To make the movement more challenging, extend one or both arms forward as you hip-hinge into the parallel position.

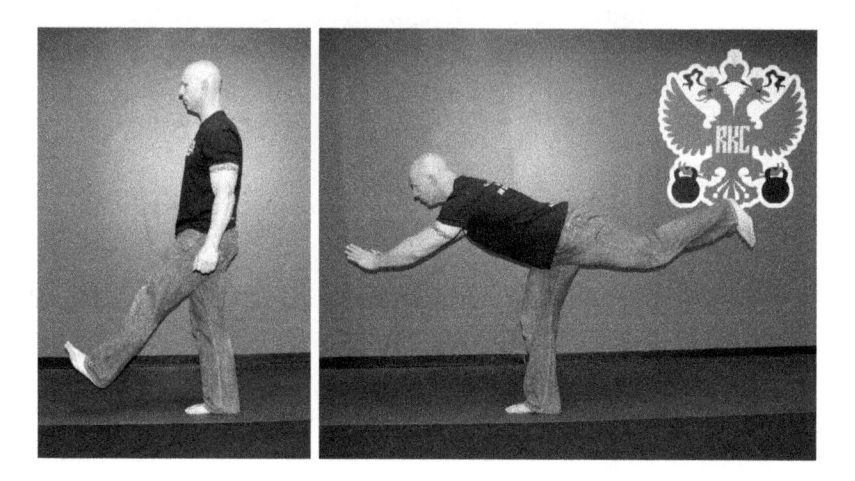

Calf raises: This is not a simple "bodybuilding" exercise. Strong calves will add to your explosive and pushing power. Your calves are also instrumental in your ankle mobility and strength. I practice the three-position calf raise variation more than the others.

You may either use a step (stair) or any raised platform that enables the full range of motion of your ankle. When you begin this exercise, it is recommended that you use two feet at the same time. Once you have developed greater strength, switch to one foot at a time.

Start on the ball of your foot with your heels in line with your toes and shins. Rise up as high as you are able and stretch as far as you can to the bottom by drawing your heels toward the floor. Hold each position for one or two counts. Perform 10 to 20 repetitions, or until you experience the burn in your calves. Stretch the calves out by pressing your toes against the step and rocking your knee forward. Repeat the same movement with your heels out and toes together for position 2, and with your heels in and your toes out for position 3. Start with one set and build up to three of each position. To make the movement more challenging, do one leg at a time by hooking the nonweighted foot behind the knee of the weighted foot. The knee of the weighted foot needs to be locked. You may also hold a kettlebell in one hand or simply slow the movement down and/or hold the top and bottom positions longer for added difficulty.

Jumps

Squat variations help you develop hip and leg strength. How do we address the explosive power required to knock an opponent silly with your kicks? That's where your jumping and bounding training comes in.

Vertical leaps: Set your feet about shoulder-width apart. Bend your knees until your reach parallel (or as close to it as you can) and bring your arms back, and rock slightly onto the balls of your feet and explosively drive your feet into the ground as you thrust your fists upward. On the descent, be sure to bend your knees and return to the original starting position. Once there, immediately begin the next repetition. Start with sets of 10 reps and build to 25.

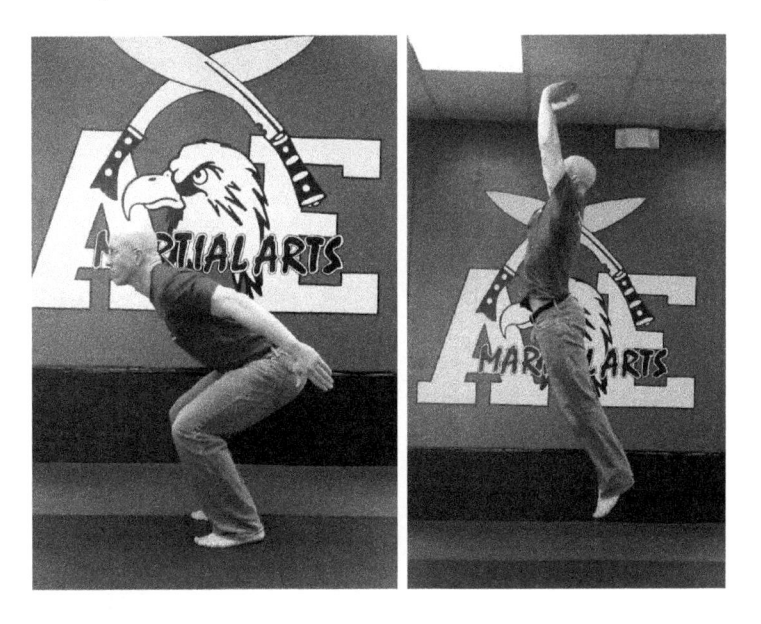

Single leg hops: Stand tall and then raise one knee up as high as you are able and hop forward by pushing off of the base foot. Land on the same foot and repeat this movement. Start with 10 to 15 repetitions on one foot and then repeat on the other. Try three to five sets each leg and then increase as you build your strength and endurance. We also do this for time or distance as well.

Lunar leaps: No, we are not doing impersonations of the legendary pop star Michael Jackson,[14] but we will be performing an extremely beneficial movement. We will be practicing lateral bounding. Imagine you were on the surface of the moon. Shift your weight onto one foot and leap forward and slightly to side, at approximately a 45 degree angle. Pause on the foot that you land on and without putting the other foot down, drive off of that same foot and repeat the 45 degree angle leap to the other side. Again, landing on the foot previously in the air. You will be both landing and pushing off of the same foot, alternating with every other step. Your pause on each foot between your landing and take off should be at least one full count. Keep the image of "bounding on the moon" in your mind while performing this exercise. Start with 10 to 20 repetitions on each leg for two to three sets.

Power skips: When you were a young child, you may have skipped around during play. Kids tend to do this naturally. What you will do is drive one leg off of the floor as you thrust the opposite knee and elbow into the air. As you land, switch sides. The power part comes in when you thrust off of the floor and upward with as much power as you are able. Do this for 30 to 60 seconds.

Leap-ups: Start with your knees slightly bent and then bring your knees up to your chest (or as high as possible) quickly. Land with

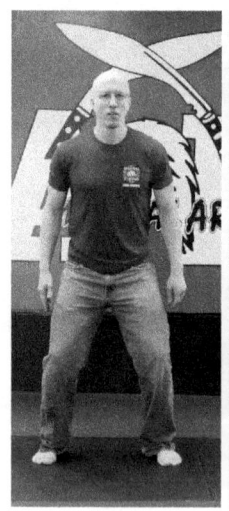

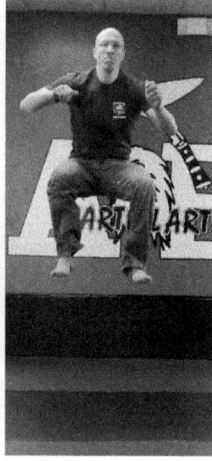

---

[14] Michael Jackson, a.k.a. the King of Pop, prior to his demise, used to perform the Moon Walk. This was one of his signature moves.

your knees slightly bent and repeat this movement for 10 to 20 repetitions for 3 sets. It is important to land on the balls of your feet and not on your heels and to minimize the time your feet are on the floor between reps.

Box jumps:
There are a variety of boxes and heights that you may use. Whether you choose metal, wood, plastic or foam mats, be sure that they provide a stable base and will not topple over. If you do not have the means to secure any of these, bleachers or a bench bolted to the ground are excellent substitutes.

Bend your knees and set your arms back as you shift onto the balls of your feet. Explode upward and shoot your hands forward as you launch yourself onto the raised surface. Land with bent knees and then jump backward off the platform. Keep your knees bent as you land to absorb the shock and prepare you for the next repetition. Some workouts go for speed, and others you will want to slow the pace a bit, especially when you are jumping onto a higher level. When training for power, do sets of 10. When considering speed, do your sets in 30- to 60-second increments.

You will begin with your hands out to the side, palms out and your feet approximately shoulder-width apart. Bring your knees up to your chest as quickly as possible as you raise your palms to the ceiling. As you land on the balls of your feet, immediately repeat the motion. You want to minimize the amount of time that your feet are in contact with the ground. Perform sets of 10 to 20 repetitions.

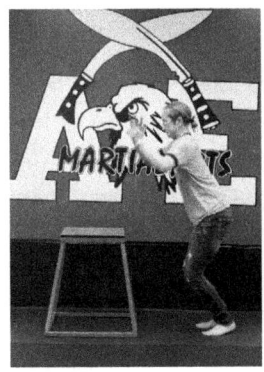

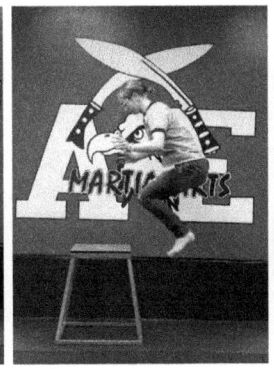

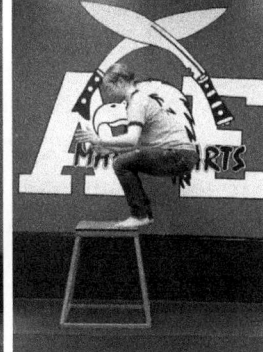

Calf thrusters: Place your hands on your hips and quickly rise onto the balls of your feet. Keep your head level and your back straight and you go up and down. When you do this for speed, execute 100 reps per set. When you are going slowly, do 25 to 50 repetitions per set.

Upper Body Strength: Pushing, Pulling and Neck (Isometric and Dynamic Tension)

PUSHING

Push-ups and handstands are essential to you building a strong frame. Please be certain to be able to execute a strong plank prior to attempting push-ups. I see far too many people trying to perform a push-up and their elbows are flaring, their backs are sagging like horses ready for the glue factory, they are dropping to their knees and moving their heads around as if they were bobbing for apples. Simply stop and work on your planks. Knee or "girlie" push-ups will *not* make your push-up better. These push-ups are an insult to women and should not be employed. Master your plank and then start with wall push-ups and gradually decrease the angle with various levels of incline push-ups until you have your hands on the floor cranking out your solid push-ups!

There are some fantastic progressions for push-ups and other bodyweight exercises in the convict conditioning series. I would strongly recommend employing these progressions for maximum bodyweight strength development.

Push-ups: Push-ups are my favorite of all bodyweight exercises. If there is a floor available, you can train. You want to achieve full-body tension with all variations. Tighten your core, buttocks, etc. You also do not want to flare your elbows. On most push-ups, have your elbow pits facing forward, grip the floor with your fingers, and drive the lower outside of the heel of your palm. Actively pull yourself down to the floor or at least to a fist's distance above. Maintain a neutral spine; do not lift your head up too high or allow it to droop downward.

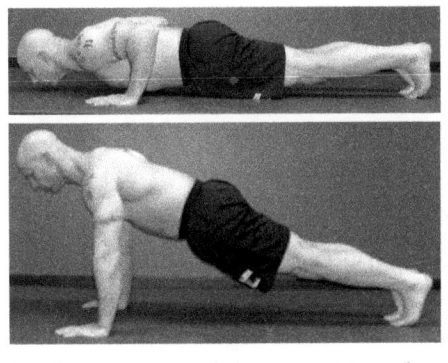

Standard (RKC) push-up: Palms flat on the ground, spread your fingers wide and grip the floor. Corkscrew your palms into the floor so that your elbow pits are facing forward. Actively pull yourself down to the floor and exhale as you push yourself up. Inhale at the top and repeat. Each direction of the repetition should consume one full count.

Ten-second push-up: Begin as you would for the RKC or standard push-up. Using a timer, clock, or simply by counting, take 10 seconds to lower yourself to the ground, touch, and count 10 seconds on the way up. Full-body tension is employed, as well as full range of motion. The goal here is to be moving for the duration of the exercise, only pausing momentarily at the bottom and the top. Start by doing 2 to 3 repetitions and work your way up to sets of 5. There is also a 5-second version of this movement.

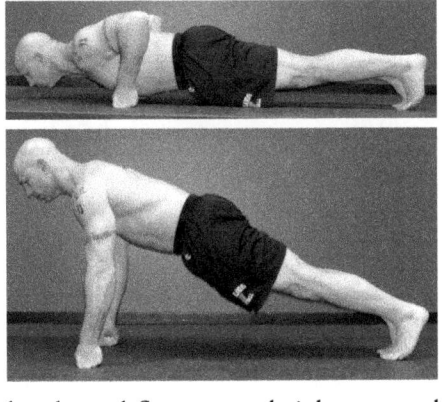

Knuckle push-up: Place your front two knuckles on the ground. Make certain that you don't rock backward and have the last three on the ground. Your two front knuckles (index and middle finger knuckles) need to be aligned with the radial and ulna bones of your forearm. Perform these on a hardwood floor or on bricks to condition and develop calluses on your knuckles.

Wide-grip push-up: Place your hands wide apart, beyond shoulder width, and keep your fingers pointed forward. Be sure to keep your elbow pits facing forward. It's a little more difficult to do with your hands set wide apart.

Triangle (or diamond) push-up: Set your hand directly below your chest with the thumbs and forefingers so that they are touching to form a triangle, or diamond, on the floor.

Fingertip push-up: Position your fingers on the floor so that only the tips are in direct contact. As you become stronger, subtract fingers from the floor. There are many people that perform one and two finger push ups.

Archer push-up: Begin as if you are going to perform your standard push up variety. Shift side to side as you extend the one arm and place most of the weight on the other as you straighten it out. You are using a swooping of your chest to the floor as you do the exercise.

Walk-the-plank push-up: Perform a push-up and then move one hand (right) to the other (left), shift the one hand out (left), and repeat the "walk" and push up sequence. Once done, repeat the movement in the opposite direction.

Medicine ball push-up: There are several variations of push-ups that one can perform with a medicine ball. You may place your hands in the middle of the ball and do close-grip or triangle push-ups. You may also have one hand on the ball and the other on the floor as you execute your push-ups. You may also slide the ball in and out with one arm or roll the ball form hand to hand as you do your push-ups. Have some fun with it. When doing the stationary types, start with sets of 20 to 30 repetitions, with the moving ones, begin with 10 reps on each side.

Furniture slider push-up: Purchase a couple of furniture sliders from the hardware store, or do what I did. Carpet installers left a set of plastic kneepads in my garage after an install. I started playing around with them and got a great workout by taking turns sliding one hand either out to the side or straight out in front. Begin with 5 repetitions in either direction.

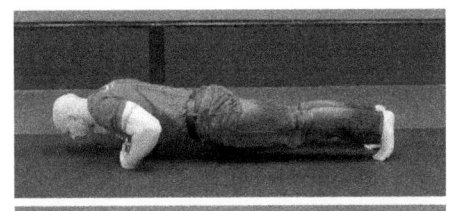

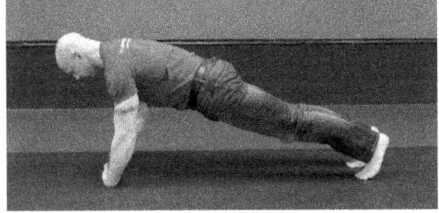

Back-of-the-wrist push-up: Bend your wrists toward your inner forearm and put your fingers together as if you were trying to pick a cherry. Place the back of your wrists on the floor and assume the push-up position. Keeping the back of your wrists planted, begin. These may be painful for beginners, but they are a great conditioning method for your wrists and forearms. Start with 5 to 10 repetitions.

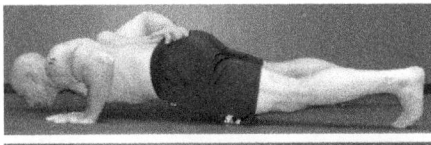

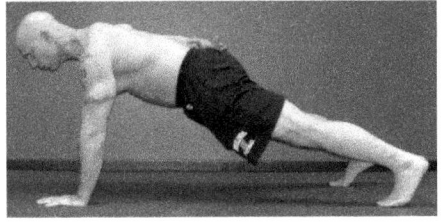

One-arm push-up: If you have been practicing your push-ups without your elbow pits forward, and if your lats have not been engaged, you will not be able to perform a one-arm push-up. If this had been the case, revisit your push up technique.

We do our one-arm push-ups on either our palms or our knuckles. The knuckle version is more difficult. Stabilize yourself on one hand and place the other behind your back or on your hip. Actively pull yourself down so that the shoulder of your suspended hand touches the floor. Full-body tension is an imperative. Single-arm pumps are a good way to prep you for the one-arm push-up. Also, you may only do partials while you are working on getting the full push-up in. The closer your feet are together, the more difficult the push-up is to perform. This goes for most variations.

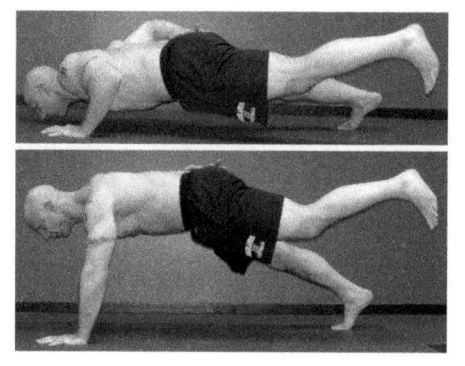

One-arm/one-leg push-up: This is one of the most difficult push-ups from the supine position to perform. A great deal of core and contralateral strength is required. Start in the push-up position, migrate to one arm, and then lift the adjacent foot off the ground. Actively pull yourself down so that the shoulder of the suspended hand touches the floor. Once this has occurred, drive your body upward by employing full tension in your body and contracting your muscles as you return to the top position. Do one to five repetitions each side.

Plyometric push-ups: There are several variations of the plyo push-ups that you may choose from. While performing any of the listed, it is important to "pop" your body off the ground and to maintain its plank position. Drop down and explode up. On these push-ups, we are not utilizing the active negative, so make certain that you are proficient at the standard push-ups before attempting any of the plyometric versions. The variations are determined by your hand position. Here are a few of my favorites: standard width on your palms, close or triangle, wide, knuckle, single-arm, and back-of-the-wrist. We also practice changing the position of the hands midair. For example: Start on your palms, switch to knuckle, and then to wrists every repetition. Begin your training with 10 repetitions. The higher you "pop up," the more difficult the push-up is. There are some people that can pop from the floor to a full standing position.

HANDSTANDS

Handstands are an incredible strength-developing exercise. I do handstands virtually every day. There are many, many handstand variations. We're going to address three.

However, I will advise you to practice crow stands prior to your handstand training. They will help you build the strength and balance required for handstands.

Crow stand: Kneel on the floor and spread your fingers out as wide as you are able, allowing you to "grip" the floor. Set the inside of your knees on the outside of your elbows and administer enough tension for you to maintain this position with only your hands on the ground. In the beginning, you may have to put your toes on the floor to balance yourself. Start with 10-second holds and build your way up to one minute. Once you are able to do a full minute, you have developed significant strength, balance, and tension to embark on the vertical position.

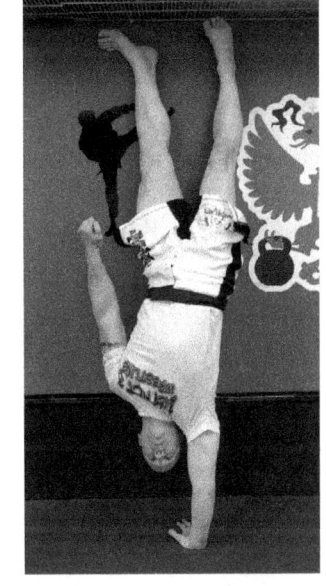

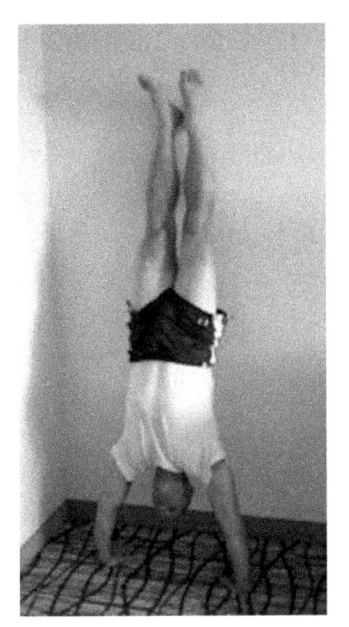

Face-the-wall handstand: Start with your hands on the ground and your feet toward the wall. Now, "walk" your feet up the wall and assume as vertical a position as is comfortable for you. Try to hold this position for 5 to 10 seconds before crawling back down. Once you are able to have an almost completely vertical position with your face very close to the wall and can hold it for 30 to 60 seconds, you are ready to attempt the next progression.

Wall handstand: Place your hands on the floor approximately 6 to 10 inches away from the wall. Grip the ground firmly, straighten one leg, and use the other to kick up to the vertical position. Use the non-kicking leg to steady yourself against the wall. Lock out your elbows and pack your shoulders, making your neck long. Focus your eyes on the wall on the other side of the room rather than on the floor. Dorsiflex your feet to aid in the creation of tension.

Gradually begin to pull one foot away from the wall. Once you are confident with this, pull the other one off as well, until you are freestanding in your handstand.

This is also a great time to practice wall push-ups. These will help you develop additional strength, tension, and balance in this position. Try to bring your head to the ground before you go back up. If you want more of a challenge, do these push-ups from a raised platform(s), parallel floor bars, or even kettlebells. This will enable you to get your head down lower.

Freestanding handstand: There are several methods to use here, and this is my favorite: Spread your fingers out and grip the floor with your hands. Bend your elbows and extend one leg out behind you. Attempt to get your face as close to the floor as possible and press yourself up as you perform a gentle kick upward with the leg that is on the ground.

Fixate your eyes on an object (usually a wall) across from you as opposed to looking at the floor. Drive your palms into the floor and create tension all the way through your heels while adopting a straight body. When it feels as though you are going to topple over, that is the position that you will steady yourself from. Bear these words in mind practicing. You will also experience this feeling when you are practicing your wall handstands as you take your feet off the wall. Try to hold yourself up as long as you possibly are capable. Generally, when first performing the freestanding version, one can only hold this position for a few seconds before losing their balance. You will eventually build your strength and balance in this position.

It is important to note that you will lose your balance and fall. The two methods of failure recovery that I have used are the roll-out and the pirouette. The pirouette is the preferred method. It requires less space than the roll out, and if the landing surface is not soft or has obstructions, injury may result. Additionally, practicing the pirouette helps you develop better balance. The rollout will require you to tuck your head, bend your elbows, and roll across your back while bringing your knees up to your chest. When practicing pirouette, shift your weight from one hand to the hand of the side that you are falling to. As you bring one hand off the floor, keeping your feet together, bend at the hips and rotate 90 degrees as you set your feet on the floor.

When your handstands become solid, you are able to determine when you'd like to come down. I like to "pop" out of the position. I start by bending my elbows and quickly pushing off of the ground and then snapping my hips as I drive my feet into the floor and come to a full, upright position. This ending is very akin to how gymnasts finish their floor exercises.

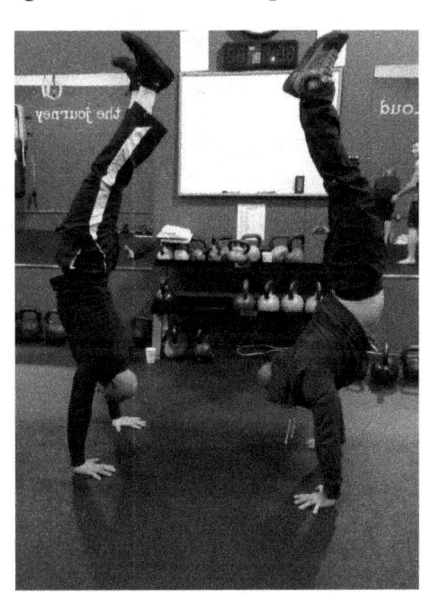

Pulling

Pull-ups, rowing motions, and partner lifts are the most effective means to develop pulling strength, sans equipment. Pulling is essential to fighting and lifting or carrying. Our pulling strength determines if we are able to move an opponent around, grab, hold, and lift them.

Pay particular attention to your elbow health. Make certain that you warm up your elbows and arms prior to any heavy pulling exercises. If you overdo your pulling training, your elbows will be the first to let you know. Gradually build; do not rush to advanced movements and large rep sets until you have properly prepared your joints and tendons. Soft-tissue injuries are common.

PULL-UPS

There are endless pull-up variations with different difficulty levels, but these are my favorite to do. I chose these versions because with proper training, most people will be able to perform some version of the listed. Additionally, by increasing the rep count or by performing the movements slowly, even the advanced practitioner will be challenged. Additionally, most of the movements lend themselves to grip width adjustment, yielding further variation to your training.

Pull-ups are an incredible barometer of strength, especially when considering strength to body weight ratios. If you cannot lift yourself off of the ground, you are either too heavy or not strong enough for your weight. When considering abdominal strength, pull-ups are a fantastic indicator. Have you ever seen anyone who can perform 20 pull-ups and has weak abs? I haven't.

Plank pull-up: Position yourself under a bar and utilize a thumbless grip. Have your arms fully extended at the bottom and assume an upside-down plank. Your toes should be dorsiflexed, and your body should have full tension. Pull yourself up so that your chest touches the bar. That complete motion constitutes a full rep. If you cannot complete a full rep, either change the angle of the bar to make it easier and/or hold the top position at full muscular contraction to develop more strength. Holding the top and bottom positions of your pull-ups is a great way to both develop and enhance your strength.

Tactical pull-up: A pull-up is generally categorized by pulling your body up so that your chin significantly clears the bar. Your palms facing forward so that the back of your hand is facing you. On the tactical version, you adopt a thumbless grip, pack your shoulders, tighten your abs, and pull yourself up. There is no, nor should there ever be, any "kipping" (gesticulation of the body to offer momentum to aid one in getting over the bar) of the body when performing pull-ups. Kipping does not promote strength development, but it is useful when performing a muscle-up. When considering pull-ups, the tactical pull-up is the standard.

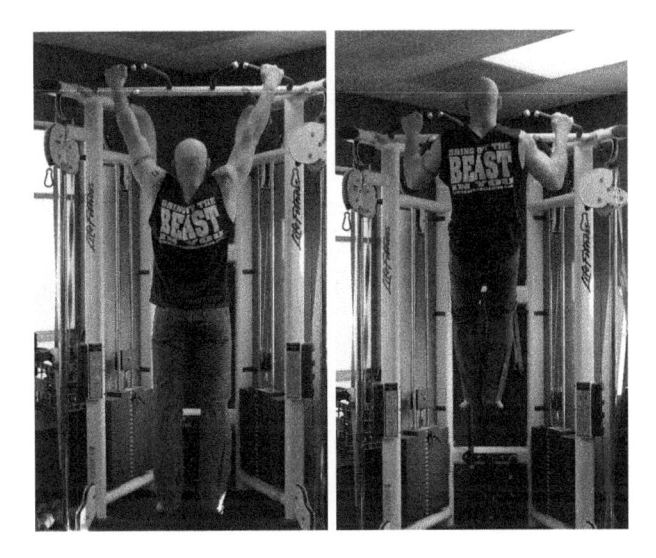

Chin-up: The chin-up is simply a pull-up with your palms facing you. I find these a little easier to perform due to the increased incorporation of the biceps muscles. This motion is also a little friendlier to the elbows. All other aspects of the pull-up remain consistent.

Wide pull-ups: I like to utilize the thumbless grip on the wide pull-ups, just as I do with the tactical pull-ups. This exercise is more difficult than the aforementioned versions due to the widened grip. The outer lats are taxed quite a bit with this movement, and it helps to widen your back.

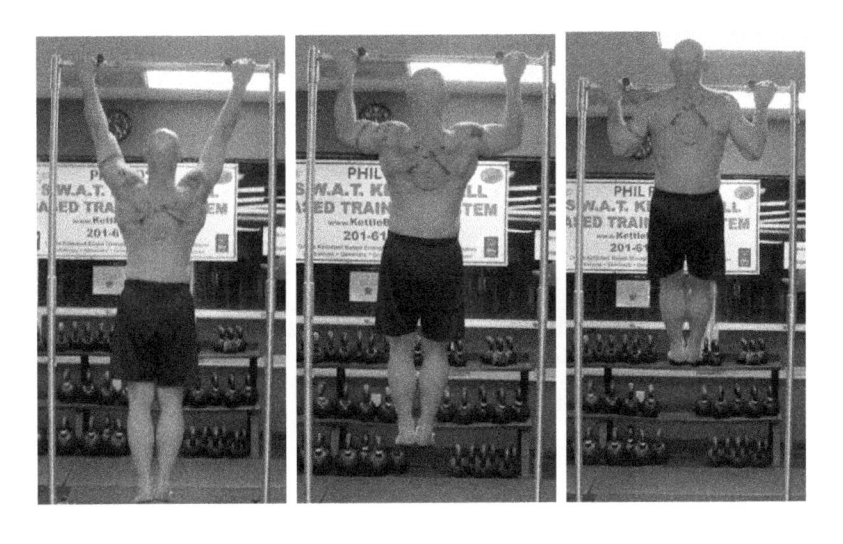

Towel pull-ups: Take a towel and fold it so that it takes on the shape of a rope and drape it over a bar. Grip tightly and pull yourself up. This adds an element of instability to the movement and develops your grip strength.

You may also use a towel in a hotel room to practice. Place the towel on the top edge of the bathroom door (it's usually a very sturdy door), take a thumbless overgrip, bend your knees so that your feet are off of the floor, and pull yourself up.

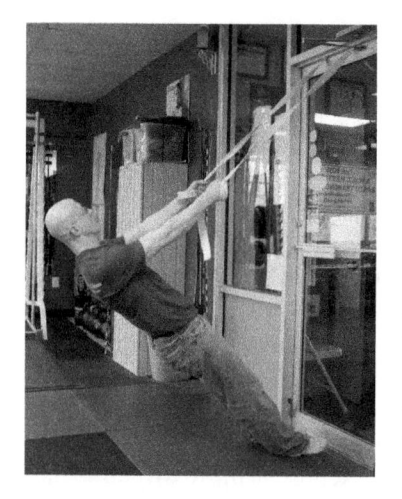

Karate belt rows: These may be done with a door or tied to a bar and with one or two arms. If you are practicing the door version, tie a knot in one end of one or two belts. Put it, or them, over the top of the door and then close the door tightly. Lean back and pull yourself upward. You may loop handles in the belt on the gripping side if necessary. I tend not to do so, though; the loops make it easier to grip, thus robbing you of additional grip training.

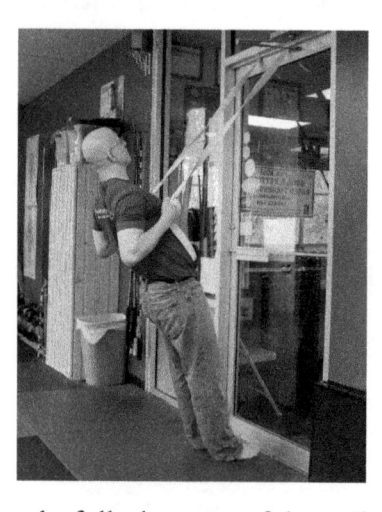

When using a bar, on a Smith machine for example, make a slipknot with the belt. Loop it over the bar, sure it up, and lean back. The bar version allows you to train with a variety of levels.

Always use the full range of motion while training for these (and most) movements. When performing the one-arm rendition, keep your shoulders square. This will aid you in developing greater core strength and allow you to take full advantage of the unilateral movement, thus making your body work harder by recruiting more stabilizers.

Lat pulls: Lie flat on your stomach and reach forward as far as you are able, keeping your hands in line with your shoulders. Bend your knees so that your lower body looks like a frog swimming and bring your legs together as you pull yourself up to your hands. Repeat.

This movement is best performed on a mat or a smooth floor as opposed to a carpet. Start with 10 to 15 pulls in accordance with your fitness and strength levels.

Neck Strength

The development of a strong neck is essential to survival. Look at the size of the necks on collision or combat athletes? They are huge. Why is this? The neck is the shock absorber for your brain. The stronger that you neck is, the less shock your brain will suffer and the fewer traumas your body will have to endure. This holds true not only in combat but in case of a fall or car accident.

Dynamic resistance 4-Way Neck: Tilt your head all the way and place your palms on your forehead. Providing counterpressure with your hands, move your head all the way forward for a count of 10. Now place your hands on the back of your head and repeat the movement in the opposite direction. After you have done back and forth, tilt your head all the way to the left and place your right hand on the right side of your head and then move your head all the way to right, counting to 10 once again. Repeat the movement to the left side. It's important to note that you should use a full range of motion and keep steady pressure for the full count of 10 in each direction.

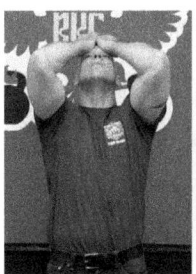

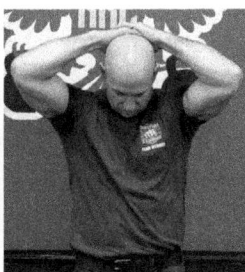

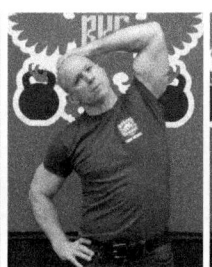

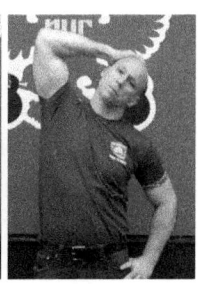

Back-pressure neck: Stand with your heels close to the wall and place a folded towel on the wall and behind your head. Apply pressure backward into the wall for a count of 10. Relax for 2 seconds and perform 10 repetitions. Perform 3 sets of this movement.

Partner Training

If you do not participate in external resistance training through kettlebells, sandbags, barbells, and the like, to maximize your lower body strength in particular, recruit a partner to work with. *External resistance*, defined as any other weight than that of your own body, is needed to develop your highest level of strength. If you don't have equipment, use your training partner. It is also best to have a partner close to your size and weight, especially when you first embark on partner training. This is not always available, so you'll need to work with what you have.

Partner squats: Direct your partner to climb onto your back, as if you were going to play chicken fights. Loop your arms around their legs at knee level and actively pull yourself down. Only pull yourself deep enough so that you are able to get up! If you bottom out, simply have your partner get off. The amount of repetitions that you do depends on the strength that you have developed during your solo squat training. However, starting with 5 to 10 repetitions is a place to begin. If you can only do 2 or 3 reps per set, you will want to improve your strength in your solo squat work and/or incorporate trust squats.

Trust squats: This exercise does not involve additional weight, but it enables both parties to safely achieve a deep squat, thus expanding their range of motion by going well beyond parallel. Start by facing your partner and then grasp their hands, right to right and left to left.

Straighten your arms and lean back as far as possible with your feet approximately one foot from your partner's and shoulder width apart. Actively pull yourself down in unison with your partner. Keep tension in your body as you drive your feet into the ground and propel yourselves upward. You do not have to be close in weight to your partner to do this exercise. If you don't have a partner, use a karate belt in a doorway. Perform this for 20 repetitions each set.

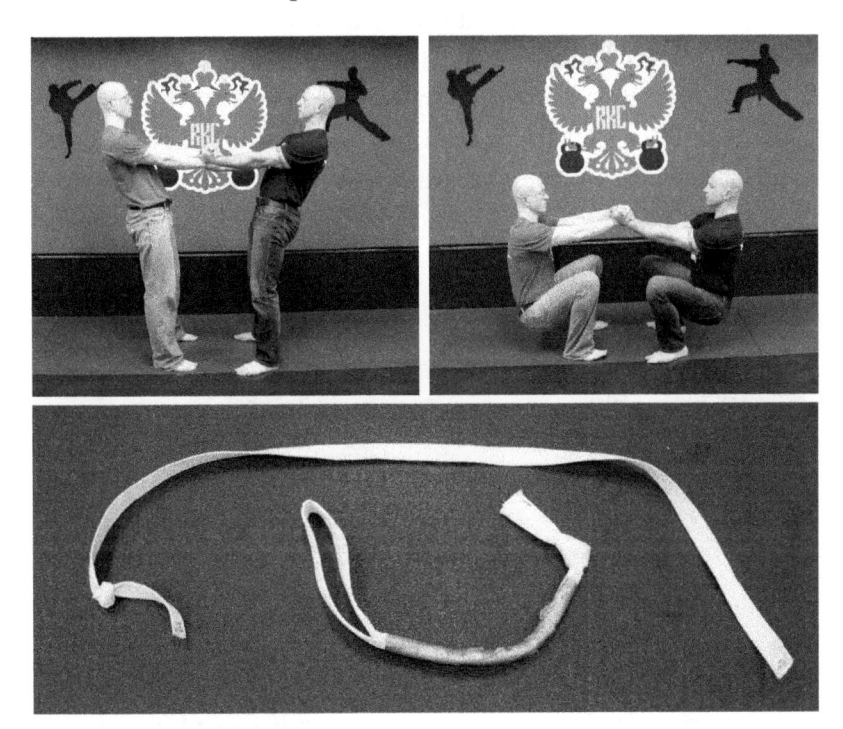

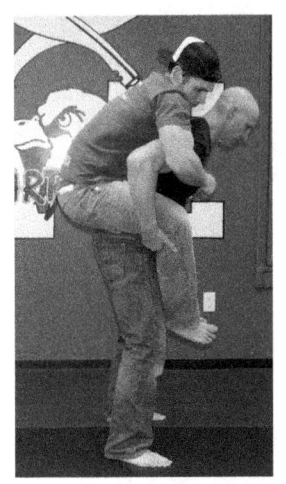

Piggybacks: Assume the position that you did in the partner squats and run with your partner on your back. Perform laps alternating with your partner. It is recommended that you run in a straight line.

Making cuts and turns with someone on your back may result in injury.

Standing lifts: There are a variety of standing lifts that you may perform. These are fantastic for developing the coordination and real, functional strength from having to make adjustments for the shifting in weight of your partner. They also develop explosive power and hip pop necessary to rip an opponent off of the ground.

Body slam lift: Facing your partner, thread your left arm through their legs and situation your right arm over the left side of their neck. Lift and tilt them toward the right side so that they become parallel to the floor and perpendicular to you. If you were to finish the slam, you would continue the movement until the opponent's feet were above your head. You would then pile drive their head into the ground. However, we are using this lift to create strength at this point. Repeat this for five repetitions each side, each set. Add more reps as you become stronger.

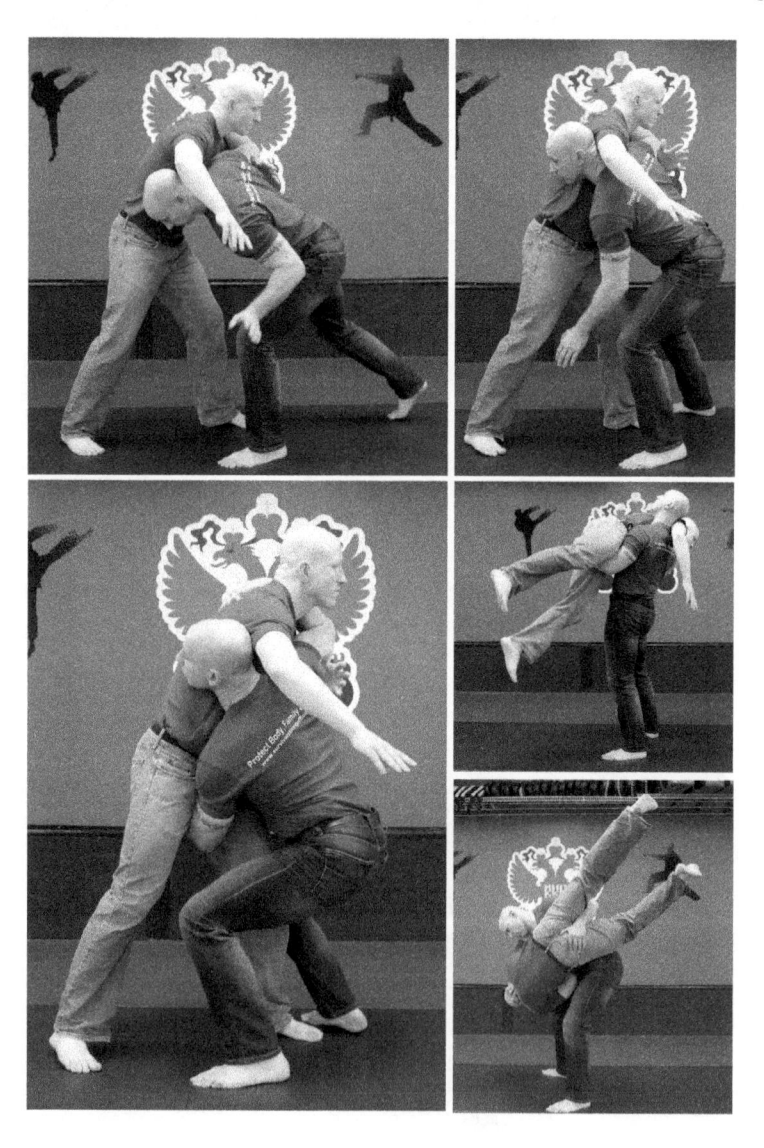

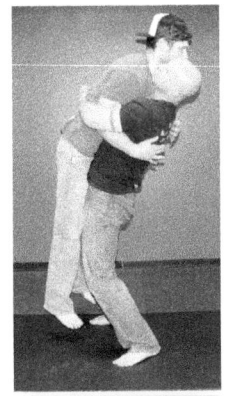

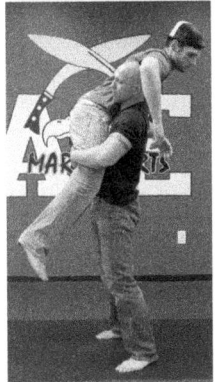

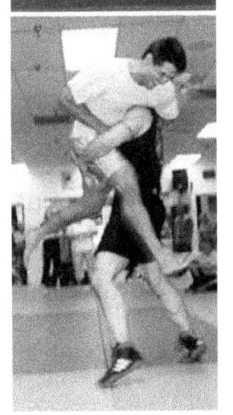

One-arm bear hug lift: Trapping one of your partner's arms, grasp them low about the waist. If you have their right arm trapped, your right hand should be facing palm down on your Gable grip. As you sure up the grip, roll your wrist toward you and into their floating ribs, step in and lift. You don't have to hurt your partner; just use enough power to make sure you have the technique is solid.

Double leg lift: Face your partner and put your head to one side as you shoot[15] in for a takedown. Pin your inside ear to your partner's body, arch your back, look upward, and lift them off the ground. Repeat this process, alternating sides. Practice this drill with the clock set to 30 seconds and alternate with your partner. Increase the time to a minute when you become more conditioned.

Donkey calves: Start by hinging your hips so that your upper body is at a 90-degree angle. Support yourself with your extended arms on a bench or another sturdy surface. Have your training partner sit on your low back, facing toward your head. Perform calf raises from this position. There are three basic positions to use. Toes pointed in, toes pointed out, and toes pointed straight ahead.

Partner deadlift carries: Have your partner get on their hands and knees on a matted surface. Approach them from the back, straddle them, and wrap your arms around their waist and use the gable (or thumbless) grip. Lift your partner up and move them forward. If they are too heavy

---

[15] Shooting for a takedown: This is a common wrestling term applied to the act of lowering your level, making a deep step forward, and grabbing either one or both legs of your opponent. You will now lift them, drive them backward, or turn them so that they wind up on the ground.

for you to move them on your own, have them assist you by pushing off of the ground with their hands and feet.

Partner drags: Have your partner lie flat on their back. Grasp a martial arts belt firmly in their hands, elbows flexed. Face your partner so that your feet are about one foot away from their head. Using two (or one if you are very strong) hands, grab the belt and pull your partner backward. Repeat this movement for as long as you are able.

Ploughhorse: Have your partner wear a martial arts belt. Position yourself directly behind them. Grab their belt with one or two hands while you are behind them. They will adopt a front stance (70 percent of their weight on the front leg and 30 percent on the rear one) and step forward as you are applying tension in the opposite direction. You want to apply only enough to make it difficult for them to walk forward.

If the person holding the belt is very strong, use one arm to hold. If you need two hands to apply more backward tension, do so.

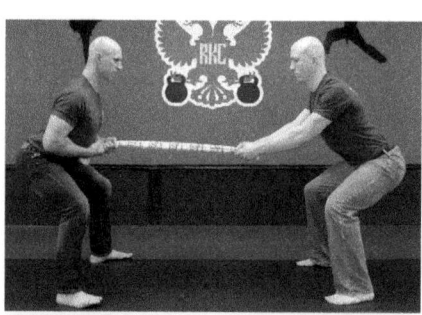

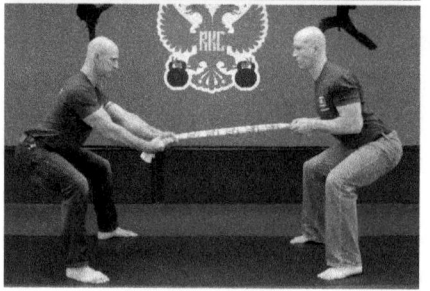

Towel tug-o-war (lat pull/s): Take a standard-sized bath towel and fold it longways until you cannot create any more folds. With both of you facing each other, bend your knees, bend at the hip, and maintain a neutral spine as you grasp the towel. One person has their arms bent and the towel close to their body. The other has their arms fully extended.

Next, you apply tension as both of you pull on the towel. The one with their arms extended is permitted to towel close in to their body as the other extends their arms. Even though both parties are pulling, just enough tension is applied to allow for a 5-second pull in each direction. Repeat 5 to 10 time repetitions in each direction. Maintain the neutral spine and "athletic stance" for the duration of the movement.

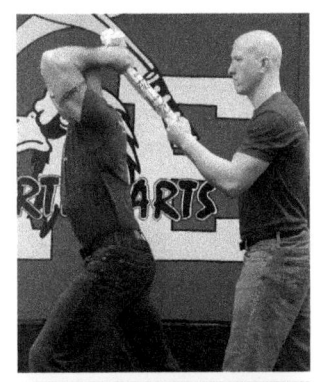

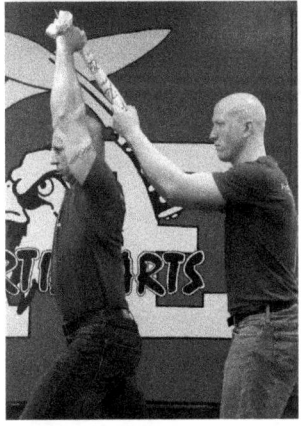

Towel triceps: You'll need one towel between you and your partner. Configure it as you have done for the Tug-O-War. The person working their triceps will grasp the two ends of the towel, elbows bent so that their hands are behind their head and their elbows are pointed upward. A "U" will be formed by the towel and will be positioned in the middle of their back. Adopt a staggered stance with one foot back for added balance. The partner will be behind and grab the towel at the bend. They will apply tension so that it takes effort for the person with the two ends to completely lock out their elbows. On the decent, the elbows must be unlocked and then the person pulls the towel down as resistance is being applied. Repeat this movement 3 to 7 repetitions per set. There should be minimal body movement during this exercise.

Leg throws: An old time gym favorite! Be certain to keep your lumbar spine "bolted" to the ground. Accomplish this by contracting your upper abdominals and forcing your hips to the ground simultaneously, as you assume the supine position. Next, your partner will stand with their feet at your head and they will be facing the same direction as you. Reach your arms upward and behind you and grab their ankles. Now raise your feet up quickly and once your legs reach the 65 to 75 degrees, your partner will push them downward so that your feet wind up approximately six inches off of the ground and then you bring them up quickly again. You may also have your partner throw your feet to the either side. Start with 10 repetitions and direct your partner to only apply as much downward thrust so that your feet go to six inches off of the ground before you bring them back up. To make this more difficult, have your partner push down on your thighs directly above your knees as opposed to pushing your feet. Once you become stronger, work your way up to 30 repetitions per set.

Dog stance: One partner assumes the dog stance position on all fours. The other sits on their back while facing the opposite direction and hooking their feet inside the thighs of their partner. The top person leans backward as far as they can go. Simultaneously, the bottom person (in the dog stance or "referee's position") uses their head to push against the low back of their partner both as the top person goes up and down. Perform 10 repetitions and then change positions.

Partner plumb: Face your partner, and then one of you applies a Gable grip to their partner's neck and pinches their elbows close together. Start slowly and then build the speed and tension as you shake and move your partner about. Do this for 15 seconds and then switch partners. Repeat this three times each. Once you become adept at this movement, you can add time and increase the sets.

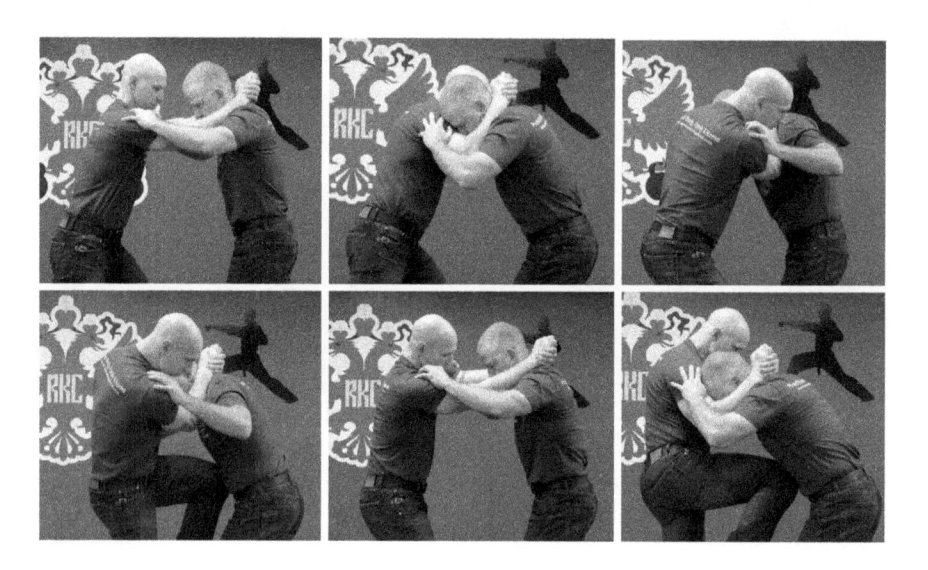

Isometrics and Dynamic Tension

Sampson press: Stand in a sturdy doorway. Place your arms from your palms to your elbows on the inside of the doorjamb and press outward. It is important to tighten your whole body as you push outward. Hold the full-tension position for 10 to 15 seconds. Repeat 3 to 5 times.

Reverse Sampson press: Begin as you would in the Sampson press, except place your arms at your sides with your palms facing you. Place the back of your hands against the doorjamb and tension your body as you press outward with the back of your hands. Hold this position 30 to 60 seconds with full-body tension. Repeat this 2 to 3 times per workout session. Upon completion, it's fun to step out of the doorway and allow your arms to go upward on their own!

Biceps and triceps: Stand tall with your feet shoulder-width or a little less apart. Pack your shoulders and engage your lats. Put your hands together with one hand palm down and the other palm up. Keep them fairly close to your body. Push down with the top hand as you are providing resistance upward with the palm up bottom hand. Perform the same movement in the opposite direction, thus working the triceps on one arm and the biceps of the other. Perform this movement for 5 repetitions, 3 seconds up and 3 seconds down, and then switch arms. Be certain to employ full-body tension while executing this movement.

Squat and hold: Stand with your feet shoulder-width apart. Applying full-body tension, assume 5 different positions during the full range of motion. The positions are as follows:

Top – Keep your knees locked out.

1/3 down – Bend your knees slightly so that you are halfway between standing and mid-squat.

1/2 way down – Bend your knees so that you are halfway between standing and the bottom of your squat.

2/3's down – Bring yourself below the parallel[16] position.

Full bottom – Lower yourself to the utmost bottom of your squat. Be sure to avoid the tail tuck.[17]

Hold each position for a 5-second count. Move from position to position. Mix it up; they don't need to be done in order. Start with 15 to 20 repetitions per set.

Lying squat: Lie flat on your back and dorsiflex both feet. Place your hands on the floor at your sides and lift your head off of the floor by contracting your lower abs and bring your knees up toward your chest or as high as you can possibly go. Have your training partner grab your instep with a hook grip, and then pull your legs until they are straight. Don't offer 100 percent resistance; you will get pulled across the floor! Once your legs are straight, repeat the process in the opposite direction. Perform 3 to 5 repetitions per set.

Endurance: High-stress situations demand massive anaerobic and aerobic capacity. During a street confrontation, you will experience an incredible adrenaline dump. The better condition you are in, the better your chances will be in processing the onset weakness, shortness of breath, and tunnel vision. Also, you may have just gone through a hard day (or night) of work and may be exhausted. If you are in better condition, you will be able to handle daily fatigue better.

---

[16] Parallel, in terms of squatting, is defined as the hip joint passing the top of the knee.

[17] Tail tuck: This occurs when your lower spine loses it's neutral position and your tail bone (or coccyx) dips under your hips. Under load, this compromised spine is open to injury. You should only go as low as you are able without allowing your lumbar spine to round into a tail tuck.

What are some of the best training methods to employ?

Skipping rope is the single best aerobic activity for a fighter. We begin every training session with 3 to 5 minutes of skipping rope. You need not perform double-jumps, crossing the rope, or other fancy rope tricks to gain the benefits from jumping rope. Why is jumping rope so good? For starters, you can do it anywhere. If it's cold or snowing or too hot outside, it doesn't matter. You can jump indoors. The coordination of moving your hands and feet in rhythm with each other. The shifting of weight from one foot to the other prepares one for moving and striking.

Burpees facilitate anaerobic conditioning and also helps us to train the sprawl.[18]

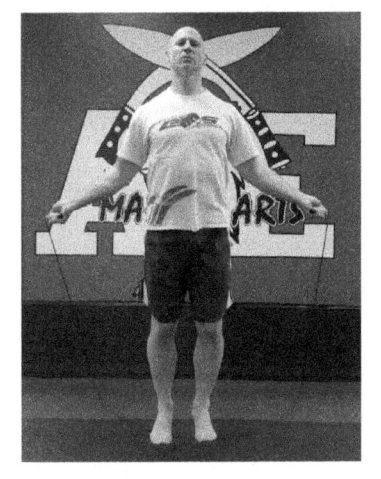

Bag work is the best combination of skill building and endurance training. The additional bonuses of power development and body hardening. We have routines listed in chapter 14.

Grappling is possibly the best man to men's strength-building endeavor you can participate in. Pushing, pulling, balancing, reacting to the movements of another human as you vie for position develops incredible strength and body awareness. Grappling also contributes to the hardening or callousing of the body. Wrestlers and grapplers are notoriously tough due to the grinding nature of their training.

---

[18] Sprawl: This is a maneuver used to defend one's legs against a single- or double-leg takedown. Typically used by wrestlers for defending a shot on their legs. It's more difficult in each direction. Look toward your left hand and do the 10 repetitions of the following 5 kicks.

Mirror or Shadow Training

The sprawl and brawl drill is a great way to conduct a solo MMA (mixed martial arts), warm-up or endurance-building regiment.

Stand in front of a mirror and practice your movement (footwork, slips, bobs, weaves, parries), kicks, punches, and combinations and every 10 to 15 seconds or so, drop to a sprawl and pop back up. Throw a knee every time you come back to your feet. Most likely, your opponent's head will be at your knee level after your sprawl. It's recommended to perform 2-minute rounds with 30 seconds of active rest.

Shadowing boxing, kickboxing or defensive tactics all may be practiced while in front of a mirror. Practice your movement and strikes in a series of combinations while imagining executing them on opponent. Set the timer and explode into the techniques. Your practice should be pointed and have purpose. Repeat specific maneuvers for a chosen amount of repetitions or specific duration. The techniques, combinations, and tactics are listed in chapters 9, 10, 12 and 13. Use the same time criterion as used in the above.

The *wall drill for kicking* is the single best exercise for perfecting your kicks and developing the power of your higher kicks. I will let you know something; this drill does *not* get any easier with practice. You simply develop better kicks. Start by placing your right hand on the wall, your right foot about a foot away from the wall and your left up, level with your head and facing the opposite direction so that you are perpendicular to the wall. All of these kicks are to be done slowly. A solid 2 to 3 seconds per kick, longer to make the drill more difficult.

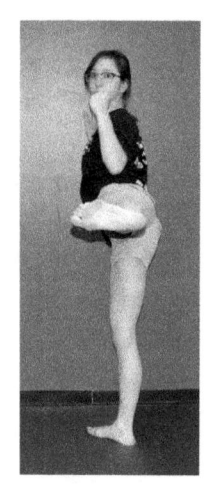

Side leg raise: Dorsiflex your foot, keep the leg that you are lifting in line with the base leg and lift it as high as you are able *without* bending your back.

Don't focus on the height of your kicks; concern yourself with your alignment. After the tenth repetition, hold leg in the up position for two counts of 10.

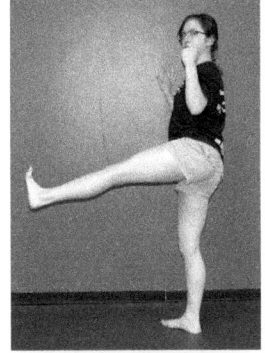

Forward crescent circles: Move your foot forward and bring it up as high as you are able. Once you have reached the peak, start to bring your foot to the back, keeping your leg up as high as you can, especially when your foot passes the halfway point of your body and goes behind you. The circles should be slow, deliberate, and at the full potential of the movement.

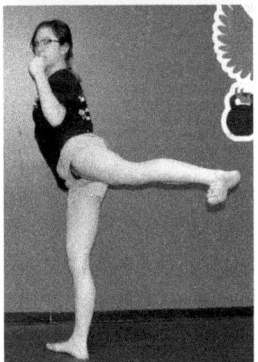

Backward Crescent Circles: This is the same movement as the previous with one exception, start the movement backwards with your heel leading the way as opposed to your toes.

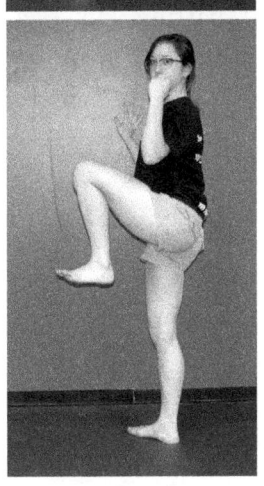

Side kick: From the starting position, bring your knee up high so that your heel is in line with your base leg. Turn your foot on the floor so that your toes are facing the wall and rotate your hips, thus turning your foot and pointing the toes of the chambered[19] leg to the ground. Slowly extend your leg outward as if you were driving your heel into your target. Return your kick slowly to the starting position. Repeat for 10 repetitions and hold in the out position on the tenth repetition for two counts of 10.

---

[19] Chamber: A leg "in chamber" has the knee up and leg drawn back and poised to kick. Fists may be chambered for punches as well.

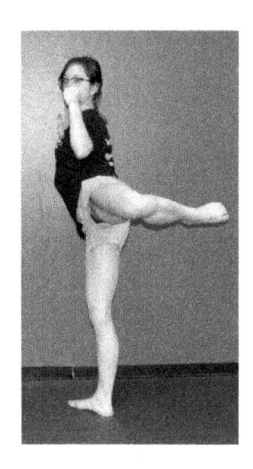

Roundhouse kick: Pull the kicking knee back until it is aligned with your hip. Plantar-flex your foot so that your toes are pointed. Extend your leg, but be sure to keep your knee in exactly the same spot. Bring your foot out and back to full extension and full flexion for 10 repetitions. On repetition number 10, hold your foot in the extended position for two counts of 10.

Repeat these movements with the other leg.

Body Conditioning

You need to forge your body into a rock-hard form. Your goal is to create a well-conditioned, durable, calloused, and resilient body.

This should be done to the extent to which you turn your body into a machine that is able to withstand an attack and return an onslaught. To what degree you develop this ability depends entirely on how much effort you are willing to put into it. One key aspect to achieving a high level of condition is to toughen the body to trauma overtime. This includes the entire body—hands, arms, shins, thighs, torso, etc. A great deal of this will be accomplished with actual sparring. However, to maximize the toughness of the body, specific hardening drills are necessary. This is called *callousing the body.*

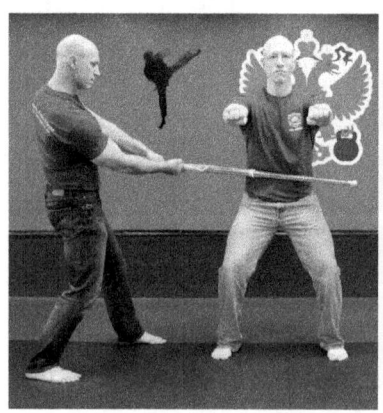

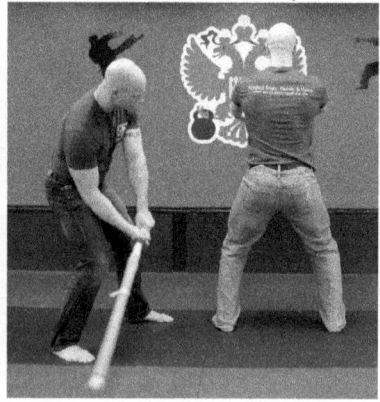

Conditioning of the shins, knees, elbows, hands, wrists, and fingertips is imperative for having a body that is strong and able to withstand an attack. You need to forge your limbs into "steel implements." The use of sand, rice, pebbles, and even crushed glass, will toughen your fingers, hands, and skin. There is a partner forearm-toughening drill that works wonders as well.

Use of a Makawara,[20] a brick wrapped with rope or buckets filled with sand, pebbles, or even crushed glass. Strike with your front two knuckles, the edge of your hand, palm, and fingers. Always begin lightly, and then increase the power of your strikes gradually as you become more conditioned. If you are using the buckets, strike downward into the bucket filled with material. Start with sand, progress to pebbles, and then on to crushed glass if so desired. This will toughen the skin and strengthen your hands for striking. This may take several months to years to build the desired callousing and bone density. If you become overzealous, you will injure yourself and prolong your conditioning process until you are healed.

The Wing Chun wooden dummy is great for toughening of the body. Forearms, palms, feet, shins. There are a variety of books and videos on the techniques for training on the dummy. The downside of this training is the size of the piece of equipment and mounting it. I haven't used one in thirty years. The other prescribed methods of body conditioning described in this book will be more than sufficient and take up less space. You would be better suited allocating the space and fund toward a 100-pound Muay Thai or boxing heavy bag.

When working with a partner, one of the best conditioning drills that you can treat yourself to is the two-position forearm-conditioning drill. Stand facing your training partner in a fighting stance, and both of you put your right foot forward. Place the backs of your forearms so

---

[20] A Makawara comes in one of several configurations. You wrap wood in cloth or rope. Make certain that the surface you strike has some give. *Do not* mount it on a wall. The energy will get transferred back to your shoulder, elbow, and wrist.

that they are against each other. Simultaneously, bring your forearms down so that your fist is at knee level and then bang the back of your forearms together. Immediately bring them back to the original position and bang them together again. Perform this process for repetitions or time. The amount of time or number of repetitions depends on your conditioning level and your partner's. Adding in more hip movement and harder strikes as you become stronger and more conditioned. As with all of these body conditioning exercises, start slowly and increase the speed and power of the callousing technique as your body becomes more accustomed to the trauma.

My all-time favorite for shin conditioning is using a fencepost wrapped with foam, carpet, or rope. We have two kicking posts outside our studio. One is wrapped in foam, and the other is wrapped in 3/4" rope. If you only have space for one, then I suggest wrapping it with a thick pile carpet.

If you do not have access to a kicking post, there are other methods to prepare your shins for combat. You may use a rolling pin and run it up and down your shins. Couple this with light taps from a rattan stick up and down the full length of the shinbone.

Additionally, your heavy bag work will contribute to the hardening of your shins, as well as your knees, elbows, and hands.

How does this work? You will experience microbreaks in your shins. They will heal, thus resulting in a thicker, denser shin. I personally know that this works for three reasons. Many of my training partners have complained about how "hard" my shins are. My shin kicks and cut kicks have yielded favorable results in competition and street application. The third, most tangible, occurred when I experienced a trilateral spiral fracture. Upon reading the X-ray in the emergency room, the physician came to me with a paled look on his face. He had thought that I had some type of "strange disease," or cancer. He went on to explain that he'd never seen anything like this before and was extremely concerned. I told him to relax and then assured him that what he saw was normal for the activity that I partake in. He was relieved. He also became one of my students and has been since 2002!

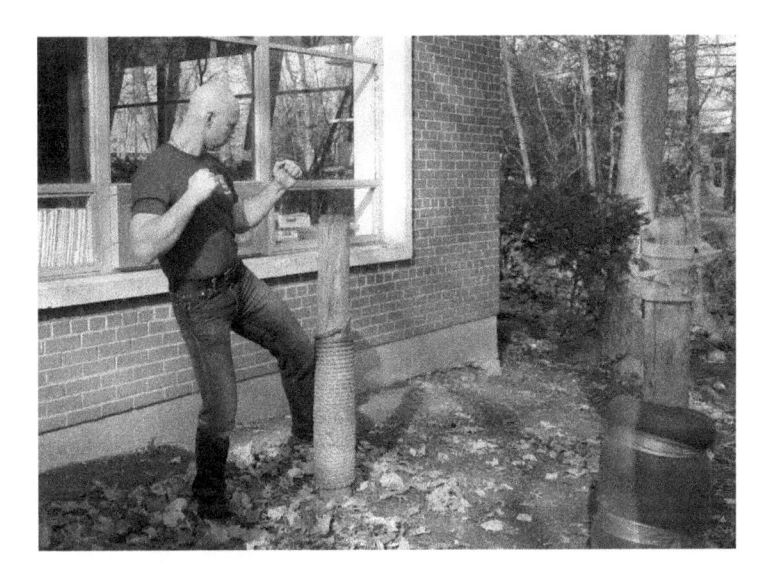

Do not start your training with hard strikes; this will injure you. Progress slowly with light, controlled strikes. As with all body conditioning, if you allow yourself to get carried away, you may get injured, and then you will miss training. Again, build slowly and condition overtime. Body conditioning and callousing is a marathon, not a sprint.

Grip Strength

The development of a strong grip is quite possibly the most important attribute to have as a good fighter. The ability to grab, hold, crush, and pull is tantamount to your ability to defend yourself and fight. Your grip is significantly enhanced through many of the exercises contained in this book; however, pointing out the importance of grip strength is essential.

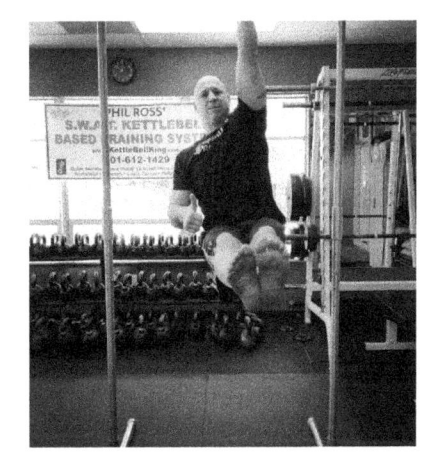

Grip strength is especially important. You will need to grab, twist, hold, and crush. We have a great deal of exercises listed earlier in this chapter, especially the exercises using a belt or a towel. Some additional training methods will include the following: Fingertip push-ups are great. Squeezing hand grippers or a tennis ball is fantastic as well. Spearhand-thrust into a bucket of rice or sand, then grip, twist, and pull. Crumple a newspaper one sheet at a time. Hang. Simply jump up, grab on to a bar, and hang. Use two hands, one hand, bring your legs into an L-sit position. Hang for a time in the various configurations. Start with 30 seconds and then increase. If you are able to support your weight for 2 minutes or more while hanging from a bar, then you've accomplished some good grip strength. Obviously, the heavier you are, the more difficult the task, but this movement, as many bodyweight movements are, is a good indicator of how much you should weigh. There are many other methods, but these are some of my favorites, and they are the most economical and easily accessible.

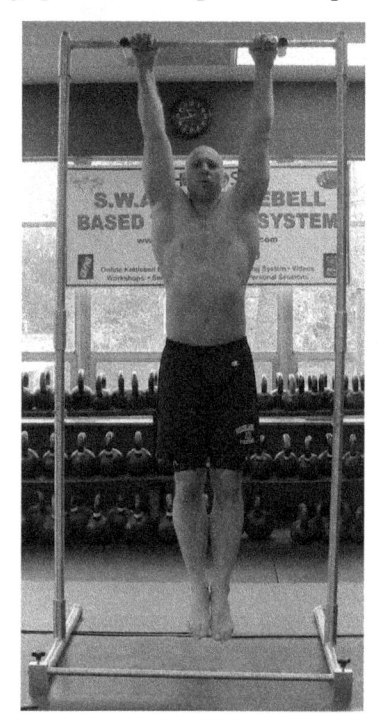

WRIST STRENGTH

Grappling will do a lot to condition the wrists, but specific exercises can be very beneficial for not only making them strong but also flexible and resilient. As mentioned earlier in this chapter, knuckle push-ups and back-of-the-wrist push-ups are great for wrist strength and range of motion. The various wrist stretching exercises, palm up with a straight elbow, palm down as well. We also use a variety of wrist rotations and stretches. Some of the best stretches for the wrists and forearms involve placing your hands palm down on the floor or a wall. On the wall, have your fingers facing the ground so that the underside of your wrist is facing upward. While kneeling on the floor, have your fingers facing you. For either of the positions, shift your weight toward your fingers while keeping your palms flat to the surface. Rock back and forth, changing the amount of pressure. Perform the exercise for a minute or so for each hand. While on the floor, do both hands at once.

Another great strength/conditioning/flexibility exercise is the wrist lock drill. Not only do you gain the aforementioned from this training drill, but you also learn how to move with a wrist lock and position yourself properly to respond once you have gotten away. Start by facing your partner. Reach out and grab his/her wrist; then you respond with a wrist lock. They, in turn, will go with the technique by either turning or rolling and re-grabbing you with a wrist lock. Repeat this process of locking, grabbing, re-grabbing, and countering for 30 to 60 seconds per round. The specifics on executing several wrist locks are listed in chapter 8, titled "Grips and Locks."

When you become more advanced, use tools, such as bamboo shinai, and eventually, wooden dowels to toughen and condition these areas. Though not normal to mainstream training, they have proven to be very effective.

Physicality is extremely important for both your body and your mind. You will need strength and endurance to be able to defend yourself at the highest level under the worst circumstances. No one has the ability to choose when they will be attacked or faced with a dire situation in the street. Victory favors the prepared. You may have just gotten off your shift at work and are completely exhausted, and then you get attacked. If you are in condition, your chances of survival are increased. If you are too weak and fatigued to respond, you will perish.

Listed below are a few examples for training sessions that we use on a regular basis. We address speed, agility, endurance, strength, mobility, and flexibility in these sessions. Feel free to design your own based on the information in this book.

Training Session Examples
ENDURANCE CIRCUIT

Jump rope for 2 to 3 minutes, perform bo staff stretching, free hand stretching, or a combination of both for 10 to 12 minutes. Be certain to include bridges in your warm-up.

Jump rope: 100 Skips
Push-ups: 10 to 25 reps
(various types and difficulties)
Jump rope: 100 skips
Standard squats: 25 reps
Jump rope: 100 skips
Pull-ups: 80% of Max
Jump rope: 100 skips

Split squats: 15 reps each side
Jump rope: 100 skips
Dips: 10 to 15
Jump rope: 100 skips
Abdominals
Wheel of death: 5 reps
Leg thrusts: 30 reps

Repeat this circuit three times.

STRENGTH CIRCUIT

Take your time and make certain that you have 30 to 60 seconds of rest between exercises. Low reps, 1 to 5 for beginners, and 1 to 10 for more advanced practitioners. The reps should be based on 70 to 80 percent of your max per exercise. Remember, our goal is strength development, not cardiovascular endurance.

Jump rope for 2 to 3 minutes and make certain that you focus on warming up your joints thoroughly to prepare yourself for the task ahead. You will be stressing your joints with these more difficult movements:

One-arm push-ups
Single leg (pistol squats)
Pull-ups
Back bridge (full or tabletop)
Handstands (to your level)

Air lunges
Hanging abs
Plyometric squats
Calf raises
4-Way Neck

Repeat this circuit 4 to 5 times.

Strength and Endurance Bodyweight Circuit

Jump rope for three minutes and loosen up your body from the ground up with ankle rotations, small knee circles, hip rotations, shoulder circles back and forth, wrist rotations, and neck stretching. With the rope jumping, this should take 7 to 10 minutes.

Set your timer for 50 seconds of work and 10 seconds of rest between each movement. Work to your "reasonable max" (not to burn out), but push yourself. If you can't do the movements for full 50 seconds, use a regression. Example: Let's suppose that it takes you 30 seconds to do 6 pull-ups, and there is 20 seconds left in the set. Perform plank pull-ups for the remaining 20 seconds. Do 5 rotations of the below-listed exercises for a total of 45 minutes. Spend 3 to 5 minutes on your cool-down and stretch.

1. Handstands
2. Dips
3. Hanging abs/abs
4. Push-ups
5. Squats
6. Bridges
7. Lunges
8. Pull-ups
9. Calves

Cool down and stretch.

5
WEAPONS OF THE HUMAN BODY

The human body, in all of its frailty and target areas, has some built-in weapons. The key is to condition them and know how to apply them properly. Use the information as prescribed in chapter 4 to accomplish this. We'll start from the bottom and work our way up describing the available weapons and how to use them best. The specifics on the execution of the actual techniques will be addressed in chapter 9.

THE FOOT

The foot has several basic areas and positions suited for attack. First is the heel. I put the heel as number one, because use of the heel as a weapon takes very little skill and is a great loosening up or distraction technique, as well as a fantastic finisher. It's also a great counterattack to employ when grabbed from behind. To use the heel, it's best to dorsiflex the foot and stomp downward. This position creates the most tension in the foot and focuses more force per square inch on a smaller area. The primary techniques to use are stomps, shin rakes, mule, and push kicks.

The ball of the foot front kick is a thrusting technique that can be delivered to virtually any part of the body from the shin to the chin, as opposed to the front snap kick, which is only good when used to strike the groin or the chin.

The instep of the foot is a great spot to strike with when delivering a roundhouse kick. The instep is located between the toes and the ankle. It is best to have the area between the arch and the ankle as the focal contact point with the desired target.

The Shin

The use of this area for striking was made popular by Muay Thai, but has been in use for many, many years and by a multitude of cultures prior to the recent Thailand-inspired fame. The Irish have a martial art called speachóireacht.[21] Chinese martial arts, Bando and many more use the shin as a weapon as well.

A properly conditioned shinbone is like a baseball bat. We achieve this by a gradual, conditioning process. Start slowly and gently at first. You will not condition your shins overnight! Try to avoid causing your shins to bruise, bleed, or get severe bumps. Discoloration and soreness is to be expected. However, do not take it to excess; if you injure yourself, you can't train.

Over time, you will create microfractures in your shins. They will heal and result in calcium deposits. As they multiply, the shin becomes harder and denser. You have now forged a formidable pair of weapons! The primary attacks using the shins are the cut kick, shin kick, and rip kicks.

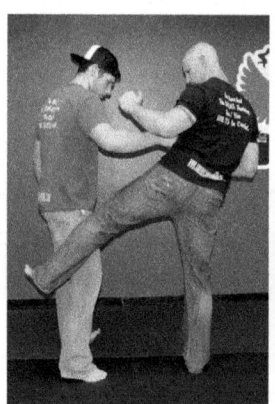

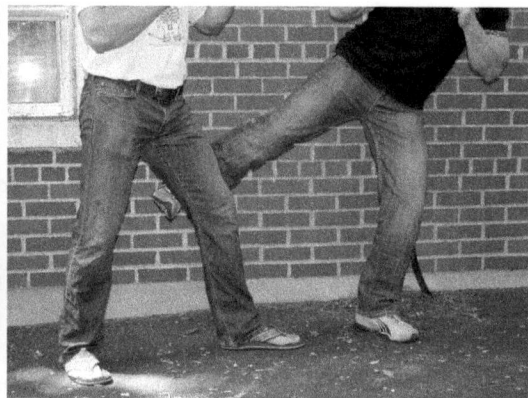

---

[21] Pronounced "spacker-okt." It's the term used for kicking techniques. Used in Gaelic football and dancing.

The Knee

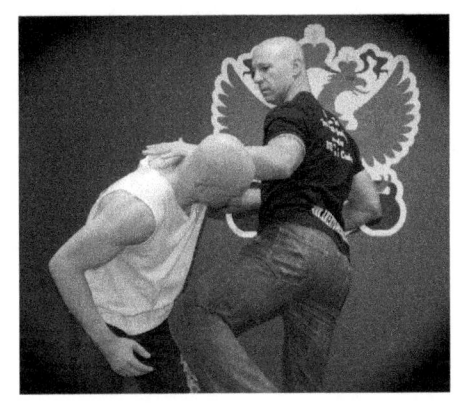

The most powerful strike that the human body can deliver is the *flying knee*. Being hit by it is comparable to being hit by a car traveling 35mph, as per the tests conducted by a *Fight Science* study conducted in 2006.[22] The flying knee may not be practical for most people to use, but simple knee strikes are very easily administered to the femoral artery (inner thigh), the peroneal nerve (outer thigh), bladder, solar plexus, kidneys, ribs, and groin. Once you've doubled your adversary over with a well-placed strike (or strikes) to the aforementioned soft-tissue areas, strikes with the knees to the face and head are easily delivered. Whatever you do, keep throwing the knees until your assailant drops to the ground, giving you ample time to escape.

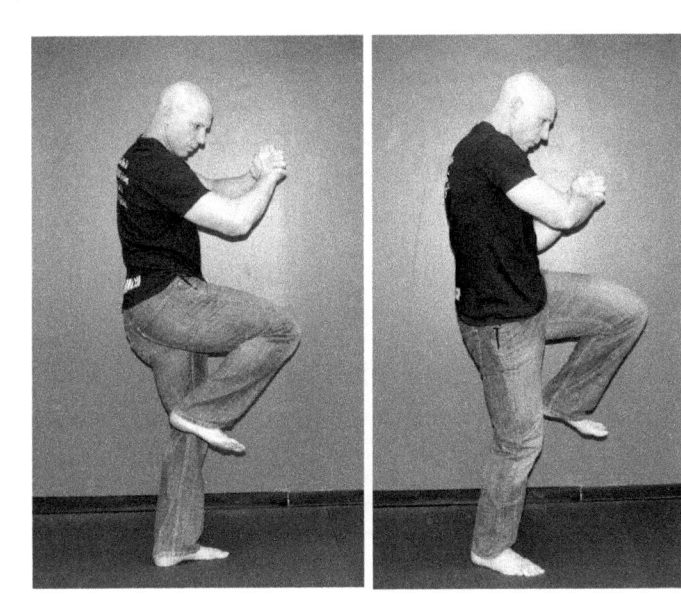

---

[22] *Fight Science* was a show produced in 2006 by John Brenkus.

There are several manners to secure a grip on your opponent when administering knee strikes. One method is referred to as *the plumb*. To use the plumb or Thai clinch, grab your opponent with both hands behind the neck. Do not interlock your fingers. Instead, use a palm-to-palm, also called the Gable grip. This grip is the most effective grip available. Several years ago, the top Division 1 NCAA wrestling teams conducted tests on the various hand grips, and the Gable grip (palm to palm) won, hands down, pun intended.

Another method comes into play when you are on the side of your opponent and they are doubled over (bent at the waist). Take one arm and place your hand on the back of their neck with your forearm positioned against their jaw. The other arm is threaded under their arm with your hand placed on their back. From this position, you are able to levy knee strikes to their face, ribs, stomach, and the peroneal nerve of the leg closest to you. This position also makes it difficult for your opponent to turn into you to grab you because you are controlling their head. There are two other distinct advantages to this position. You are able to see the surrounding area and you are positioned to throw your opponent either to the ground or into another assailant.

The *springboard knee* is simple and extremely powerful. The strike is delivered at close range. Stomp one foot hard into the ground and then "spring" upward as you drive the other knee into your opponent's body. More power is garnered by this method due to the plyometric nature of delivering this strike.

The *flying knee* is the most powerful, yet the landing percentage is not as high as the other methods for delivering the knee. When you literally launch yourself at an intended target, you gain sheer power from the movement and speed generated; plus, you eliminate the friction with the ground. This is a risky move, and you stand a greater chance of missing. I would only recommend this strike if you catch your opponent completely off-guard or as a finishing technique once they have sustained a significant amount of damage and they are unable to move quickly.

THE HIP AND BUTT

On the surface, the hips and buttocks seem like unlikely weapons, but the applications are many. Use your hips and buttocks to smash into your opponent to break their balance or to create space for you to deliver other strikes or to facilitate an escape. When grabbed from behind, smashing your butt into the attackers groin is an effective distraction or space-creating technique.

THE SHOULDER

The shoulder is a great, unorthodox striking weapon of the human body. When you find yourself in the grappling and trapping ranges (covered in chapter 8), smashing your shoulder into you opponent's face is extremely distracting. The shoulder is also a good lead-in on a takedown. Drive your shoulder into the solar plexus, stomach, or chest as you perform your takedown. Follow this to the ground as you drive your opponent to the floor. When you find yourself slightly crouched and under your opponent's chin, explode upward and drive your shoulder into their chin.

THE ELBOW

The elbow is an extremely devastating weapon. Jon "Bones" Jones[23] has mastered the art of the elbow in the sport of cage fighting. He has destroyed opponents with slashing downward elbows, upward elbows, elbows from the ground and pound,[24] spinning elbows, etc...The elbow is very, very hard and close to the power base of the body. Experiment on a heavy bag. Throw a punch at it and then hit the bag with an elbow and see which strike yields the greater amount of power. You may never throw another punch again! Additionally, the thick elbow bone is much

---

[23] Jon "Bones" Jones is the current UFC Light Heavyweight Champion. He has devastated many foes faced in the Octagon with his elbow strikes.

[24] *Ground and pound* is a term applied to the activity of delivering strikes form the position where one fighter has a full mount (straddling their opponent with one knee on either side) and is raining down blows on the downed fighter.

more durable than the multitude of bones (27, to be precise) available to break in one's hand.

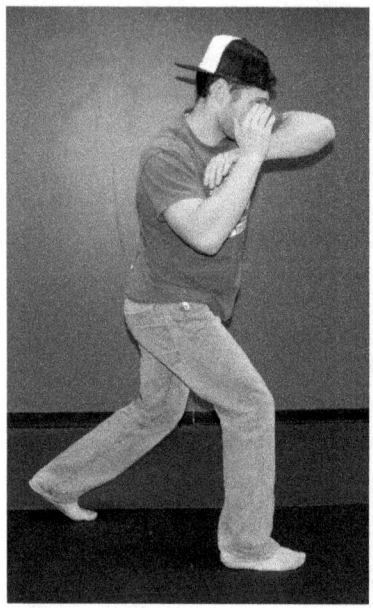

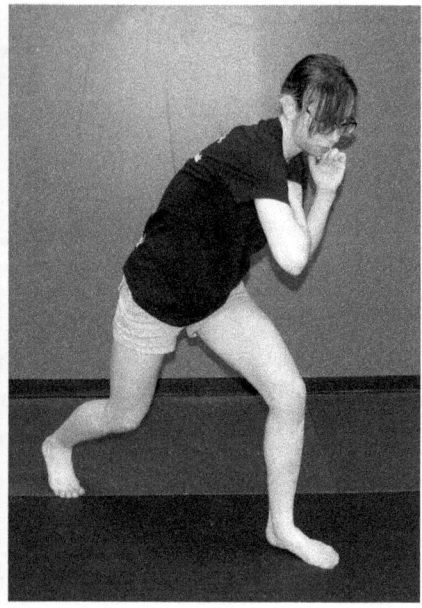

The Forearm

Ask any football player if they like using the forearm as a method to strike or block and how well it works. One of the core movements for an interior lineman is the forearm shiver. Step into your opponent with one hand open and the other fist clinched while you deliver a stiff forearm shot to the chest. The forearm and side of the wrist can be used to choke or levy pressure on an opponent. Blocking and deflecting blows as well as striking to the clavicle and neck of your adversary is met with favorable results.

The Wrist

As an implement of striking, the wrist is often overlooked. Proper execution of a stick punch yields one of the most powerful strikes that can be delivered by the upper body. Back in the early 1990s, the power meter striking pads were very popular. *Karate International Magazine* was hosting a very large karate tournament in the New York Metro area (Hackensack, New Jersey). I entered my student into the Impact Pad Striking competition. He was a seventeen-year-old new black belt who weighed about 175 pounds. There were approximately 30 adult black belts in the competition. Several were master-level instructors, many of them quite a bit larger than my young black belt student. They attempted Reverse Punches, Ridgehands, Boxer's Cross, etc... My 17-year-old, 175 pound student beat them all, by quite a margin with the Stick Punch technique. The judges and other participants were in utter disbelief (and a few Master's were a little irked) and made him perform his strikes a few more times. He still won with the back of the wrist stick punch. Handily. In one sparring competition, I witnessed a fight where one combatant almost tore another one's jaw off with the stick punch. Roy "Big Country" Nelson knocked Cheick Kongo with a stick punch in their televised UFC bout.

The back of the wrist may be used at close quarters as well. We routinely break boards with the back of our wrists at very close distances of 1 to 3 inches. Not only can offensive strikes be delivered with the wrist, but it's great for blocking and deflecting blows as well.

THE FIST

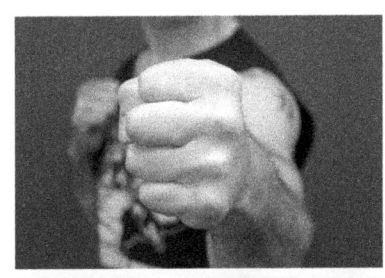

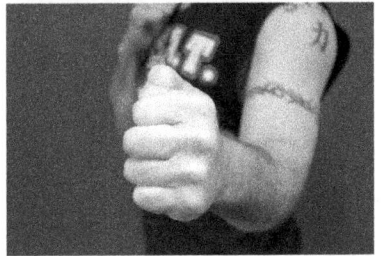

The fist is the universal demonstration of power, might, defiance, and defense. The clenched fist is almost an autonomic response when angered or threatened. One of the most powerful upper-body strikes is the straight cross. The whole martial art of boxing was developed with only the fists as weapons. You may have noticed that I referred to boxing as a martial art. It is. A uniform and a ranking system is not a necessary precursor for being considered a martial art. *Martial* is derived from "warring," therefore applied to all combat sports and training.

The Hand

The hand assumes a multitude of configurations for striking and defending. Open palms for both thrusting and slapping techniques work best for striking the "hard" targets such as the head. Open hands for parries and redirecting strikes coming at you while you are defending yourself.

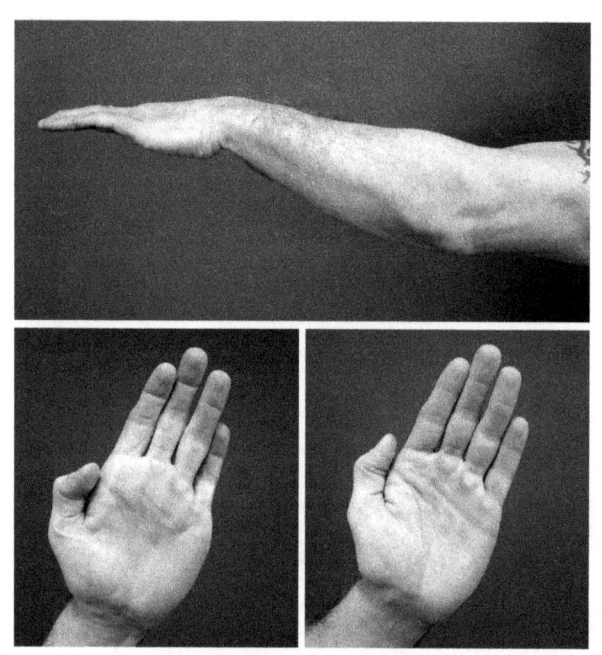

Proper hand position on the left (strong) and improper on the right (weak).

The Fingers

The finger techniques may not "finish" your opponent off, but they will certainly provide the opportunity for you to. Fish hook, finger jabs, flicks, eye gouges, and being applied to pressure points and nerve centers. Attacking the eyes with your fingers yield the greatest results—permanently or temporarily blinding your assailant enables you to escape or provides a distraction for you to deliver a more lethal counterattack.

The Head

Head butts delivered by the front, side, and top of the back of the head are both shocking and potentially devastating. Also dropping your head down to deflect a blow directed toward your face.

The Mouth

Mike Tyson does not have the corner on the use of bicuspids for fighting. There are many targets that one can assume the role of Hannibal Lecter with. You may sink you teeth into one of several available fleshy areas to inflict damage or to create a release from a grip or hold.

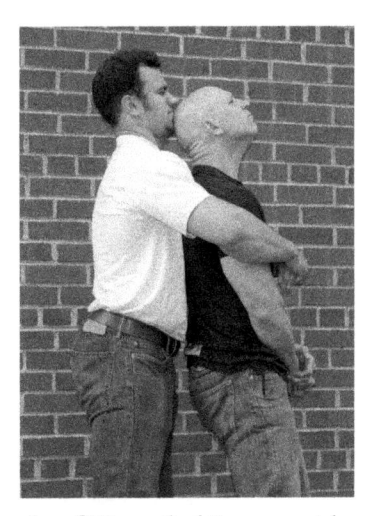

6
TARGETS OF THE HUMAN BODY

Unfortunately for us, we humans have a cornucopia of vital and semivital targets to attack. Fortunately, the human body has a great deal of target areas to direct attacks to. What is a blessing is a curse as well. Knowing our target areas enables us to both protect ourselves and exploit the weaknesses of our assailants.

Most of our vital and semivital target areas are located on the centerline of our bodies. We need to both protect ours and attack the opponent's at the same time. Let us peruse the available areas to focus our attacks on. Starting at the top:

VITAL AND SEMI-VITAL TARGET AREAS OF THE HUMAN BODY

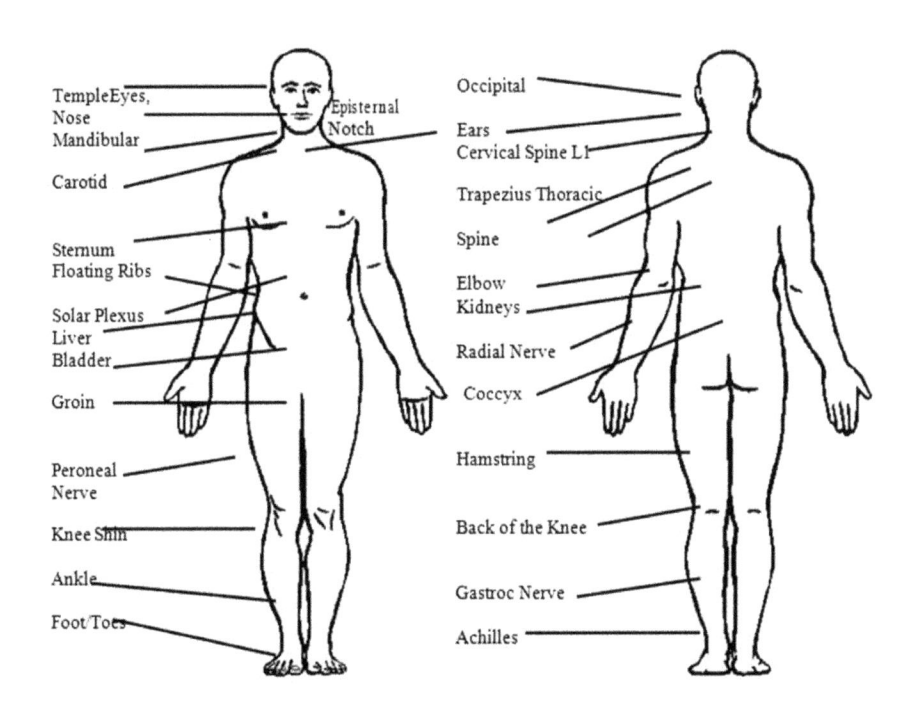

Temple, Eyes,
Nose
Mandibular
Episternal Notch
Carotid

Sternum
Floating Ribs

Solar Plexus
Liver
Bladder

Groin

Peroneal Nerve

Knee Shin

Ankle
Foot/Toes

Occipital
Ears
Cervical Spine
Trapezius Thoracic
Spine
Elbow
Kidneys
Radial Nerve

Coccyx

Hamstring

Back of the Knee

Gastroc Nerve

Achilles

101

The Eyes

A poke, gouge, punch, scratch, or strike will either permanently or temporarily incapacitate or blind your opponent. The toughest guy in the world has eyes that are no stronger than a baby's. Animals instinctually squint during combat to help protect their eyes, knowing their vulnerability.

The Ears

A cupping slap, especially a dual one, will disrupt the balance and cause a great deal of pain, potentially perforating the eardrum. The dual slap is also an excellent entry technique to gouging both eyes with your thumbs. Almost a two-for-one deal! An authoritative single slap to the ear can knock out an assailant or render them incapacitated. In the worst case, delivering a slap to the ear is quite effective and will act as a significant disruption technique.

The Nose

This is one of my favorite spots to strike for several reasons. Its located smack dab in the middle of the face, striking the nose hard can cause it to break and allow blood to flow, and smashing the nose will cause your opponent's eyes to water. The whole notion of "sending the nose back into the brain" is a lot of garbage. The nose will fracture and collapse, and the cartilage will bend well before anything reached the brain.

The Throat

It matters not how big, strong, or nasty you are, you have a throat. One cannot develop muscle to cover and protect the front of the windpipe. It's a great target. The best techniques to use on the throat are the scissor punch, axehands, and the thumbs. If you strike the throat with a scissor punch, you can crush the windpipe, precipitating blood to fill the area, essentially causing the opponent to drown on their own blood. You are also immediately set up to grab the windpipe and crush it. To properly grab the windpipe, use your index and middle fingers and your thumb. Try to make them meet each other behind the windpipe, squeeze, and pull.

There are also a variety of less lethal attacks to the area. Jamming a thumb or index and middle finger into the episternal notch will invoke the gag reflex and acts as an effective distraction technique.

THE NECK

Some people have necks the size of a Rottweiler's, so direct attacks to the thick areas of the neck will not work on everyone. However, the carotid arteries running up either side of the throat are a great target. If someone were to grab you with a front bear hug (arms-free version), take your thumbs and drive them into the carotid arteries. This will send a nasty shock and cause their grip to release. I've also found that the more muscular someone is, the closer the nerves are to the skin's surface. This makes the application of this technique more effective.

There is an area of the neck that strikes in MMA, karate and boxing have outlawed. It's the area directly below the skull where the spine and the skull meet. An attack to the C1[25] can result in paralysis or death. Even if you do not kill the opponent, a knockout or temporary disablement is imminent.

THE TRAPEZIUS

The once famous Spock shock[26] is a fictitious technique and only works on TV. The best way to attack the traps is with a downward hammerfist

---

[25] C1 is the first cervical vertebra, and a blow there can result in paralysis or death.
[26] The Spock shock was a fictional technique made famous by Dr. Spock from the original Star Trek TV series. Dr. Spock would pinch his adversary's trapezius between his thumb and forefinger, thus knocking him unconscious.

or a chop. Attacking from the rear works best. If you attack the front, the collarbone is more easily accessible.

The Sternum

This is located in the center of the chest and often referred to as the breast bone. There are nerves very close to the surface of the skin here. Striking with a closed fist may result in cracking the sternum and potentially stopping the heart. An open palm strike is less lethal, but will also stop an assailant in his tracks. Your striking technique must be strong and sound if you are to gain the desired result with either of these techniques.

The Abdomen and the Trunk

The solar plexus, liver shot, the kidney and floating ribs, and the bladder are the primary targets of the trunk. The solar plexus, or the xiphoid process, is located directly below the sternum and is where the soft tissue begins on the abdomen. Striking this area with a closed fist will take the wind out of your opponent.

The liver is located on the front, lower right side of the body. A well-placed shot will drop an opponent. My favorite techniques to this area are knee drives and a short vertical punch or an uppercut.

The kidneys are located in the back on either side of the lumbar spine. Elbows, knees, and vertical punches are my techniques of choice when addressing these areas.

The floating ribs are the last ribs located at the bottom of the rib cage. Only one side of the rib is attached to the rib cage. Vertical strikes, knee drives, and side bear hugs with the wrist cutting into the area are very effective attacks.

The bladder is generally a weak area on most people. The muscle wall is thinner than that of six-pack abs located directly above. The bladder is located two inches below the navel and above the groin. This is the area common to hernias. Any of the thrusting attacks with the knee or foot, or an uppercut with a balled fist works well here. Your opponent may even wet themselves as they double over in pain after sustaining a well-placed power shot!

The Spine

The complete central nervous system is encased in the vertebra of your spine. Spinal cord injuries are debilitating and are potentially lethal. The spine will include the area from the bottom of your skull to the end of your coccyx (tailbone). The most devastating areas to strike are the C1, as described before; the T1, where the thoracic and the cervical sections meet and the coccyx.

We have previously addressed the C1 region; the T1 area is between the top of the shoulder blades. Downward elbow strikes work best here. The death elbow technique is a downward elbow strike focused on this spot.

A knee drive from behind delivered to the coccyx is extremely effective. A kick to this area does not offer near the impact as the knee offers.

The Groin

Everyone has groins, and they all hurt when struck. It is quite evident that a strike delivered to a male's groin is more devastating, but a well-placed kick, strike, or knee to a female's genital region can cause some significant pain and act as an effective distraction. Kicks, open-hand strikes, fist strikes, or a slap, grab, and twist are all effective attacks directed to the male.

The Thighs

There are many areas of the thighs to attack. The ones that provide the best results are peroneal nerve and the femoral artery. A well-placed shin or a cut kick delivered to the outside of the leg approximately mid-thigh will cause the leg to buckle, or worse. The spot to strike is the space between your quadriceps and hamstrings. There is not much muscle between the skin and the bone in this area. A strike there will pinch the nerve between your shinbone and the femur of your opponent. So you are essentially crushing their peroneal nerve between their own femur and your shinbone, incredibly effective.

The femoral artery is the main artery that supplies oxygenated blood to the lower body. Kicks, strikes, slaps, and "horse bites"[27] are very effective when directed to this sensitive area. A roundhouse kick with the foot or instep is more effective than that of a shin blow when directed to the inside of the thigh. The snapping strike delivers more damage effective on this area than a "thudding" attack.

The Knees

To destroy a knee requires a blow with only 30 pounds of pressure directed against the joint of the knee. It takes less to cause significant pain and temporary incapacitation. Front kicks, side kicks, cross stomps, and oblique kicks work best when attacking the knee. Roundhouse kicks work well to the inside of the knee, but for destruction, the thrusting kicks against the joint will yield the desired result.

Roundhouse kicks or cut kicks delivered to the inside of the knee are very effective. Generally, the result is not as devastating as the attacks levied to the outside and the front of the knee, but these strikes can cause some damage and disrupt or distract your adversary.

The Shin and Calves

A well-placed ball of the foot front kick when applied to either the shin or the calf is a great distraction technique, and may even temporarily disable your assailant.

---

[27] A horse bite is a pain compliance/disruption technique. Levy a slap followed up by a grabbing and twisting motion of the hand with the captured flesh.

Have you ever banged your shin into the coffee table in the middle of the night? Man, does that ever smart. Now imagine a well-placed kick with the tip of a boot or a hard shoe. You can just imagine the effectiveness.

The spot to attack in the calf is located directly below the lower insertion point of the gastrocnemius muscle where the sural nerve and the muscle meet. This is a great spot to attack someone from behind as you immediately grab your opponent by the trapezius and yank them to the ground.

The Ankles and Feet

A well-placed strike to the talus or a stomp to the foot and the toes can provide temporary incapacitation or, at the very least, act as an effective disruption technique.

The talus is found where the instep of the foot and the ankle meet, the section of the foot where the crease forms when you bend your ankle. A ball of the foot or a kick using the point of a boot or shoe tip to this area could dislocate the ankle. Whether that occurs or not, the strike is still very effective and difficult to defend against.

Foot and toe stomps are painful, effective, and easy to apply. Period. A case of "turf toe"[28] can sideline a 245-pound NFL running back! Dorsiflex your foot and drive your heel into the top of the target's instep or toes. These stomps will effect the nerves and potentially crush any number of the 26 bones of the human foot.

---

[28] Turf toe is a sprain of the big toe at the joint where the toe meets the foot. Extremely painful.

Stance

How should one stand?

There are many different stances to adopt. Most of the stances used in most martial arts classes are useless for actual combat. The "crouching tiger, hidden dragon" type of nonsense will get you killed in a real fight. However, these stances are beneficial to strengthening your legs and helping you develop balance and learn how to root with the ground. Please bear in mind that these type of stances are simply a transitory means to move from position to position.

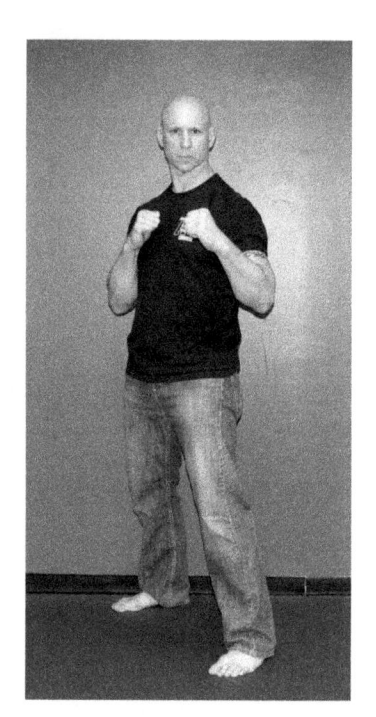

You are better served to position yourself in a boxing or kickboxing stance we refer to as a *walking stance*. Start with your feet together and simply walk. Stop at full stride, put your hands above your head, and then drop your elbows so that your fists are next to your jaw. Turn your body slightly sideways. Once you have become comfortable with this stance, you may vary it in accordance to the distance from your assailant and the aspects of the terrain.

Once you are in your stance, you will either have your left or right foot forward. Bruce Lee[29] espoused fighting with your dominant side forward, but maintaining the ability to switch. Traditional boxing proclaims that your power hand should be the rear hand. There are valid arguments for both.

Personally, my belief is that you should start with whatever side you feel more comfortable with and then work the less dominant side. I

---

[29] Bruce Lee was potentially the most influential martial artist of all time. He broke the mold of the traditionalists and promoted learning different styles to produce a superior, ever-evolving fighting system.

like to start with my left side forward. I am left eye dominant, and my left foot delivers better kicks than my right, yet my right hand hits harder than my left. Since the first thing that meets my opponent will be my left foot, I prefer to have my left forward.

However, when you throw a kick with your back leg and move forward, your stance will be changed. So it would behoove you to be able to fight from either side.

Stances and Fighting Positions Explained

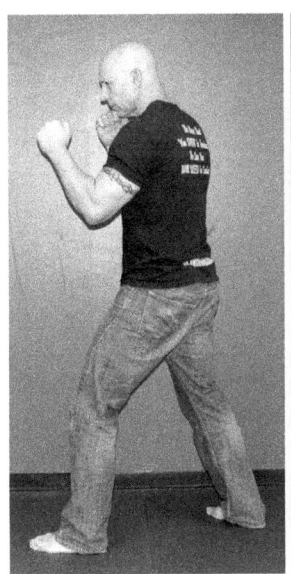

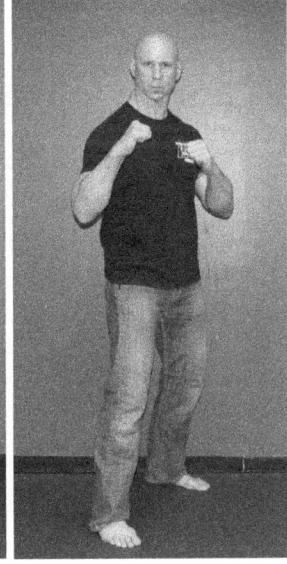

Orthodox: Right hand and right foot are in the back and the left hand and foot is forward. People are predominantly right handed; therefore this is the most popular stance.

Southpaw: Your left hand is in the back, and your right hand and foot are forward. The term *southpaw* originally came from the game of baseball. Due to the alignment of one of the original New Jersey baseball fields, the lefties' dominant hand faced the southern side of the stadium. Hence the term "Southpaw".

Now, if both fighters are in an orthodox stance, they will be *chest to chest*. If one of them is in an orthodox stance and the other is a southpaw, they will be *mirror image*. It is important to train with different stances and different looks.

When you are fighting someone with a different stance than your self, it's important to "own the outside." What I mean by that is if you are an orthodox fighter facing a southpaw, your left foot needs to be on the outside of their right foot. This keeps you farther from their power hand and gives the advantage to your power side.

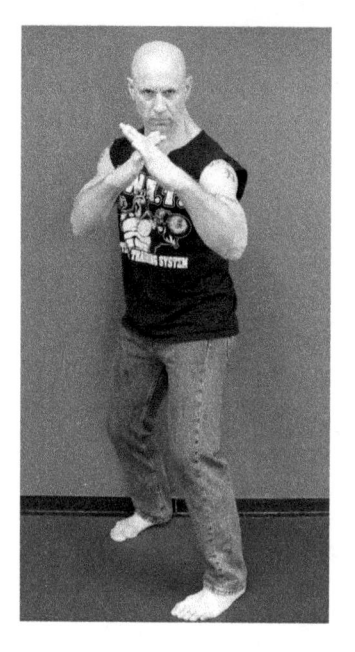

X-stance or cross stance: You start out like you would for your walking stance, and then you make it more compact. This is an unorthodox fighting stance and may throw your opponent off.

Round your shoulders, lower your head, and have your hands in an axehand configuration and crossed in front of you. Turn your toes slightly inward and bring your knees closer together, drawing your genitals back so that they are provided some protection from an initial attack. This stance may be practiced from both the orthodox and southpaw posture.

7
GENERATION OF POWER

There are three main components, and they must be accomplished to maximize your striking and throwing power. This training sequence must be followed to achieve the highest level of implementation, no exceptions. *Technique, speed,* and *power.* Too many practitioners try to apply too much power and too much speed to the techniques prior to learning how to perform the movements properly. They ultimately cheat themselves of power and speed—plus, they leave themselves exposed to counterattacks.

Focus on proper technique execution. To achieve ultimate power and speed, you have to master the techniques. Work your movements slowly, at first paying particular attention to the position of your body during the execution of the movement. The adage, "Fast is slow and slow is fast", holds true. If you do it fast, you'll learn it slow. If you do it slowly, you'll learn the movements quickly. Practice your movements slowly until they flow. This holds true for combinations as well.

Efficiency of movement and no wasted motion. Take your time and master the basics.

TECHNIQUE, SPEED, AND POWER

If I sound redundant, it's on purpose. These tenets must be followed to the letter if you are to be successful. Fast is slow, slow is fast. Practice proper execution of your techniques, and speed will come. Efficiency and fluidity of movement is crucial to successful implementation of your technique. Once you are able to perform your strike, block, movement, throw, submission, or combination with technical fluidity, you will become faster and faster. Once speed has been added to the technique, power naturally will come. Remember, speed kills. You will not have speed without technique. You will not have power without speed. All these attributes of fighting technique must be added in order.

Hips

All power is generated from the hips. Pick a sport, any sport (even golf, which is an activity, not a sport) where real movement is critical. Watch an NFL running back carry the football and elude defenders as he runs downfield. Observe a professional baseball player drive a ball over the deep wall, witness a knockout blow delivered by the middleweight champion. The limbs are mere delivery mechanisms for the power and movement generated by the hips. Torque, explosive power, and incredible force are generated from our hips.

For eons, the Asian cultures have revered the notion of ki/chi energy. *Chi* (from Chinese), *Ki* (Japanese). Ki, in my opinion, is not some mythical notion, or at least it didn't start that way. The center of your body is where your Ki generates from. I do not subscribe to the mystical nonsense of using someone's Ki against them, or having ki wars. I've seen far too many of these so-called masters debunked. However, the notion originated from somewhere.

I will assert that the notion of ki energy was a direct result of the application of hip power in movement. Using the hips adds incredible power to any movement. Your legs, glutes, and back come into play here. Try to throw someone twice your weight using your arms and shoulders, you will not be successful and most likely tear a shoulder muscle. If you incorporate your hips, you will be pleasantly surprised with the results.

Relaxation/Tension

If your muscles are tensed up and tight, you cannot move. Try it, flex your arm, and then see how slowly it moves. If it's completely tight and rigid, it won't budge. This is why having incredible weightlifting strength does not translate to being a good fighter. One has to relax the muscle to be able to move it. The tension and locking of the muscles occurs at the moment of impact.

Practicing tension and relaxation are crucial to developing power. Why is this? Your movements must be relaxed in order to be quick. As we have stated before, speed leads to *power*. Power enables you to deliver meaningful blows that will incapacitate your opponent.

Rooting with the Ground

The most powerful force in your surroundings is the ground. There are times, especially when delivering hand strikes, that we will have our feet planted firmly at the exact point that our strike contacts the assailant. Using the force that you generate when driving from the floor or ground increases your power, stability, and balance. Do not confuse this with immobility. This rooting is quick in coordination with the delivery of a strike. However, when training to develop this power, you will need to be stationary. Once you have developed this skill, incorporate movement.

Friction Reduction

Friction slows down your movement, period. You will notice this particularly when you kick. When executing your kicks, one needs to turn their foot on the floor. This will incorporate the power of your hip. To make this kick even more effective, add a slight jump so that your foot is off the ground. Your kick will be faster, thus more powerful.

Forward Movement

You motion forward will add power and speed to your technique. Straight line and multiple motions close the gap quicker. For example, if you throw a jab and do not step forward, it will not be as powerful as one that you make forward progress with. Even if it's only a small step, there will be a significant addition of power. Additionally, if you don't have to step in to hit someone, you are so close that you should already be hitting them! If they're that close, they'll surely be hitting you.

ECONOMY OF MOTION

The shortest distance between two points is a straight line. You lose speed, power, and accuracy when you "loop" punches. Even a hook punch or an uppercut, do not "loop." A punch follows this path: hip, shoulder, elbow, and fist. This will keep your technique in line and maximize your alignment, which will yield more power and speed.

The same is true for blocking. You should not overextend your blocks. Hands are 4 to 5 inches wide; you don't need to extend your blocks and parries much beyond your own body. Plus, when you reach too far past, it takes longer to get the limb back to the guarding position and leaves you exposed to another attack longer. We have techniques designed to take advantage of blocks that the defender overextends on.

DELIVERY MECHANISMS

Reduced surface area provides more power per square inch. Therefore, striking with the knuckles or the edge of the hand will have a greater effect than an open-hand strike, given the same force applied to the blow. Simple physics.

However, you must consider what target you are striking. Ponder the notion of yin and yang (often referred to as yin yang, yinyang, and others as well)—the dualities of nature. Hard versus soft. Dark versus light. Good versus evil, etc... The defining line is not straight but curved. Demonstrating that there is a little of each in both, while also depicting that one cannot exist without the other. You may be asking yourself, what does this have to do with striking? Well, a great deal. Have you ever seen anyone with broken knuckles or wrists from punching another in the head? That is because they used a hard implement to strike a hard surface—someone's head, for example. If you want to punch someone in the head with a closed fist and avoid injury, your hands need to be extremely well conditioned. You are better off using a soft striking implement to strike a hard area and a hard implement to attack the soft portions of your assailant.

Examples: Use a clenched fist to deliver a blow to the stomach or the kidneys. Use an open-hand strike to hit the head. Try this experiment, if you dare. Walk up to a wall and slap it as hard as you can. Your hand will probably sting a bit. Now, address the same wall with a straight punch. What do you think will happen to your hand? If you do so (not recommended), you will most likely experience severe damage to your phalanges and metacarpals.

8
GRIPS AND LOCKS

There are certain basic locks, grips, and holds that can be learned with relative ease. The biggest mistake that people make is practicing the individual movements without practicing the entry to the submission or choke. How do you get there? In a Brazilian jujitsu or grappling training, there are many excellent flow drills that teach you how to position yourself properly and move from position to position, attempting to secure a submission while avoiding your opponent's submission or prevent yourself from losing your advantageous position. This is an art unto itself and should be treated as such. We will be focusing primarily on the street application of locks, grips, and chokes.

SMALL-JOINT MANIPULATION

Finger locks can be extremely effective and very painful. The fingers are filled with nerves and are sensitive. My favorite to apply when someone pokes me in the chest or puts a finger in my face is to place my thumb against their fingertip as I grab the rest of their finger with my hand.

When grabbed, especially from behind as would occur within a full nelson attack, isolate two fingers and pull them backward in a twisting motion. This method is best applied when your opponent attacks you from behind and you put your arm over theirs as you pull their fingers backward. Grab their fingers from the back side of their hand with the pinky side of your hand facing upward. It's best to grab two fingers. If you grab one, it may snap. You want to maintain control through pain compliance rather than snap off their finger.

WRIST LOCKS

There are many, many wrist locks that are taught. We will focus on just a few techniques that work for most people in most situations. Please note that in order to "earn the right to use jujitsu", meaning locks and holds, the opponent must be "dummied up" prior to their application. Deliver powerful strikes prior to even attempting to apply a lock or hold. This is especially prevalent when performing wrist locks. We also must understand that the holds are placed on the hands, not the wrists. However, it is the wrist that experiences the pain.

It is particularly important to note that *there need to be three directions of pressure with all locks.* Two directions do not supply enough power to cause pain compliance and balance disruption. Additionally, *never* bend your back on any of these (as with most) techniques; bend from your knees and maintain a neutral spine.

The terminology of the techniques vary among styles and instructors. Below are the names as I was taught and how they are referred to while training.

Kotegaeshi (or the looking glass): This position is accomplished when you gain control of the opponent's hand by twisting it so that their fingers are facing upward with your thumbs directly in the middle of the back of their hand. You will grab the inside of their palm at their thumb with one hand and their pinky with the other. You apply pressure by pulling your fingers toward you, pushing your thumbs toward them as you step to the outside and rotate on an angle downward and towards their thumb. Also, be sure to keep their hand on your chest. This will add pressure to the wrist of the assailant. If you are quite a bit smaller than your opponent or don't have a great deal of comfort with the technique, the application of the chest pressure will be invaluable.

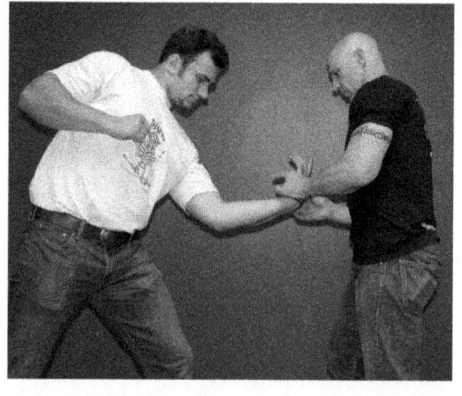

Gan Kun: One of the best ways to apply this move occurs when you get grabbed at the lapel. If he grabs you with his right hand on your left lapel, reach across with your right hand, keeping your elbow high to protect your face from getting punched. Apply an overgrip so that your fingers grab the hand at the section below the pinky, and insert your thumb into the thenar muscle (the spot between the thumb and the forefinger). Rotate your left shoulder inward as you shift back and raise your left arm high enough to clear the hand. You will rotate their hand so that their pinky is facing upward, push upward with your right thumb, and drive your left elbow downward into their forearm as you step and drag your foot backward. Be sure to keep your back straight and bend from the knees.

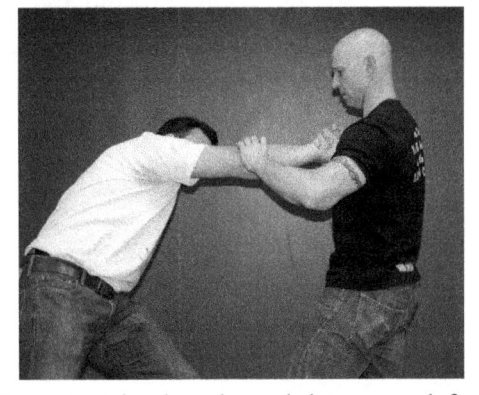

There are other versions of this move as well. All will be the same as in the above-described defense, except you will grab the assailant's arm with your left hand so that your fingers access the radial nerve. You will employ a C-grip, thumb under and fingers over, thus resembling a *C*. Rotate their wrist to the right and their arm to the left as you push their wrist toward them on a downward angle. This is also referred to as the washrag technique due to the motion like the wringing out of a wet rag.

Goosenecks: These are very popular among law enforcement and security personnel. Often referred to as "come-alongs," the gooseneck enables the person applying the technique to move or direct the other person from one place to another by using pain compliance. Hence the name *come-alongs*.

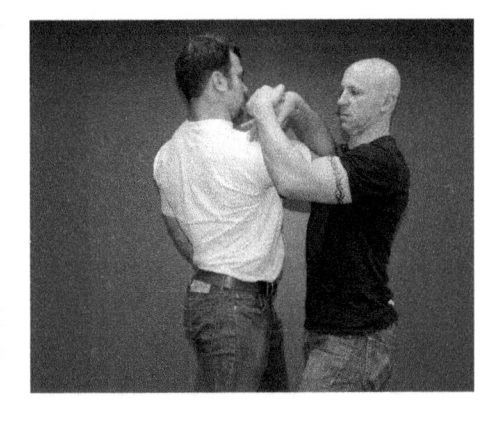

There are several variations, but they all stem from the base lock. Grab their right hand with your right hand. This is generally done from a standing position, but can done from the ground as well. Thread your left arm under their right and apply a reverse chop to their biceps insertion, causing the elbow to bend. With your right hand, you should grip their thumb with your fingers. The thumb of your right hand should be aligned with their middle finger. Pull up on their thumb, pressure down on the back of their hand with the palm of your thumb and place your left hand on top of your right as you apply pressure.

You can also hinder their movement by stepping on their right foot with your left. By being on the side of the arm that you are controlling, you have removed yourself from a potential strike from their left hand.

Walk the dog: This is another excellent come-along technique. I like this one best because you are behind the opponent. There are many ways to attain this position. We'll focus on one method. Reach for the opponent's right hand with yours. Step to their right side as you pull down on their wrist and chop the inside of their right arm with your left hand so that their arm bends on a right angle. Slide your right hand over the back of their right hand so that you are able to bend their right wrist and their elbow is in the crook of your right arm (inside of the elbow). With your left hand, grab their trap to prevent them from spinning to face you. Pull the fingers of your right hand toward you as if you were a baby waving bye-bye. This will induce a great amount of pain in your subject.

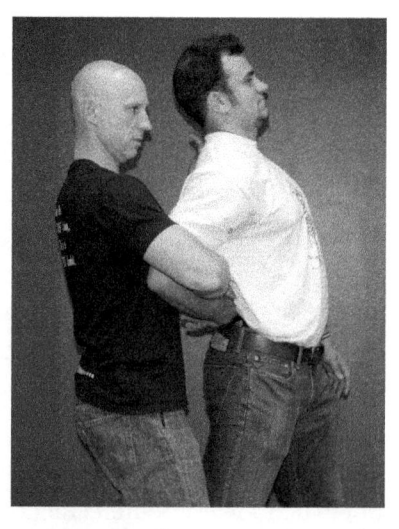

Arm locks: There are many variations of armlocks, armbars, and other associated pain compliance and submission techniques that may

be applied. The locks listed below are some of the most universal—meaning they can be utilized by the greatest majority of people.

Please note that for a street confrontation, *I never recommend that you go to the ground. Except is you are getting pummeled while standing up and striking.* It must also be understood that if the action lasts more than 10 seconds or so, the chances that fight will end up on the ground are dramatically increased. As I have stated, I'd rather keep a street fight standing, but you'd better be prepared to unleash a hellish ground game if you fall or get taken down.

The application of the below-listed movements are many. You will find the best methods of securing these positions through training with your partner. It's also good to practice transitioning from one position to another. Rarely will you ever simply end up in a lock; you will get to it through an opportunity presenting itself during a scramble.

Kimura (Double Wrist Lock): One of the reasons I like the Kimura (aka the Hammer Lock) is that it can be applied from a variety of offensive and defensive positions. If someone is behind you and has their left arm around your waist, take your left arm and go over their arm. Take you right hand and grab their left wrist, then grab your right wrist with your left hand. Next you will pivot on your left foot and step around toward the side with your right foot. During the application of the Kimura, be sure to employ the thumbless or Gable grip.

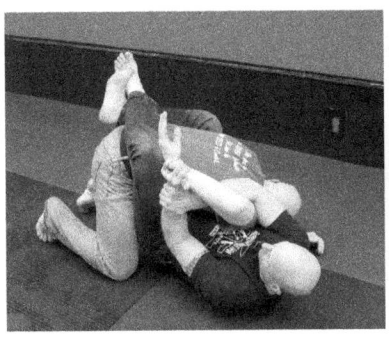

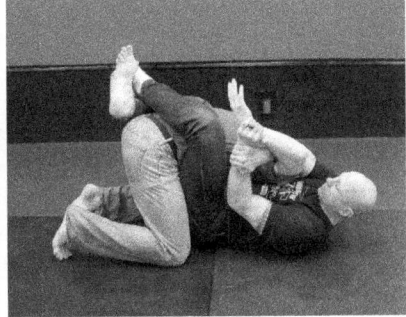

You may also apply the Kimura while on top or from the bottom while you are facing the opponent. If you are on the bottom, if you have your opponent in the closed guard[30], as you sit up and unlock your legs, position your left shoulder to theirs as you loop your left arm around their left arm. Grab their left wrist with your right hand. Thread your left arm through and grab your right wrist with your left hand. Relock your legs and scoot your hips to the right as you drive their left hand behind their back and toward their right shoulder.

When you find yourself in the top position, in either a full [31] or side mount[32], grab your opponent's right wrist with you right hand, thread your left arm around their right arm above the elbow and then under the arm as you secure lock by grabbing your right wrist with your left hand. If you are in Side Mount, slide your right knee over their belly to assume the Full Mount. Once there, pivot on your right knee as you step your right foot toward their head while running their wrist toward their left shoulder and lifting their elbow to their head.

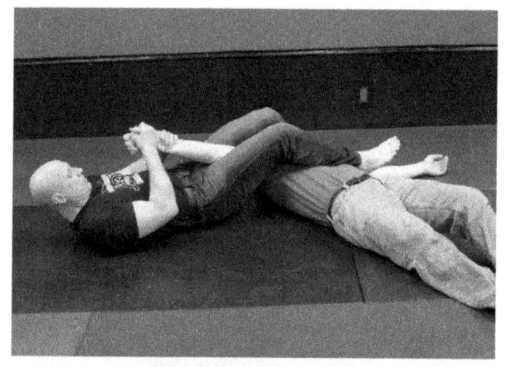

Armbar: There are many armbars that may be applied in street combat. Some are better suited for grappling competitions and not the best for the street. However, when you are on your back and faced with a last-resort situation . . . let your training take over and do what comes naturally.

---

[30] The closed guard: There are several guards utilized by Brazilian jujitsu practitioners. Closed, butterfly, spider, half Guard, X-guard, to name a few. The Closed Guard occurs when you are on your back and you have your legs wrapped around their waist with your feet locked at the ankles.

[31] Full mount: When you are straddled over an opponent while they are in a supine position.

[32] Side mount: Any position when your opponent is supine and you are on top of them in a chest-to-chest position with both legs on side of their body.

When considering self-defense, the BJJ guard (closed guard) is not a position that is recommended as a street combat position. Your groin, centerline, and face are exposed. Additionally, a strong opponent will be able to lift you up and smash you off of the pavement. However, if you do get knocked to the ground and find yourself on your back with an enraged attacker on you, you had better have an answer. Let's consider that you have been knocked to the ground, your assailant is on top of you, and raining punches down on you. What are you to do? If you happen to be fortunate enough to wrap your legs around their waist and pull them into your guard, we will proceed as follows. If they have you in a full mount position, this will be covered in chapter 13.

Now on to the move. For one, tuck your chin, contract your abs, and try to sit up as much as possible as you "swim" your arms and shift your body from side to side as you deflect punches. Secure their right wrist with your left hand and grab the elbow of the same arm with your right hand in the thumb-down (pointing toward you) position. Pivot on your back toward your right and assume a perpendicular reference and place your right leg high on their back so that their arm is located on the inside of your leg. Hold on to their arm with your right hand; shove their head to the side with your left hand as you bring your left leg over their head. Drive your heels to the ground as your arch your back, driving your hips into the elbow joint while you are pulling on their wrist. This is not a tournament; don't stop until the arm snaps.

When we apply the standing version, you have knocked your assailant to the ground. Grab their right wrist with your right hand. Deliver a front kick to the downed attacker's ribs with your right foot, thus wedging your foot underneath their back. Lift your left foot up and over their head and bring your heel down into the left side of the head of the supine attacker. Sit your butt to your heel as you land on the ground with your head up and extending the opponent's arm. Again, apply quick, strong pressure until a snap results.

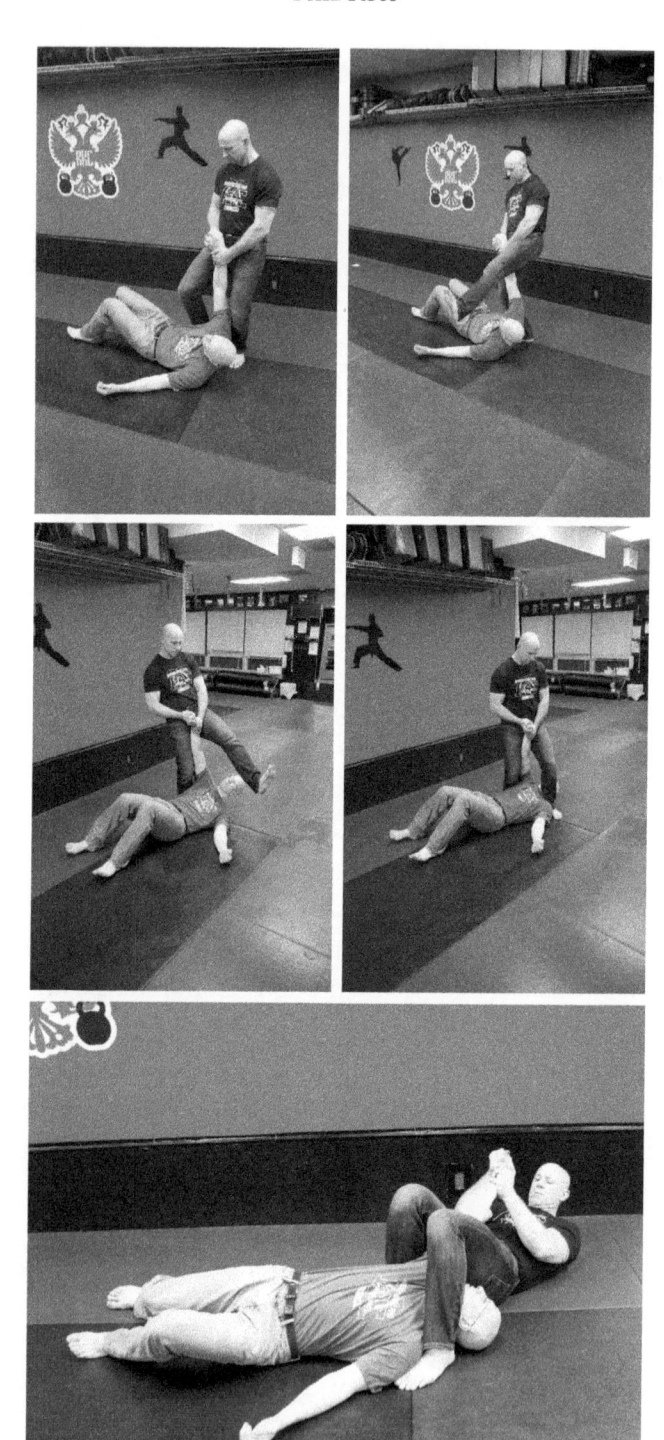

Americana (key-lock): Think of this as a "reverse Kimura." When in the side mount, if the attacker has their hand close to their head, palm facing upward, grab their left wrist with your left hand and press down hard, thus pinning their hand to the ground. Slip your right hand underneath their arm and thread your wrist through and grab your own left wrist. Roll the knuckles of your left hand down toward the ground as if you were operating the throttle on a motorcycle. Simultaneously lift your right elbow up as you drag their pinned wrist in an arc downward and toward you. Do not stop until you hear a snap.

Python grip: This is my favorite for the street. This technique may be utilized from either a standing position or with the aggressor on the ground. If the antagonist throws a right punch, block their arm with your left hand chop and loop yours over theirs at the elbow and snake your arm through. At the same time, hit them in the throat with a right scissors punch and squeeze their throat as you place your left hand on your right elbow. Straighten your right and left in unison. From this position, slam the attacker into the wall or take them to the ground. Snap their arm and/or choke them out. You can do the same move to a downed opponent, provided you are able to thread your arm around theirs as you take them down. This is not as difficult as one may think, provided you practice.

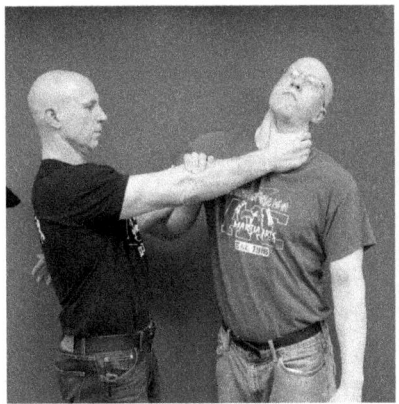

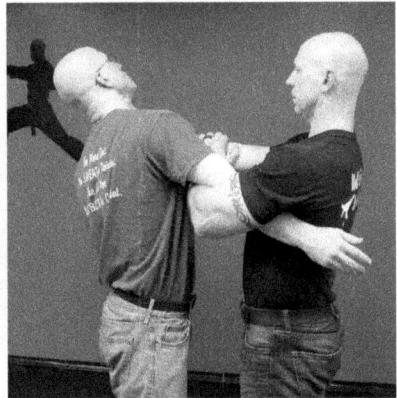

There are a few other standing locks that you may be afforded to apply from the standing position. I like these better for the street because you are not compromised by going to the ground.

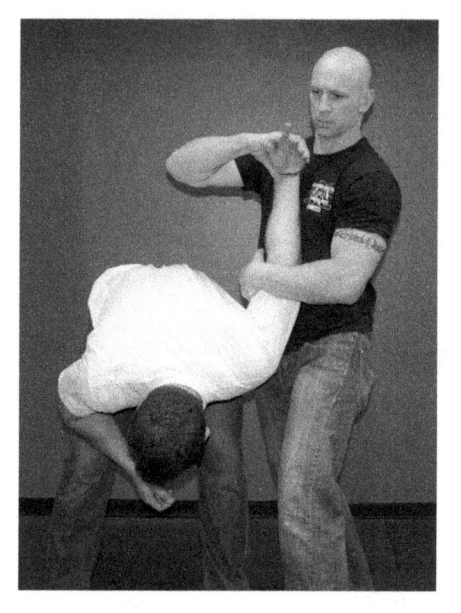

Straight arm lock with wrist: If you practice BJJ, think of it as Kimura that you straighten out and apply a wrist lock to. This position is usually attained when someone grabs you around the waist from behind. As with all self-defense movements, employ one of the loosening-up techniques, foot stomps, shin kicks, groin strikes, etc…If you are attacking his left arm, hook your left arm around his elbow and grab his left wrist with your right hand. Step 180 degrees toward the left with your right foot, and as you straighten his arm, pin it at the elbow against your chest with your left arm. Bend his right wrist downward. Apply knees to the head if necessary.

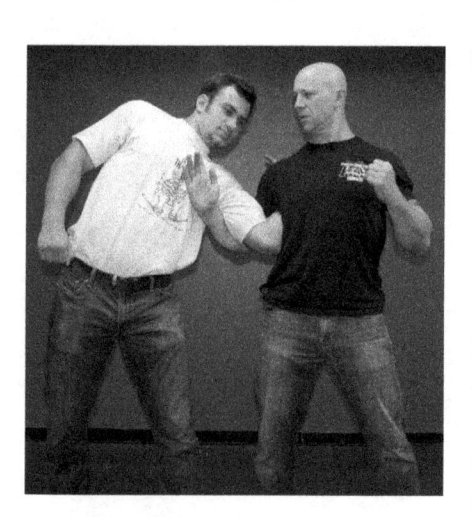

Standing whizzer: This position is a temporary one. You will need to begin striking or take the opponent to the ground once you've initially applied the hold. One of the best ways to get into the position is when the attacker grabs you by the shoulder. If your left shoulder is attacked, immediately place your left arm over their arm and scoop your elbow behind theirs as you point your elbow to the ceiling and put the back of your hand against their chest. You will need to launch your counterattack now. Knees to the their midsection and groin, move into the python grip position or chin-jab them to the face.

Choke Holds

No one loves MMA more than I do. It's the best sport on the planet, bar none and no holds barred (pun intended). Some of the chokes take too long to apply in a "street: life or death" predicament. You don't have 5, or even 3, seconds for a choke to take effect. A street choke needs to provide immediate results. Imagine if the guy has a knife in his pocket or boot and your choke takes 3 seconds to garner results. He could easily draw the knife and stab you several times in 3 seconds.

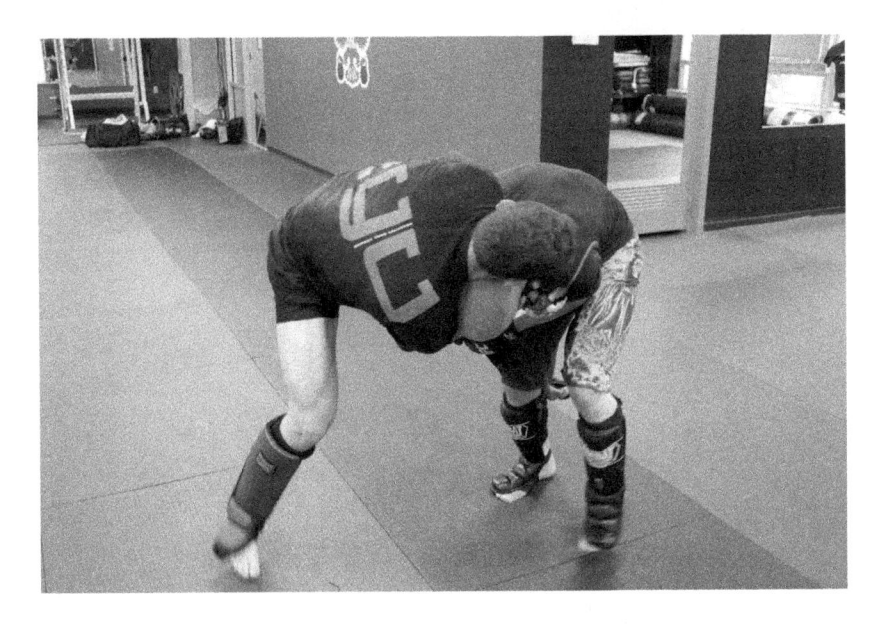

The notion on *no gaps* is never more evident than when considering chokes. You do not want to leave any wiggle room available to someone that you are applying a choke to. You will only rid yourself of these gaps when you practice these chokes over and over, and over again while gaining feedback from your partner.

I have been practicing these chokes since the mid-1980s, so my terminology is based on what the chokes were referred to back then.

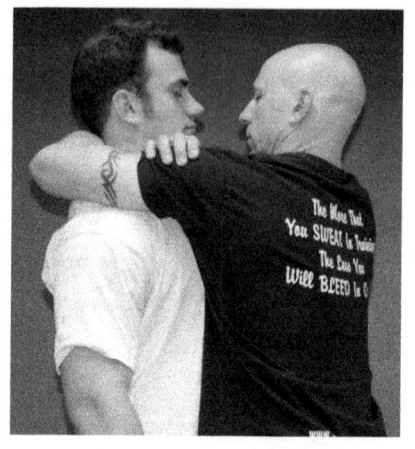

Two-point choke: This choke is very similar to the Ezekiel choke. I will typically employ this choke when someone has me in an arms-free bear hug from the front or off of strike defense. Slide your right arm on a 45-degree angle up with your palm down. The hard edge of your wrist needs to be against their throat and your fingers reaching back over their right trap. Shoot your left arm under your right hand and then quickly wrap it around their neck. With your left hand, grip your fingers into the crook of your elbow. This choke may or may not result in your aggressor losing consciousness, but it's a great distraction and allows you to deliver head butts to their nose and mouth, as well as knees to their groin and bladder.

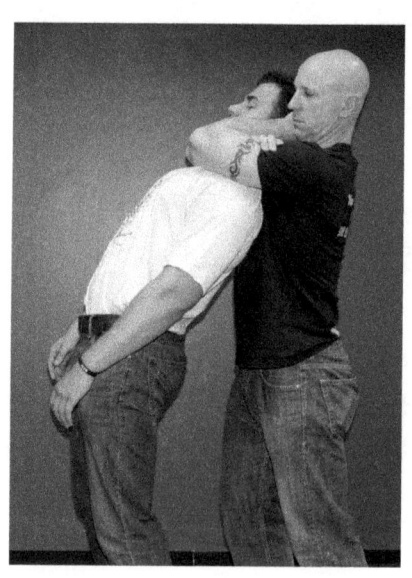

Three-point choke: Our next choke is often referred as the RNC (rear naked choke) and is applied from behind. You will want to begin this move with a left biceps punch to the left side of your assailant's head as you wrap your left arm around their throat. Be sure to have your arm under their chin as you slide your arm back so that the back of your hand is against the right side of their face. This position is extremely important because with your hand in this position, it ensures that your wrist is planted firmly against their trachea. Next, slide your right arm over their right trap with your palm up. You will secure the choke by grasping you right bicep with your left hand, and then bend your elbow to allow placing your right hand on the top of the left side of their head. There should be no gaps whatsoever. To finish the assailant off, roll your left wrist into their throat and upward, drive your right elbow down into their chest as you push their head on an angle down and to the right by curling your wrist. Done properly, the result will be an immediate loss of air and a crushing effect on the trachea.

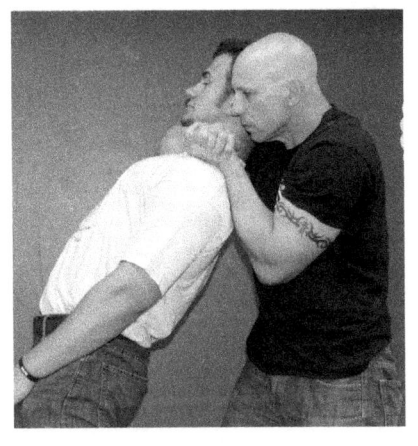

Four-point choke: The most devastating choke of them all. This is my preferred method to choke someone from behind. The entry is shorter and quicker than on the 3-point choke. With the thumb of your right hand facing up, ride downward along their right clavicle and then snake your hand onto the left side of their face and position the back of your hand against the left side of their face. Your right hand will be palm down and set to meet the left.

Now with your left hand in a palm-up position, secure a Gable grip as you place the top right portion of your head to the back of the left side of their head. Situate your left elbow in their back as you pull your right elbow back behind their shoulder, and then roll your right wrist upward and inward into their throat. This will provide you with four points of pressure. Applied correctly, the choke will yield the desired result in less than 1 second. Yes, I did say 1 second or less. This choke is the quickest, nastiest, and most devastating method of applying a choke from the rear position.

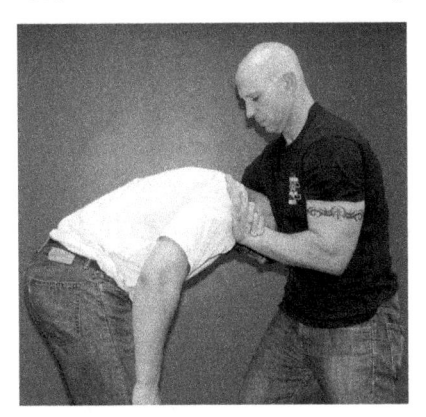

Front choke, standing: If you have struck you opponent in the groin or have done a head snap and brought them down so that they are bent over at the waist, it's a good time to apply the extremely effective choke. Loop your right arm over their neck so that your bicep is against their face and the back of your wrist is against their throat. Your hand should be dorsiflexed, thus bringing the back of your hand against the side of their face. Smash into their shoulder with your left hand and then grab your left wrist with your right hand. Apply pressure by dropping your right elbow and shoulder downward, pushing into their shoulder with your left hand and driving your hips toward them in an upward and inward motion. Be cautious with your training partner, this movement places a great deal of stress on the neck.

Leg Locks

Leg locks are a great deal of fun and very devastating, but extremely difficult to apply in a street situation. Unless you have taken you opponent down and remained standing, you have to be on the ground to administer one. As discussed before, going to the ground in the street is not recommended. This limits the amount of choices that we are able to utilize because we must remain on our feet. Additionally, certain footwear makes it difficult to apply a pressure lock; the twisting ones will be effective or using a foot lock to then deliver strikes to the legs and groin, apply the Italian Gas Pedal or forward roll.

Achilles lock: There are several methods to get to the position where we can implement the Achilles lock. One is to a downed opponent that tries to upkick you. Another is when you apply a single-leg takedown. The other most likely to happen will result from an opponent throwing a kick at you. Secure his right leg by wrapping your left arm around his leg so that his foot is in your armpit and the back of your arm is against his Achilles. Thread your right arm under your left hand and then place it on top of his leg at the shin. Roll your shoulder back and down, then roll your wrists into the technique as you extend your arms. This is referred to as the python grip. Next, kick him in the groin with your right foot as you arch upward. Sweep the remaining leg and step on it when it's on the ground. Now to finish him, hold this grip and execute a forward roll directly on top of the downed attacker. This will wreak havoc on his hip, knee, and ankle.

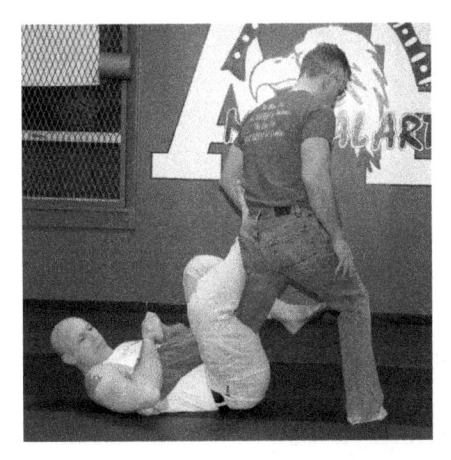

Heel hook: Let us assume that you begin from the basic position of the Achilles lock with the assailant on the ground and you in control of his right foot. With him in the supine position with his toes pointing upward, slide your left arm placing the crook of your elbow firmly on his heel. Bring your left hand over the top of their foot with your palm down while you firmly grasp your right hand, employing the Gable grip. Pivot on your right foot and step in a semicircle toward the downed opponent with your left foot while you twist their ankle. The knee will receive the brunt of the damage.

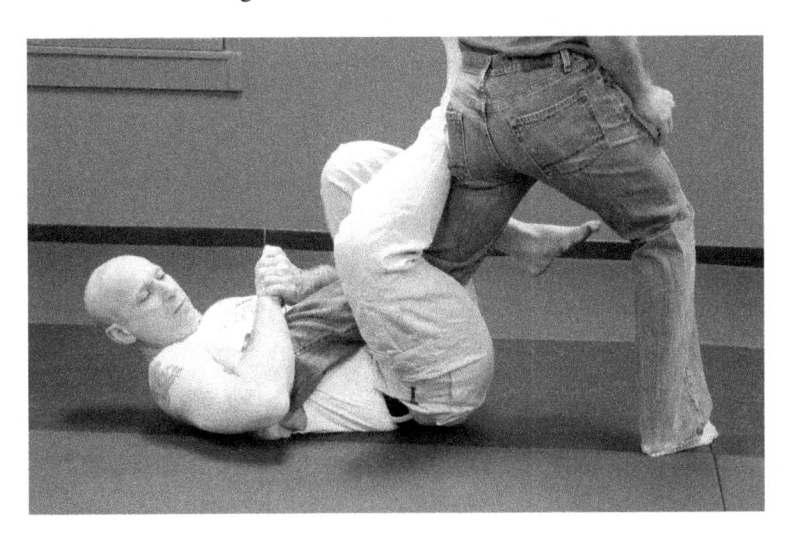

BREAKING GRIPS AND LOCKS

There are a plethora of manners in which you may be grabbed. Especially if you are a smaller individual, larger perpetrators will attempt to grab and control you. As we have stated previously, we have to earn the right to use jujitsu, so delivering strikes to vital and semivital target areas is your first response to being grabbed. That being said, we will consider the universal principles when defending ourselves.

Small Circle (jujitsu): Was developed by Professor Wally Jay[33] and focuses on small joint manipulation and the application of small circle movements to gain an advantage in leverage. This is based on the principle of using as much of your body to control a small portion of theirs. By bringing a limb, joint, or hand close to your body and away from theirs, you have created a power and balance advantage for yourself. Here is an example: If someone grabs your left wrist, they are most likely going to pull you toward them. Let them and then strike them in the face with a palm heel strike. Keeping your elbows tucked into your body, rotate your left hand in a small circle and slip your right hand underneath, grabbing their right hand. Place the axehand edge of your left hand in the palm of their right hand and pressure down. Next, step off on an angle to their right side with your left foot and then your right, all the while you are controlling wrist. It is important to note that the hip drives your power 100%. This should be an effortless motion, not matter what the size differential.

Grab, re-grab: One the most effective methods of practicing your grips, locks, and escapes is with the grab, re-grab drill. This is a flow drill. Start off slowly and then add speed and power to your practice. Start in the standing position. One partner grabs the other by the wrist, hand, or collar. Apply one of the wrist lock techniques, Gan Kun, Kotegaeshi, or one of the variations. Your partner will "go with the flow" and move in the direction that you are taking them. They will counter with a wrist lock of their own; now you are to move with this pressure and perform and counterlock. This lock-counterlock continues until the drill is over. We usually do it for time, 2 to 3 minutes at a clip. This will exhaust your grip, so be prepared to work. When you have two people who are

---

[33] Professor Wally Jay developed small circle jujitsu based on small-joint manipulation and applied leverage. His teaching blend well with other systems of combat.

very experienced at this drill, it's amazing to watch them roll, counter and apply one lock after another with speed and fluidity.

Leg lock defense: I love the fact that MMA has become mainstream. It's a dream-come-true for me. Back in the early 1980s, we yearned for a venue such as the UFC to compete in. You younger guys (and girls) have no idea of how lucky you are!

As with all great things, there are some drawbacks. Untrained knuckleheads see this stuff on TV and in their video games and try to emulate it. There is one positive aspect in our favor—it's reasonably difficult to successfully apply a potent leg lock. Again, we will focus on the principles. You need to go into the technique by bending your leg, dorsiflexing your toes, and moving toward the assailant. If you attempt to pull away, you will only succeed in making the lock tighter. Once you have accomplished this, secure a top position and rain down strikes on your opponent.

9
ENTRY AND SINGLE TECHNIQUES

As conveyed to me by one of the American pioneers of jujitsu, Dr. Tony Palminteri, "You have to earn the right to use jujitsu." What does that mean? In a nutshell, there is no way you are simply going to walk up to someone and apply a lock to them. It just won't work. They will strike you and resist. The idea is to accomplish your goal while sustaining the most minimal amount of damage to yourself. A well-placed strike (either by you *or* your adversary) can render one helpless. This works both for and against you. A powerful punch in the nose can turn a BJJ black belt into a white belt. Whereas a well-placed loosening-up technique will dramatically increase your chances of successfully applying a choke or lock. You won't be able to properly administer your techniques until you "dummy the opponent up."

So we need to consider our entry or loosening-up techniques. The ones below listed, along with other single strikes and techniques, are extremely effective. If you are practiced in grappling, how difficult is it to apply a lock or choke? This is why we strike first. It's far easier to apply once the opponent is loosened up. The strikes "earn" you the right to use your Jujitsu.

ENTRY TECHNIQUES

These techniques must be applied very quickly and with purpose. There can be no hesitation or holding back whatsoever. You may also implement them in multiples. There is no rule that states these techniques are only designed to be entry strikes. In actuality, application demonstrates quite the contrary. Many of these tactics may be used to temporarily or permanently disable an attacker. Your proximity to the assailant will determine what techniques are available to you.

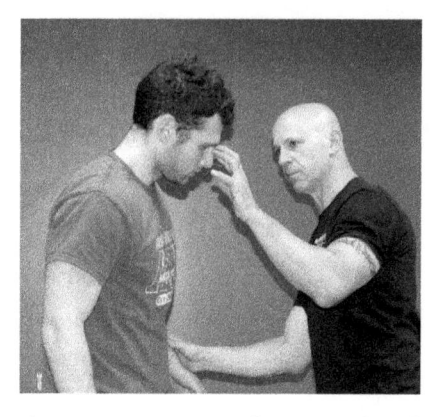

Finger jab to eyes: Extremely quick and effective. Use all four fingers and aim for the bridge of the nose with the full intention of striking the eyes. Flick the fingers out quickly while they are slightly bent. It does not matter how big, tough, or strong your opponent is—everyone has eyes, and they all feel the same amount of pain. If they are wearing glasses, rake the glasses down and simultaneously strike. All you need is to have one of your fingers hit an eye to cause temporary blindness.

Short axehand: This technique both protects your head and face, as well as serves and a powerful, unorthodox strike. This technique may be delivered via a variety of methods. You may launch your attack from a cross stance (chapter 6), interview stance, or from a fig leaf stance with your hands folded one over the other in front of your groin. From this fig leaf stance, have your right hand over your left. Apply pressure and tension to both hands, with your right hand pulling back on your left and your left providing counterpressure. You are creating a spring effect very similar to a jack-in-the-box. When you are ready, release your left hand, launch forward with your left foot, stomping hard on the ground as your axehand hits any of the targets (eyes, nose, throat, ear, mouth, carotid artery, neck, etc.) from the neck to the ear. Your striking implement will be the fleshy part of your hand located directly below your pinky. Your hand must be flexed and with tension. Practice making your hand big by forcing your metacarpalphlangeal joint (knuckles) outward while pulling your fingers back. Practice this movement—it will add strength and flexibility to your hands. It is one of the easiest and most effective methods to develop the intrinsic muscles of your hand. Axehands are the only hand techniques where the hip moves in the same direction as the strike. All other hand techniques require the rotation of the hip inward of the striking limb.

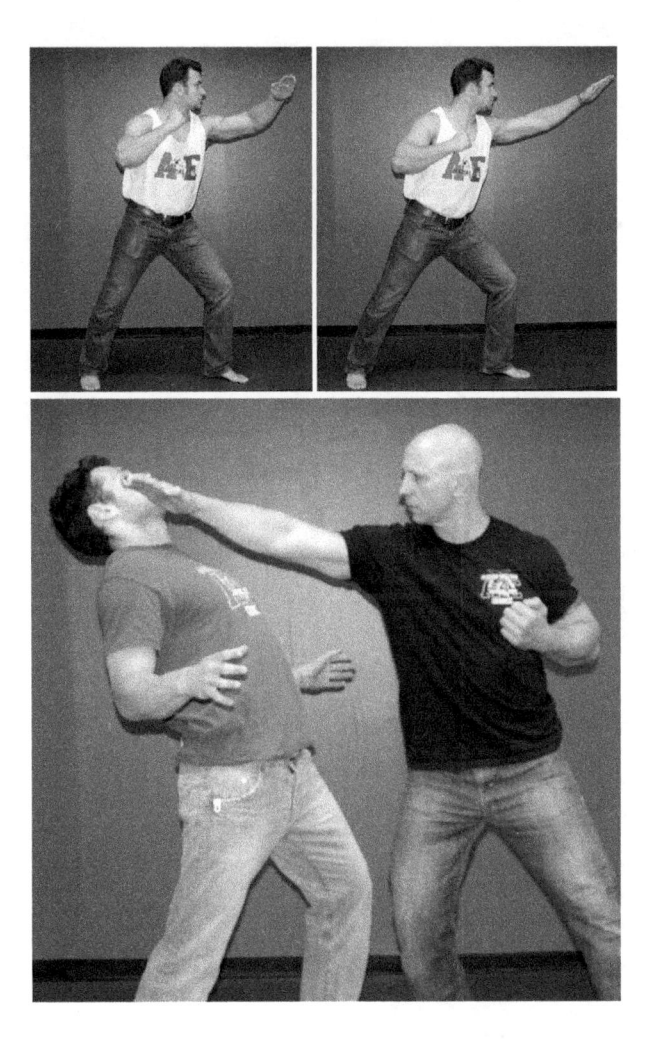

Palm heel: This technique is excellent when delivering strikes to the face, mouth, and especially the nose. The motion is very similar to a straight punch except that your hand is open, you pull your fingers back and your contact point is heel (lower section) or your palm. Since this is considered a "soft" striking area, it is perfect for striking the harder sections of the body. However, this technique is very successful when applied to the sternum, which can be fleshy on larger individuals.

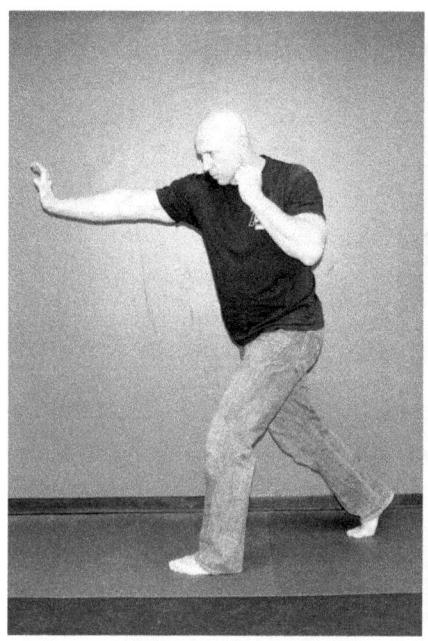

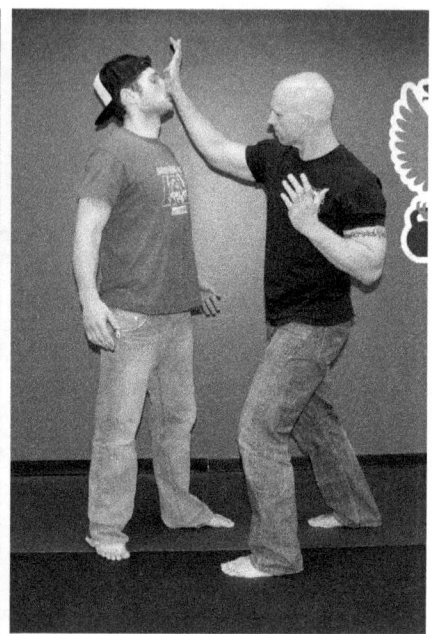

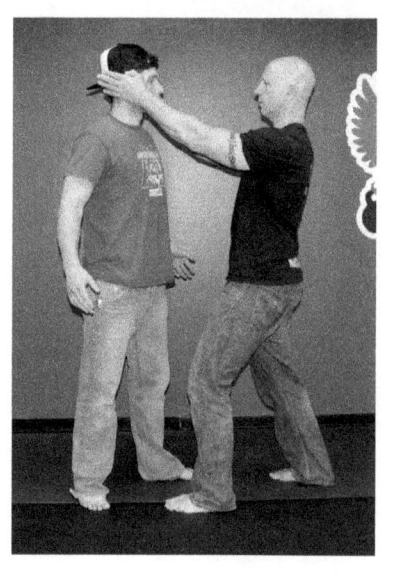

Slaps: Brought up from the hip out of the opponent's line of sight and then quickly and powerfully placed on the ear of the target. The strike is delivered with an upside-down *L* pattern, straight up and then straight across as you rotate your hip into the strike. To increase the effectiveness of the strike, slightly cup your hand, thus forcing air into the eardrum of the attacker. Slaps are a great means employed to loosen up or distract, enabling you to deliver a more potent knockout or disabling technique. Slaps, as well as other open-hand strikes, are the best methods to deliver head blows in street defense.

Head butts: There are four basic head butts to use to defend oneself. All are extremely effective and carry relatively low risk.

Forward. When face-to-face and at very close range, you will attack your opponent's nose or mouth with your forehead. Drive your head forward and down toward the target while contracting your abs and moving your whole upper body forward. Many people are under the false impression that the power of the technique comes solely from the neck. As described, the whole upper body is involved in the power generation, and the forehead is simply the delivery mechanism.

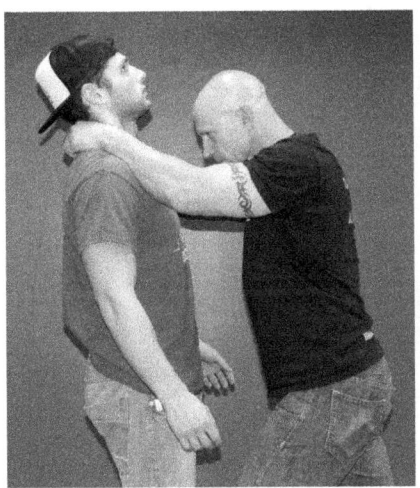

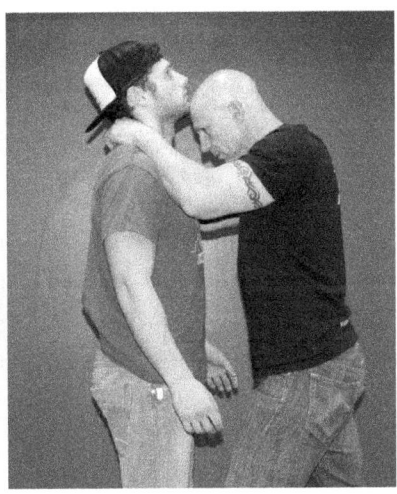

Backward. When you are attacked from behind, bring your head forward and then back—*hard*. It's tough to see where their nose is from this position, so it's recommended that you incorporate a butt smash into them coupled with foot stomps.

Upward. You may be facing each other in front of them, but with your head lower than theirs. Bring your head upward into their chin. If they are positioned properly, you can apply a forward head butt when their head comes back down. Generally, it's best to strike an open target or knock them to the ground.

Sideways. If you are bear-hugged from the side, immediately bring your head sideways bang the upper back corner of your head into their face. The targets of the nose and mouth should be utilized again. This movement, as with most head butts, will not result in a knockout, so you'll want to immediately hammerfist smash them in the groin and stomp their foot. In most instances, this will be enough for you to get them to loosen their grip so you may escape.

Additional Single Techniques

These will be your core striking techniques. You should practice these movements with regularity, focus, and intensity. The muscle memory and neural patterning will only be developed through this type of practice. Knowing how to do something and being able to execute under pressure are two completely different entities.

Consider an MMA fighter: he practices a plethora of strikes and kicks, submissions, takedowns, and combinations for hours on end. Striking pads, drilling and sparring with partners, and working on sequencing and transitions. What percentage of the moves practiced do they pull off in a combat situation? As a general rule, somewhere between 10 percent and 15 percent of the trained movements. That seems amazingly small, but when you consider the time that you have to react and the response to the specific situation, there are only so many techniques that you will be able to execute. Bear this fact in mind when training. As we have pointed out beforehand, the magic number 7, plus or minus 2.

Long axehand: Form your hand, as you would for short axehand. Next, draw your right hand back past your ear with your elbow in front of your face. Step toward your target with your right foot, landing with a stomp as you deliver the axehand to the side of your opponent's neck or head. You should make a full motion through; and while practicing in air or on a pad, bring your right hand back far enough to pass your right shoulder. As with all strikes, incorporation of your hips and engagement of your complete body in the movement is essential for maximum results. As with the short axehand, long axehands require the hip to move in the same direction as the strike.

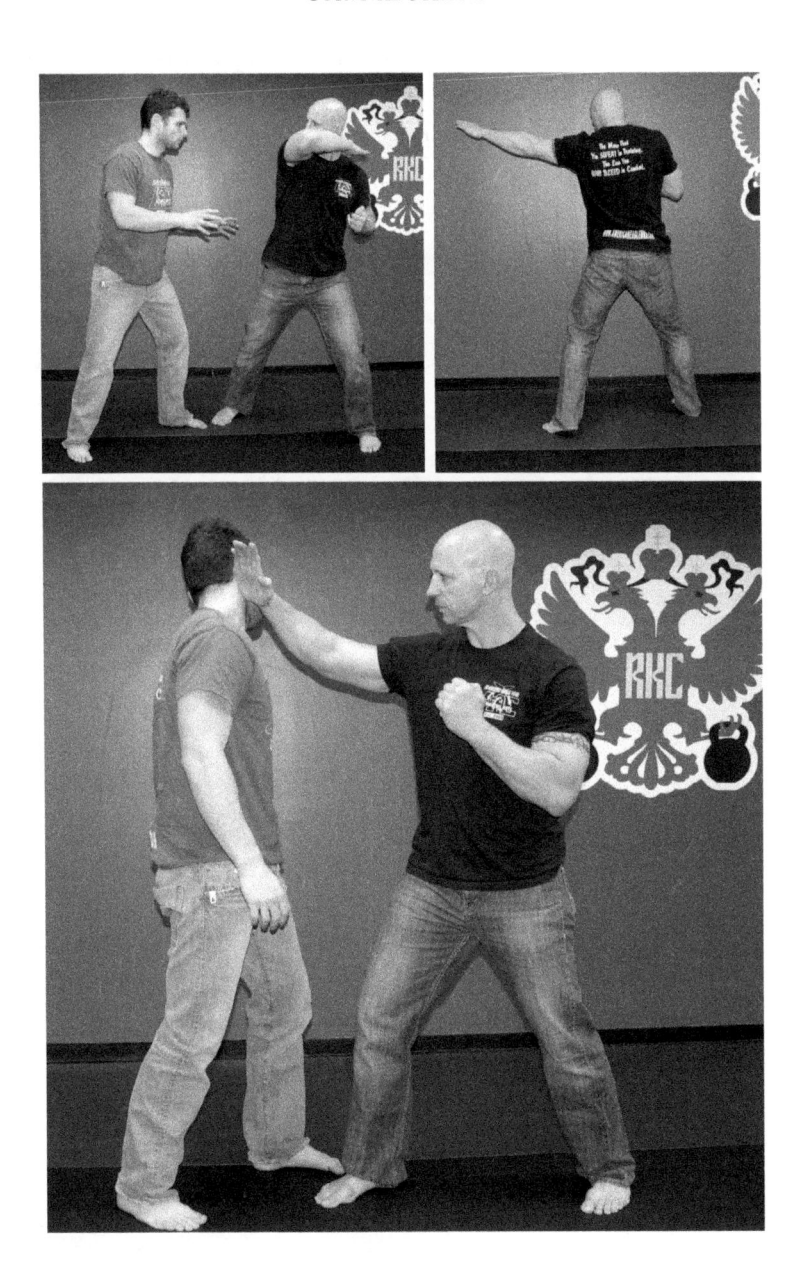

Chin jab: This is an incredibly powerful strike, generally resulting in a knockout. Your hand is positioned like it would be for a palm-heel strike, with your fingers pulled back and your hand flexed so that the heel of your palm will land first on the designated target. Your forearm slides up your assailant's chest on an angle as the radial and ulna bones drive into the chin. Follow through with the upward-angled motion snapping their head backward. This motion will induce referral shock. This quick shot will cause the brain to move in its fluid cushion and crash into the surrounding skull.

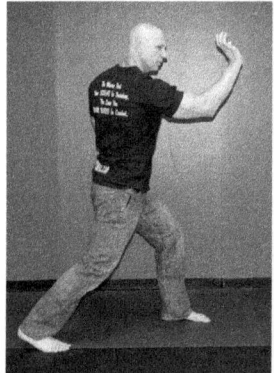

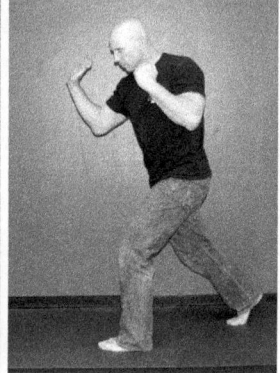

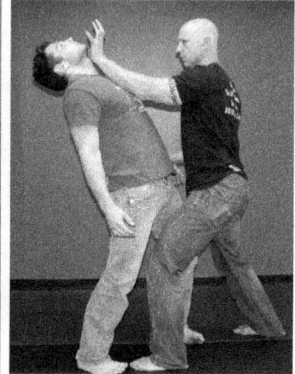

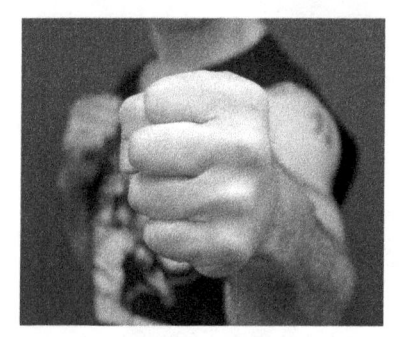

Vertical fist: This technique is best suited for bare-knuckle applications or while wearing MMA gloves. Due to the size and configuration of boxing gloves, the strike is not as effective with large, 10- to 16-ounce gloves on. The fist is clenched with the thumb at the top, and the pinky is facing the ground. Generally, this punch is delivered at close range, and the arm is not fully extended, meaning that the elbow is not locked out. This blow is delivered to the targets of the centerline: bladder, solar plexus, sternum, chin, or nose. The arm is slightly bent, the lats are locked, and the body tightens completely upon contact. Prior to that, as with virtually all strikes, the body is loose. The strike is based on the Bruce Lee 1- and 3-inch punches.

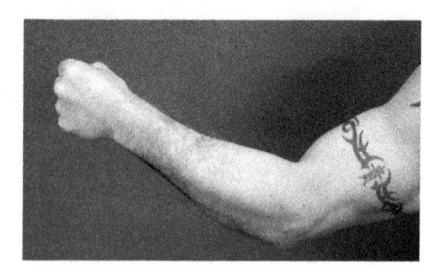

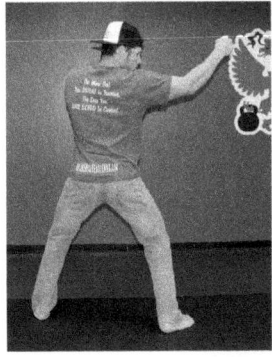

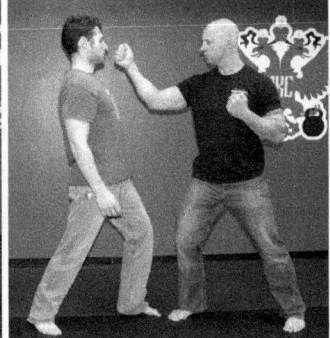

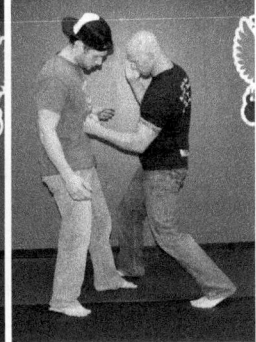

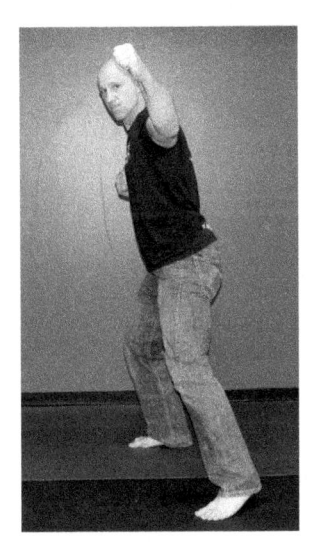

Backfist: Made popular in the 1970s by the most innovative martial artist of all time, Bruce Lee, this lead hand technique is efficient and very quick. The angle that the technique presents varies from the standard straight lead hand techniques. Keep your hand high, step in with your lead leg, rotate your lead hip inward as your fist is directed in the opposite motion and toward the target. Keep your other hand high by your head. Even though the technique is effective, it is not generally considered a knockout blow but more of a setup strike.

Scissor punch: Slightly curve and press your fingers together and separate your thumb from your forefinger as far as possible, so that the webbing of your thumb and forefinger is taut. Deliver a straight shot to the throat, striking with the crotch of your thumb and forefinger. Immediately grab the windpipe of the perpetrator and wrap your thumb and fingers tightly around, attempting to crush it in your hand.

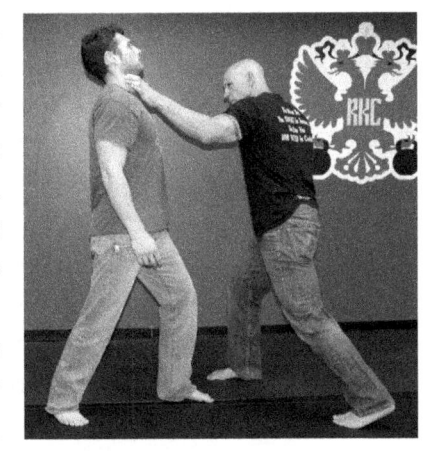

Eye gouge: The best method to apply an eye gouge is generally after a head butt, groin strike, or a double ear slap. Grasp the sides of the attacker's head and stick your thumbs into the section of their eyes closest to the bridge of their nose. Then dig your thumbs in deep and "scoop" the eyeballs out toward their ears as you grip the sides of their head tightly.

Punches: One through six. These are the 6 basic punches. This is the numbering system that we employ in our kickboxing training. There are some western boxing systems that use the same numbers; others vary slightly from this particular number system. The odd numbers are delivered with the lead hand, and the even numbers represent the rear hand techniques. The path of all punches follow his hip, shoulder, elbow, and fist. The hip generates the punch, and then it goes to the shoulder. Shoot the elbow straight forward, keeping it in line with your hip as you rotate your fist, positioning your thumb facing the floor and the back of your hand at the ceiling. Your arm is loose and quick as you step forward into the technique, only momentarily tensioning upon impact.

Retract the hand quickly to diminish *dead time*. The dead time is the period of time that it takes for your hand to get back to your head. We want to employ one of two tactics when considering the retraction of punches. You will either bring your hand to your head or your head to your hand. If you are using angle steps forward, bring your hand to your head. If you're more or less stationary, bring your hand back to your head. Retraction of the fist is extremely important. Hand to Chin or Chin to Hand. Pretend that there is a rubber band attached to your hand and shoulder. Once out, it snaps back to place set to defend and deliver another strike. Once you throw the punch, snap it back to the original position. Always use head movement. Moving targets are more difficult to hit.

Additionally, whenever you throw a lead hand technique, the lead hip rotates inward. When throwing the rear hand, the rear hip moves inward. This axiom holds true for all punches, jabs, crosses, hooks, uppercuts, back fists, etc. Except for the Axehand, the hip rotates outward in the direction of the strike.

Jab. This straight punch is thrown off of the lead hand. Step in slightly and time the landing of your step with the fist's contact of the desired target. Not only is this strike a great setup tool for your other techniques, but you can knock someone out with a good stiff jab, especially if they are moving into you. Muhammad Ali was famous for his jab, and George Foreman's first title was won almost exclusively with it.

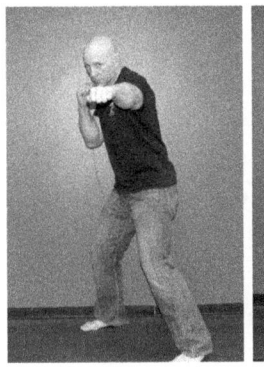

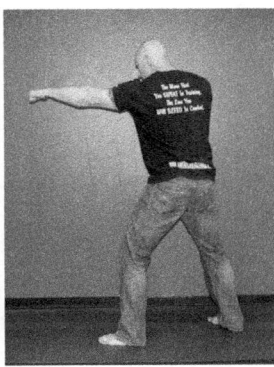

Cross. "Big Bertha," as we often refer to it. The knockout punch is also a straight punch but thrown from the rear, or reverse, side of the body. In karate, it's referred to as a reverse punch for this reason. In boxing, the term *cross* is applied because it crosses your body. This enables you to generate more power from the increased rotation of your hips. Slide the foot of the punching hand forward and slightly to the side as you deliver the strike. The rear foot moves up to keep your feet equidistant. Be sure *not* to rise up onto your toes but to keep the balls of your feet on the ground, pivoting them as the punch is thrown. Your hand assumes the same position as with the jab and the retraction strategy is also consistent.

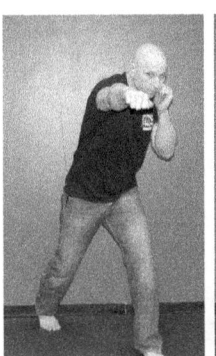

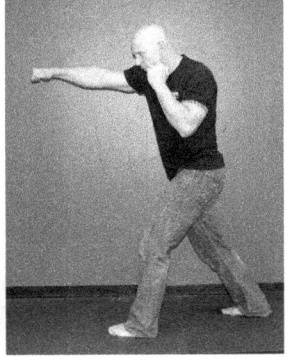

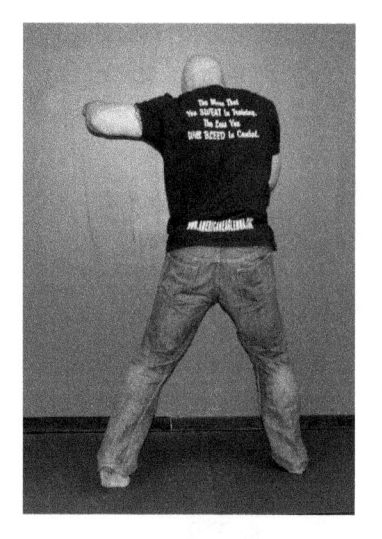

Lead hook. This technique requires more athleticism to throw than any other punch. It carries tremendous knockout power, and Joe Frazier[34] won a world title with it! It's a great counter punching weapon. To execute this punch, start out as if you were throwing a jab and then rotate your hip and pivot on your lead foot pointing your heel toward the target. Your fist should be in relatively the same position as the jab, except thumb rotated slightly down and the pinky slightly up. The elbow is bent on a 90-degree angle, your lat is locked in place, and your shoulder is packed. The punch is delivered across (into the target) and on a slight angle down. The footwork employed is generally a slight step to the outside to avoid a straight punch. A hook that lands on the side of the jaw can easily drop an opponent. By hitting the chin at this angle, more than 50 percent of your target's neck muscles are removed from the stabilization of the head.

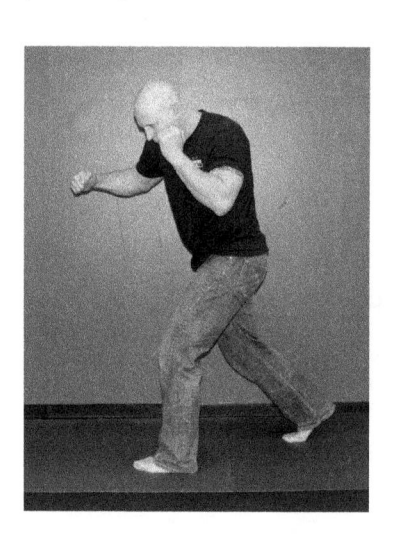

Rear hook. This athletic maneuver is an exceptionally effective means to attack the body. I like to use this to attack the floating ribs, solar plexus, and liver. You want to take advantage of your leg power when delivering this blow. Be certain to bend your knees and synchronize landing your shot as you come up. Your fist is almost vertical when it lands, the thumb is at approximately 80 degrees, and the pinky is facing the ground.

---

[34] Joe "Smokin' Joe" Frazier was an Olympic Gold Medalist for the USA and a World Professional Boxing Champion. His bouts with Muhammad Ali were epic. The movie *Rocky* was based loosely on his career.

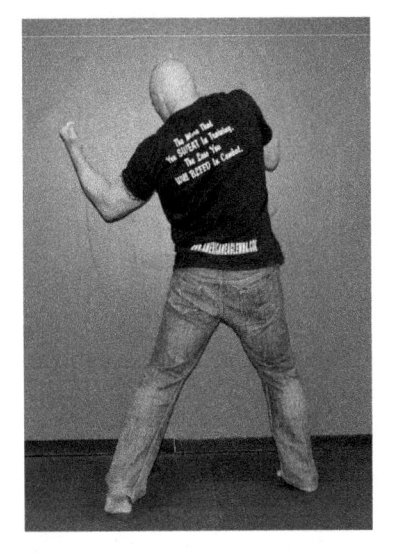

Lead uppercut. This punch is generally used to strike either under the chin or to the solar plexus. As with the hook, you want to have your arm bent at a 90-degree angle, your shoulder packed, and your lat locked. Use your legs and hips while you drive the strike upward and inward into the target. The fist is positioned with the palm facing you as you twist your hand with a quarter turn en route to impact. The uppercut also works well if someone is diving for your legs and trying to take you down.

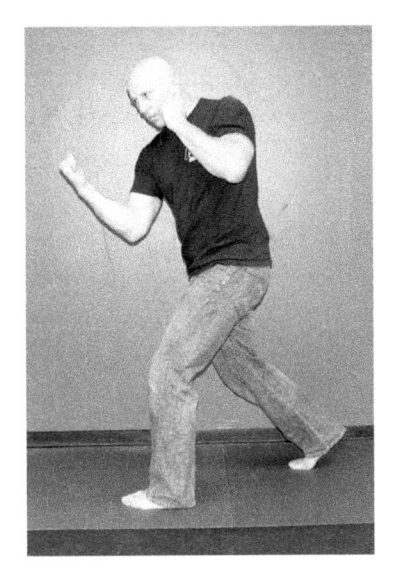

Rear uppercut. This strike is used primarily as a body shot. Throw it as you would the lead uppercut, except with more potential power because it's off of your rear hand and enlists more leg and hip power. The general targets are floating ribs, bladder, solar plexus, and groin.

Overhand right: This is a derivation of the cross. I also refer to it as the barroom punch. Think of combining a hook and a cross together. This punch is best delivered after either a jab or a jab fake. Slide your lead leg inward and on a 45-degree angle to the outside as you bring your rear foot in. The fist travels in a slight arch; it goes up and then downward. At the point of impact, your elbow is slightly higher than your fist.

Elbow variations: The elbow is an extremely effective striking technique. I like to use the elbow, if possible. Why? For starters, the elbow is closer to your power base, so you are able to deliver more power. Secondly, the chance of injuring your elbow is very slim when compared to what can happen to your hand when striking. Most elbow strikes thrown to the face and head are on a slashing nature, so you will want to keep your hand open. This will aid the slashing movement and maximize the damage when ripping the skin of the face or head. When you are attacking the body, you want to employ a closed fist. This will deliver more power to the intended target. The clenched fist will deliver more power when thrusting or smashing with the elbow.

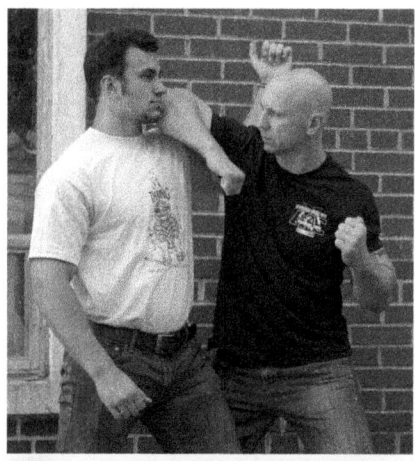

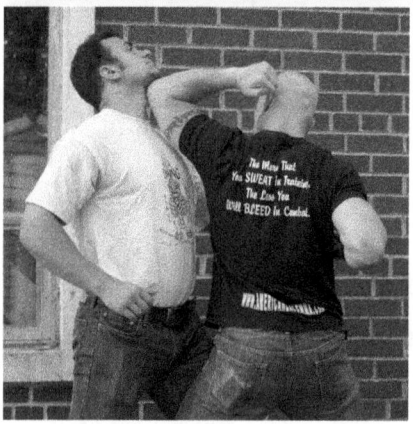

Across. If you are throwing a right elbow, step into the target with the right foot. Your forearm will be parallel to the floor with your palm facing down, hand loose as you bring your elbow across the face of the assailant. Aim for the side of the head at the temple and go all the way across the head.

Upward. The upward elbow strike is another one that we perform with a loose, open hand. This blow is directed straight upward into the chin of the attacker. This is the main target area of this technique. It's not very effective to any other targets.

Downward. This strike begins with an open hand and then ends with the closed fist upon impact. Often referred to as "the death elbow", this technique is delivered to the cervical or thoracic spine. The downward elbow was deemed so damaging, that the UFC banned its use from fighters in the top position. Once you have doubled your opponent over with a strike to the bladder or groin, rise up on the balls of your feet, twist your hips to the right, and then drop the right elbow downward, smashing it into the attacker's spine. Deliver this downward blow with speed and power as you drop your weight into it.

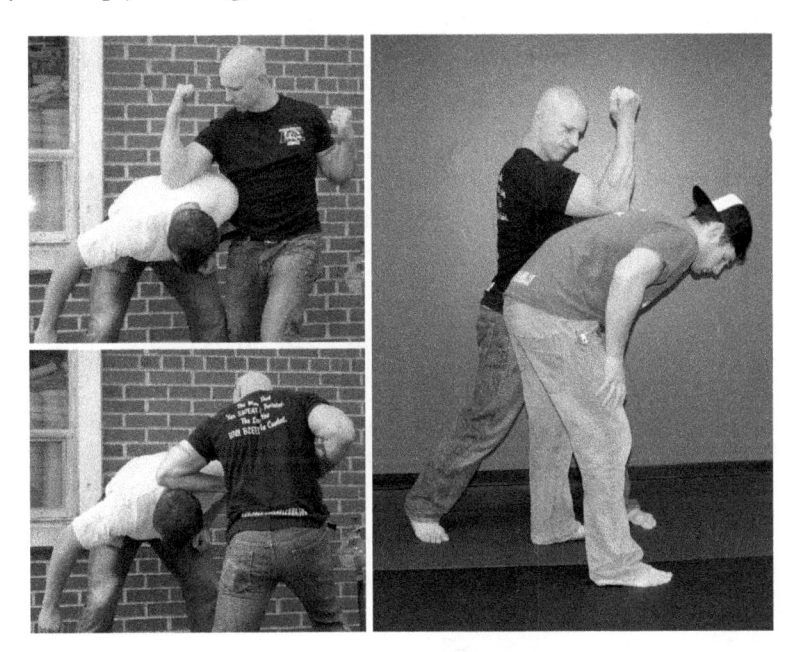

Side and back: The elbow strikes directed to the side and the back are thrown the same way. Make a fist with the hand of the striking elbow; place the open palm of your opposite hand on the knuckles of the closed fist. Step into the technique, bend your knees, and twist your hips into the strike while pushing on the clenched fist with the open hand. The elbow strikes are delivered to the ribs, stomach, or bladder.

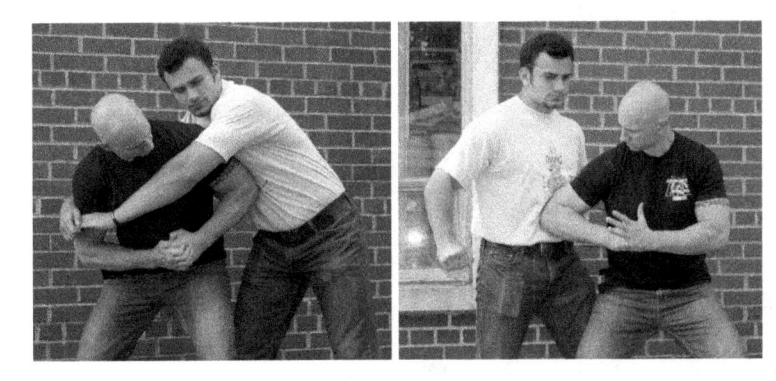

Angular. Elbows thrown on an angle, either upward or downward, are thrown with an open, loose hand. The open hand accentuates the ripping of the skin and maximizes the trauma. Loop the elbow upward and then downward and across the target, generally the head or the face. As the strike comes downward, drop your weight by bending your knees and turning your hip into the technique.

Upward, bend your knees and then partially straighten them as the elbow is thrown on an angle upward into the chin or side of the head, if the head is turned.

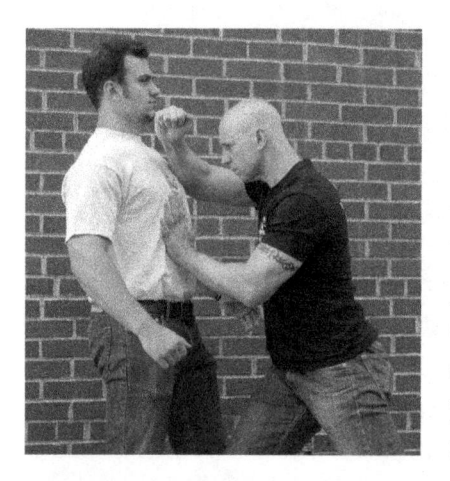

Forearm shiver: Step into your opponent with one hand open and the other fist clinched while you deliver a stiff forearm shot to the chest. The forearm and side of the wrist can be used to choke or levy pressure on an opponent. Blocking and deflecting blows, as well as striking to the clavicle and neck of your adversary, is met with favorable results.

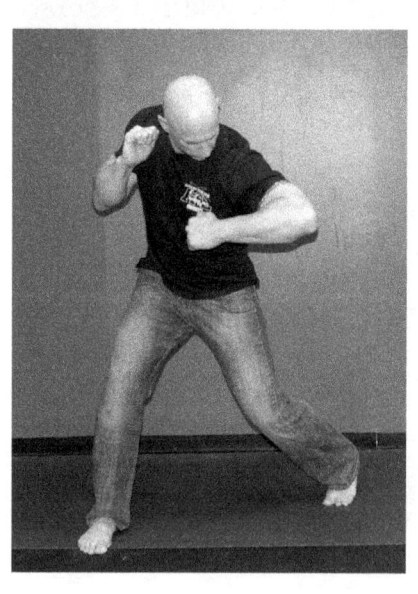

Forearm smash downward: Once your opponent is bent over, rise up on the balls of your feet, rotate your hip first up and then downward as you smash your forearm down upon their back, neck, or head. Position your forearm parallel to the ground.

Blocks

Most blocks double as strikes and may be used as a push or a shove. The blocks that we list are both defensive and offensive weapons.

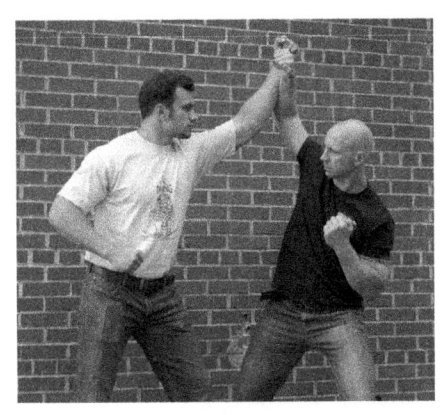

High block: Synonymous with most basic karate standards. This image of a karateka in a horse stance with one hand over the head in a high block and the other in fist in chamber at the hip. To practice this movement, take your left fist and place it in your right armpit as you twist your left hip to the right. You then rotate your hip back in the other direction as your arm is positioned above your head. Your arm is on a 45-degree angle, with your palm slightly rotated toward the ceiling. This is the typical block. You need to bear in mind that if you attempt to stand in front of someone and execute this block, you will be hit. You need to step back to allow for the time necessary to execute the block successfully. In bando, we use this block more as a means to shove the opponent back. You assume the same basic position and then lower your level and use a front stance with the foot of the blocking hand forward as you launch the forearm into the assailant.

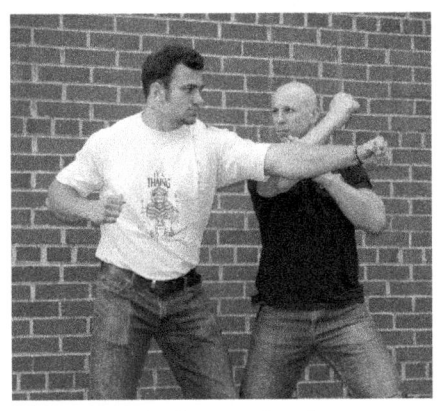

Hammerfist block: This movement, being both a block and a strike, is very evident. When performing the blocking application, you'll need to move backward. Step in and attack with the technique when you are on the offensive. Place your clenched fist up to your ear with your pinky facing the ceiling and your thumb facing the floor. Bring the hand across your face as you rotate the fist so that your knuckles are facing the ceiling and the palm side of your hand is facing you. Make certain that your fist travels all the way across your head with both the block and the strike. The hammerfist is used against a straight punch directed toward your face, and it's used to attack the side of the head or the neck of the assailant.

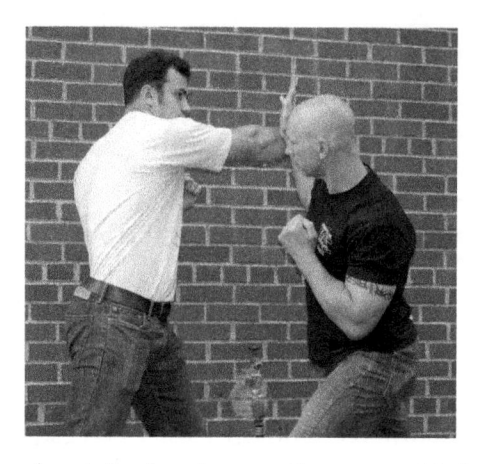

Outside middle block: This movement is primarily a block, but a grab may be employed as well. Do you remember the old "wax on, wax off" from *The Karate Kid*? Well, it's that block, more or less. Take your right hand and reach under your left arm, touching the back of your right hand against your left triceps. Twisting your hips to the right, bend your elbow at a 45-degree angle as your open hand is brought across your body. Your fingertips are at approximately eye level. Use this technique to block a straight attack to your midsection.

Knee drives: How many techniques illicit a better result than a well-placed knee strike to the groin or a lunging knee to someone's head? On the straight knees that are driven upward, the straight and springboard knees, dorsiflex your foot. This engages the hip flexors to a greater degree and enables you to lift your knee higher and faster. When performing the roundhouse knee, it's preferable to point the toe in the event that your opponent moves back; you may easily turn the knee into a roundhouse kick.

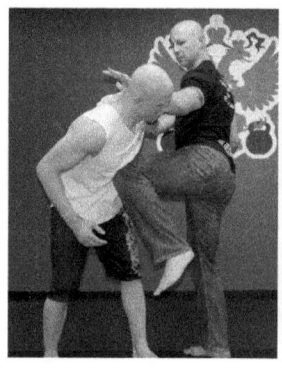

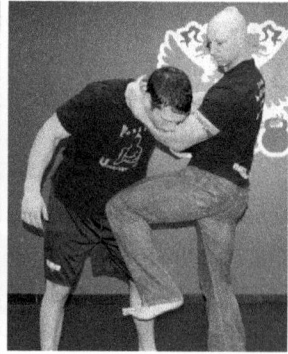

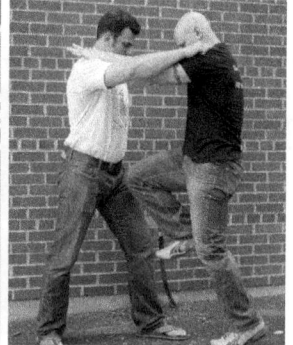

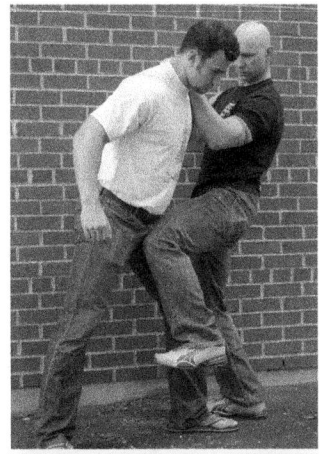

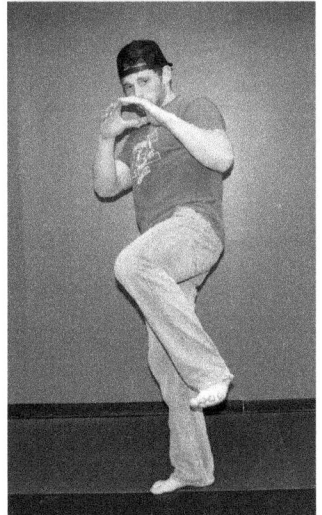

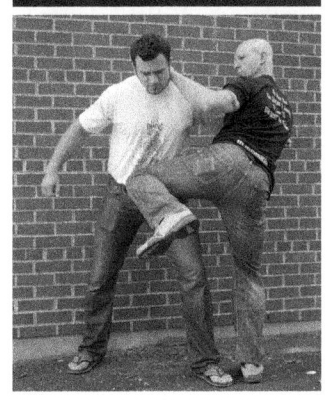

Straight knee: Deliver a quick strike upward to the opponent's groin, quadriceps, peroneal nerve, solar plexus, or bladder. You may also throw this to the face of a doubled-over opponent, usually after a knee to the groin or the bladder.

Springboard knee: This is an extremely powerful blow delivered to almost any part of the body, but primarily directed to the same leg regions of the aforementioned knee strike, groin, solar plexus, sternum, rib cage, face, or head. This strike is done after the initial loosening-up techniques and is used as a finisher. If you were to deliver the knee strike with your left knee, stomp your right foot on the ground and simultaneously bring your knee upward into the intended target. Repeat this strike as many times as possible until your assailant falls.

Roundhouse knee: We generally direct this technique to the peroneal nerve, the IT (iliotibial) band, the floating ribs, or the side of the head to a doubled-over opponent. If you are throwing a left knee, step toward your opponent on a 45-degree angle with your right foot. As you step, pivot your foot on the floor and bring your left knee into one of the aforementioned targets.

Foot Stomps

This counterattack maneuver can be applied in several combat situations. If you are grabbed from behind, if you are face to face or grabbed from the side. Draw your knee up as high as possible and dorsiflex your foot. Drive your heel down into their foot with as much force as possible. Repeat this movement as required.

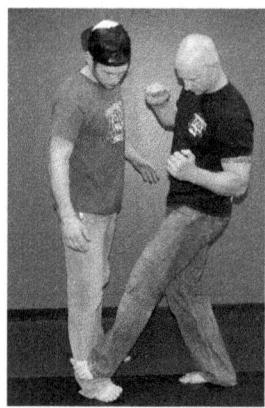

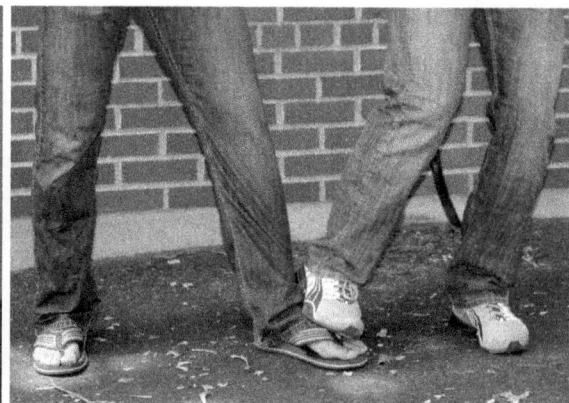

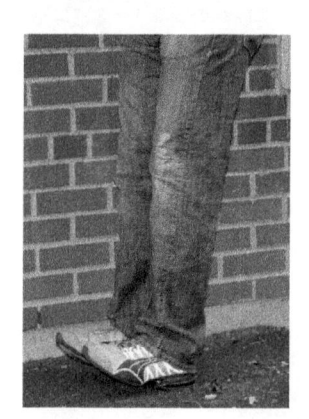

Parachute stomp: The name comes from the act of bending your knees and driving your legs very hard into the ground as you would if you were landing while using a parachute. We use this technique as a finishing blow to a downed opponent. It makes no difference if the assailant is supine or prone. Let us consider that our opponent is in the supine position: Place your feet together and jump into the air while bringing your knees up to your chest and dorsiflexing your feet as you drive your heels into the downed assailant's groin, abdomen, chest, or head. This should put an immediate end to the situation.

This next group of kicks are performed from the fighting stance or at least while you have some distance from your opponent.

Roundhouse kick: This has to be my all-time favorite kick. When I look back at all of my fights, I don't think that I had one ring fight (that included kicking) when I didn't throw a roundhouse kick. It's quick, versatile, and can be used to attack many areas. There are also many variations of this favorite kick of mine. We will focus on the *lead leg roundhouse kick*. There are four parts to this kick: the up, out, back, and down. You bring the knee up into chamber, kick the foot out, bring the foot back, and then place it back on the floor. Make certain that you turn the foot on the floor to engage your hips and maximize power. This is a chambered kick. When you first learn to do this kick, you step up with the rear foot and then lift the lead foot as you step into the kick. As you become adept at throwing this kick, you will replace the lead foot with the rear and almost "hop" into the kick. Thus yielding more speed and power due to the forward movement, the slight hop that reduces friction and the power that you will get from having your foot land on the floor as your striking foot lands on the target. You will need to plantar-flex your foot by pointing toes. The striking area of your foot will be the instep to the talus. You may direct this kick to many spots on the human body—from the shin, knee, femoral artery, quadriceps, groin, bladder, ribs, neck, and head, to name a few.

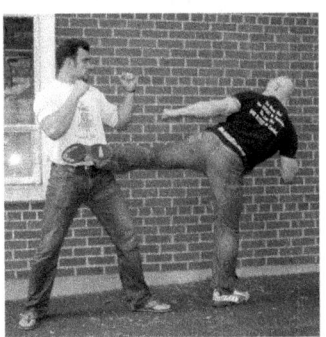

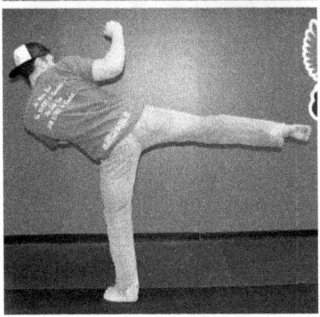

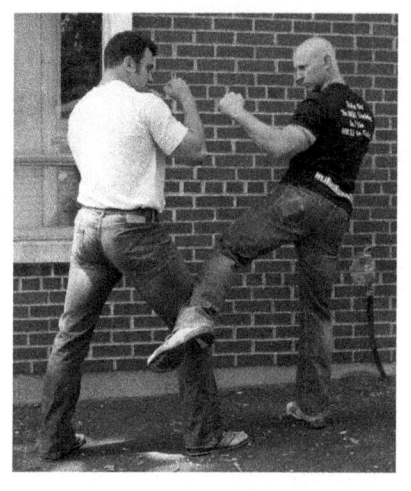

Cut kick: This is a standard as far as kicks are concerned with bando and Muay Thai. You will use the shin as the attacking implement. If you were to kick with your right leg, step on a 45-degree angle with your left foot into the opponent. Throw the kick from the hip—not a chambered kick; rather, a kick thrown with the knee locked and only slightly bent. The primary targets are low: the shin, gastroc, peroneal nerve, and the hip joint. Be cautious with the shin-to-shin kick. If your shins are not conditioned sufficiently, you may incur just as much trauma as your assailant! When you become more accomplished at this move, you can direct shots to the rib cage, and even to the head. However, for most street applications, you have no reason to kick someone higher than their abdominal region.

Shin kick: This closed-quarter kick is an excellent, hard-hitting kick that can be thrown while you are in boxing range. Bring your knee up high, dorsiflex your foot, and throw a sharp short hybrid roundhouse kick with your shin to their thigh or ribs. This kick may be extended into a ball-of-the-foot roundhouse kick, if the opponent backs up out of boxing range and into kicking range.

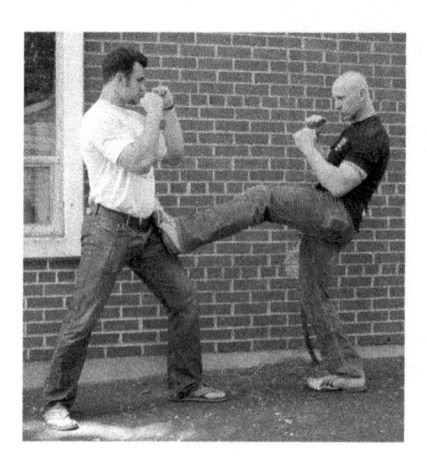

As with most of these kicks, turn your foot on the floor, rotating your hip over.

Front kick: There are a great many varieties of this kick to throw—lead leg, lunging, ball of the foot, flat of the foot, straight up with the shin, and so on and so forth. The full (rear leg) ball-of-the-foot version is applicable in most situations. This is a chambered, four-position kick. Bring the leg up, kick out, and then bring it back and to the floor. In a real situation, you will most likely be moving forward. Practice both stationary, to aid with developing your balance and moving forward, as you would do when driving your opponent backward. This is a straight kick: keep your hip, knee, and the foot of the kicking leg in one straight line. There is a slight rotation of the foot on the floor, but not nearly as dramatic as with the roundhouse or side kicks. I like the ball-of-the-foot kick best; there is a greater pound per square inch of force yielded with the reduced striking area, and you also get extra distance of your kick with the extension of the foot, and the kick may be directed to virtually any part of the body.

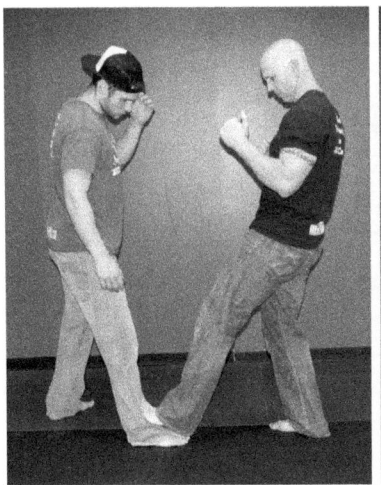

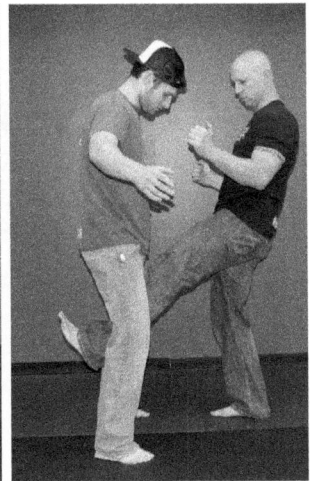

Side kick: This is a great striking technique that is underutilized in MMA competitions but is a mainstay in most other Tae Kwon Do, Karate, Kung Fu, and many other striking-based arts. I will attribute its lack of use in mixed martial arts competitions to the overwhelming presence of Muay Thai as the preferred striking art. However, there is an increasing number of MMA fighters using the sidekick in their arsenal.

There are several side kick methods: stepping, skipping, potochagi (sliding), jumping, and many more. We will focus on the stepping side kick. If you are in the orthodox position in a side stance, your feet will be lined up evenly with your left side forward and at a right angle to your target. Attack with the lead foot by stepping up with the rear foot and replacing the lead foot as you pick up the lead foot to kick. This is another chambered kick that has the up, out, back, and down. As the kick comes out, rotate the foot on the floor and turn the toes of the kicking foot downward by rotating the hip. Be certain not to overrotate your upper body. Accomplish this by counter-rotating your left arm and shoulder. Your heel, knee, hip, and left shoulder should all be collinear and direct your energy through the target, not simply to the surface. Your foot is dorsiflexed, and the area of the foot you hit with is your heel. This kick may be delivered to the ankle, knee, quadriceps, hip, ribs, stomach, chest, throat, or head. Unless you are particularly skilled at high kicks, do not kick your attacker above the waist.

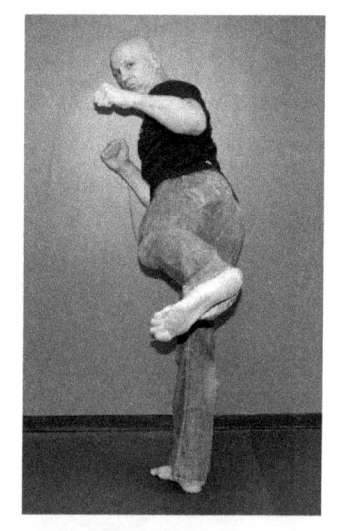

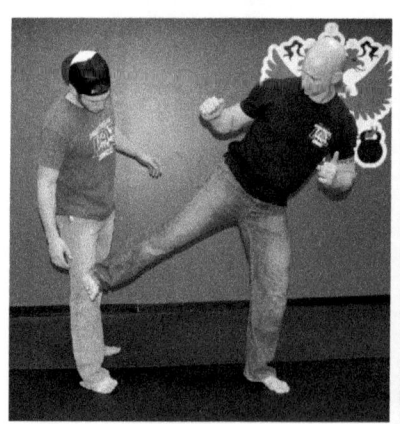

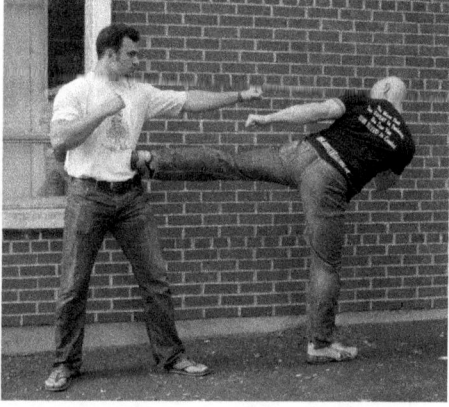

Mule kick: The delivery of this kick is how it attained its name. Imagine a mule throwing a kick with its hindquarters, and there you have your kick. Pick your knee up high and toward your chest, bend your upper body forward at the hip, thrust your kick straight back with foot dorsiflexed, and then strike with your heel. This kick is delivered to targets behind you. If your opponent is in front of you, make a quarter turn to your back so that your back is facing momentarily toward your target and then execute the kick. This move is often referred to as the *back kick* when thrown in this manner. There are many targets to hit with this kick, but it's a perfect counteroffensive technique directed to the knees, groin, and the midsection of the assailant attacking you from behind.

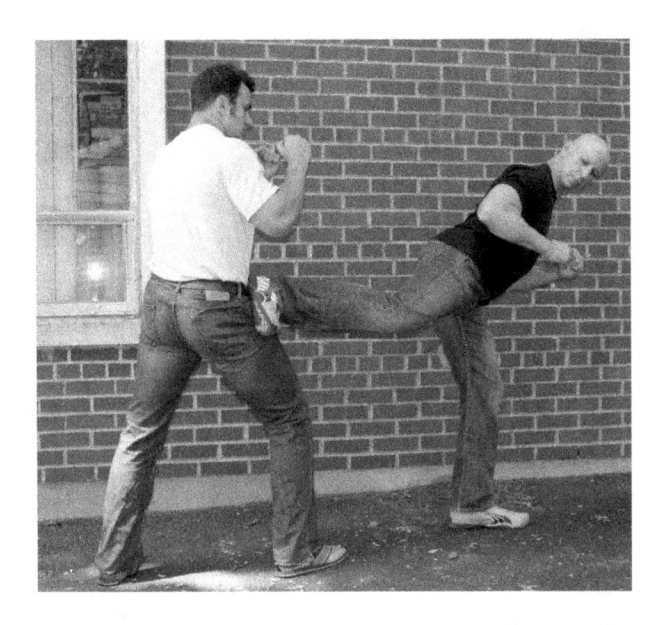

OK, we have this great list of techniques, *when* and *how* do we use them to our advantage? This will depend upon the circumstances that you are faced with. There are crucial elements that need to be considered, the most important being your proximity to the opponent, the number of assailants, who you are with, are there weapons involved, the escape routes, and the environmental conditions and constraints.

Examples
If there is ice and snow on the ground, it may not behoove you to relinquish 50 percent of your balance by delivering a kick. You could easily slip and fall, thus making defending yourself more difficult.

What if you have a child in your arms? What would you do first? You need to protect the child and yourself, plus deal with the imminent threat. You may have to put the child down on the floor behind you.

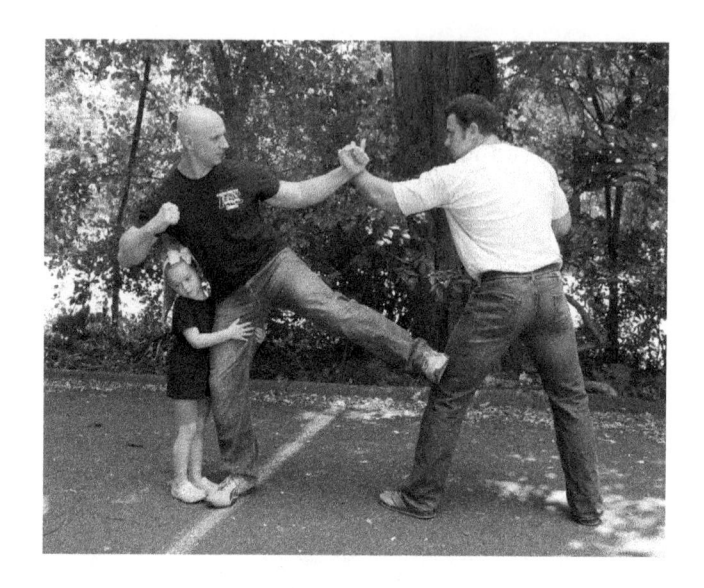

What if there is a gang of assailants surrounding you? How do you choose the first one to hit? The biggest one, the smallest one, or the perceived ringleader?

We must first acknowledge that action is *faster* than reaction. This means that if someone attacks you, there is a delay before you respond. The movement must be recognized by your eye, and then it must register in your brain, cross the synapse, and then tell your body to move in the proper manner. That's a lot for you to accomplish in the time (between 200 and 400 milliseconds) that it takes when someone initiates an attack until the time you have been grabbed or struck. Therefore, it's best to strike first. Despite what you may see in the movies, most street fights are won by the guy who lands the first blow. If you want to increase your odds of success in the street, strike first—and do so with conviction. The Bad Karate Instructor from the Cobra Kai in *The Karate Kid* did have a valid mantra, "Strike first, and strike hard, no mercy, sir!" Good words to live by if you want to survive a street encounter.

So you may think that I am telling you to run around punching people in the head. Not quite. I am, however, letting you know that unless you get the first shot in, you are at a distinct disadvantage. How do we tip the odds in our favor yet work within our legal rights? We accomplish this by positioning and anticipation.

Most people who have been in a confrontation were aware that it was going to happen before the attack occurred. We will not address those who have been set up by another person. If you did something bad in your past to the wrong person, you're probably going to have to spend a great deal of your time looking over your shoulder. In that case, you best handle your situation and bring it to a resolution. Enough said on that. So let's get back to situations that may actually happen to people simply minding their own business and/or those whose vocations require confrontation resolution.

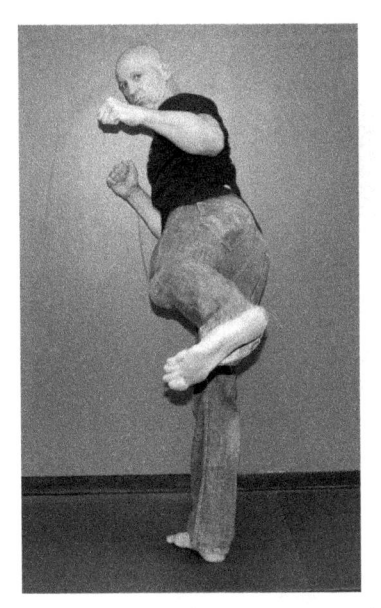

Your success in a situation can greatly be increased by the stance that you adopt when the verbal portion of the confrontation occurs. When I was a young bouncer, we had quite a few confrontations on a nightly basis. The club that I worked at was previously a motorcycle club, and we were converting it into a dance club for the college crowd. The owner and my coworkers could tell, simply by my stance, that a confrontation was to ensue. First, I would put my hands up in front of my face with my hands open. (It's quite easy for me to talk with my hands due in part to my Italian American heritage) hands up, one foot slightly back so that I was essentially in a "hidden" fighting stance. In this position, I could readily defend myself if an attack was launched. My hands were up to deflect an attack and deliver blows. My feet were positioned in a fighting stance that would allow me to move to avoid an attack and then apply a counterattack.

Practice this position and become comfortable with it.

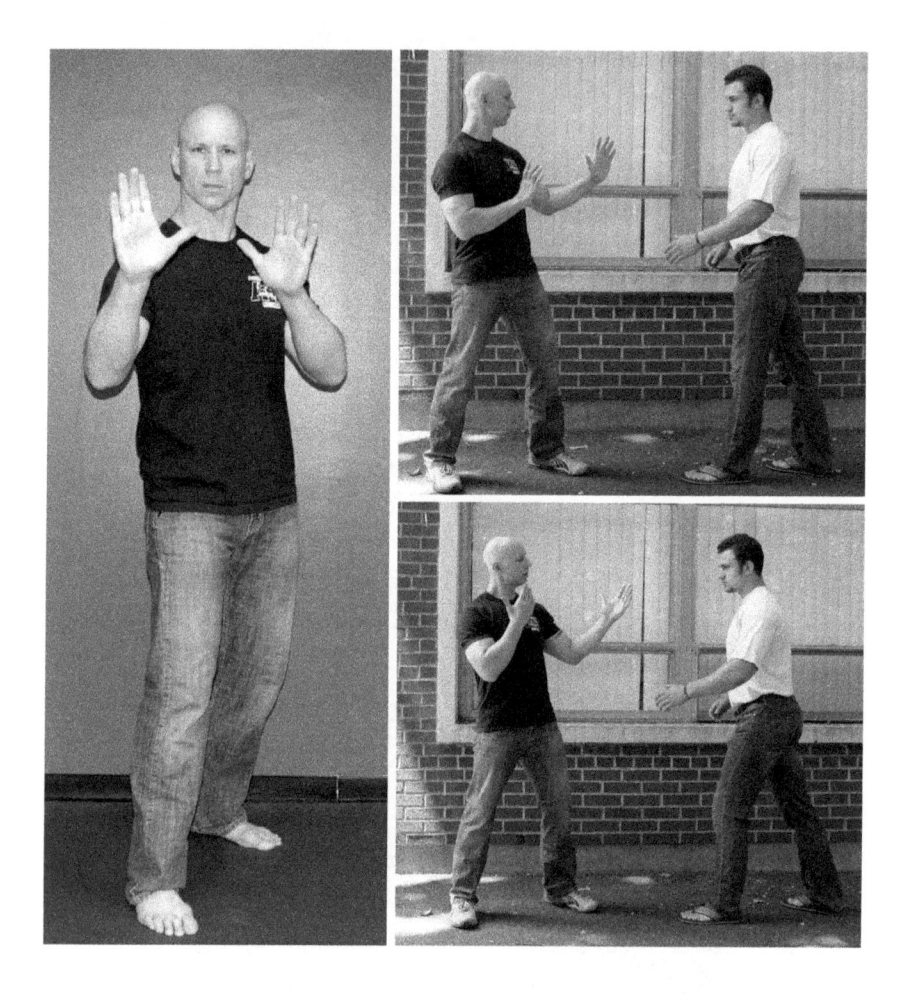

10
MOVEMENT AND ZONES

The knowledge of the various zones, your position relative to your assailant, and the availability of your tools, as well as your exposure to the opponent, are essential and one of the most ignored components to unskilled fighters.

Understanding movement, position, and ranges tilt the odds dramatically in your favor. Include and practice these skills every training session.

Please bear in mind that if the assailant moves from the green zone to a yellow zone in an aggressive manner, an assault has occurred. If you believe that you or someone you are with is in imminent danger, you may defend yourself. If you believe that your life or the life on a loved one is in peril, then you may take whatever means necessary to provide protection.

Green: This is your *safe* zone. The opponent can't reach you, but neither can you reach him without some type of overt movement.

Yellow: This is the *caution* distance. The opponent has entered your personal space. You are at the distance to strike, but also can be hit.

Red: This is the *danger* zone. You are in a hot spot. Your proximity to your assailant is too close to react. You must be fully engaged in combat at this distance. You should be striking, moving, and looking to finish.

MOVEMENT AND POSITIONING

Movement is key. You hurt what you can hit, and you can't hit what you can't touch. So *move*, and move with purpose. You will want to avoid the attack and position yourself to launch your counterattack. Practice economy of motion with your fluid and purposeful movement. Practice your footwork religiously and keep your hands up!

Pie stepping: Think of a large pizza with eight slices. Other than up and down, these are the only directions that you can move in. Any other direction is simply a variation of these eight. When practicing pie stepping, always step back to the center. Imagine the little "mouse table" on your pizza—this represents the center of the pie (the mouse table keeps the cheese from sticking to the top of the box). During practice, your direction change will occur at this point. When repeating this stepping movement, the foot that you perform your 8th step will be the same one that you do the 1st step with to repeat the sequence. Practice this in both directions.

1. Front
2. Back
3. Straight to the right
4. Straight to the left
5. Up on a 45-degree angle to the right
6. Up on a 45-degree angle to the left
7. Back on a 45-degree angle to the right
8. Back on a 45-degree angle to the left

Keep your hands up the whole time, always keeping your lead hand forward, which will require you to switch your hands according with which foot is forward. Move from one position to the next with a shuffle step. Place the majority of your weight on the stepping foot so that you would be able to throw a kick with the inside foot.

Step 1. Move forward and jam the advance of the opponent. You will back them up placing them on their heels.

Step 2. Move backward, shifting your weight toward the back foot. This will draw your opponent toward you.

Step 3. Move straight to the right side and face the center.

Step 4. Repeat to the left.

Step 5. On the 45-degree angle up and to the right. Parry with your left hand as you position yourself to the side of your opponent.

Step 6. Return to the center and do the same up and to the left side.

Step 7. Fade back and to the right, avoiding the attack on an angle.

Step 8. Do the same to the other side. While practicing, this foot will be the same one that you perform step 1 with.

Jamming: Think of this as an extension of step 1. Move into your assailant with your hands up with your forearms at a 65-degree angle as you shove them backward. This puts them on their heels and makes it difficult for them to defend themselves.

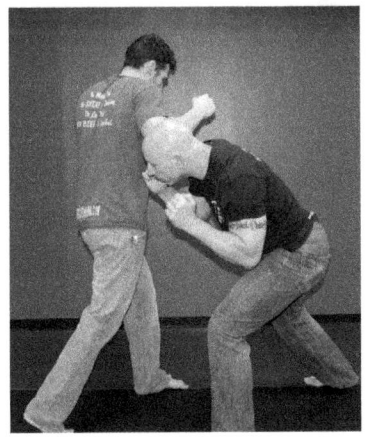

Ducks (bobs): Imagine that you have a pencil in the middle of your forehead and that you are drawing a *U* with it. If someone throws a right punch at you, bend your knees and move your head from left to right in a *U* fashion, placing your head on the outside right of the opponent. You are now positioned to counterattack, usually with a right-body shot and/or a left hook to the chin.

Angle fade (draws): There are times that you will need to fade back to draw your opponent out so that they commit to a movement. Stay slightly out of range and apply a counterstrike.

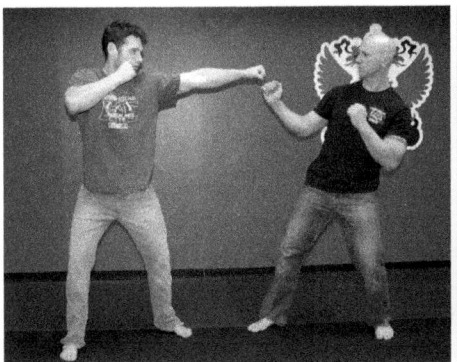

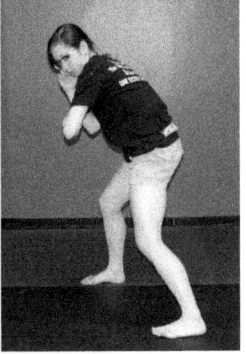

Parries: Using an open hand, slap a punch away as it comes at you. If a left strike is being thrown, parry with your right hand as you move to the right, avoiding the strike and positioning yourself to launch your counteroffensive. Generally, there are two taps of your hand with the parry, the initial and the redirect. The motions used should only be large enough to redirect the strike. If you push it too far, you may compromise your ability to defend and counterattack.

Box stepping: This stepping method is very well suited for sidestepping and maintaining your good stance. Pretend that there is a box on the floor and that you are in a fighting stance. It does not matter if you are in the orthodox or southpaw stance. If you are in the orthodox stance, move to the left, step with your left foot first, and then your right. Lead foot then rear foot. When moving to the right, right foot first, then left. Rear foot and then lead.

Whatever stance you are in will make no difference. You will step with the foot that's closest to the direction that you need to move. This will now put you in an advantageous position to strike.

11
BASIC GRAPPLING

I have made it quite clear that it is far better to keep on your feet during a confrontation, but you need to know how to grapple for several reasons. To effectively combat something, you need to know how it works. If you are trying to defend against a takedown or submission, you need to have a basic knowledge of how they are applied. As we have discussed in other sections of this book, if a fight lasts more than 10 seconds or so, the chances of it ending up on the ground increase dramatically. You had better know what to do once you are on the ground. Proficiency in grappling must be gained through working with a partner, so secure a good one. The closer you are to each other in weight and size, the better, especially if you are a beginner.

There are complete arts dedicated solely to the art of grappling. The grappling arts are the most difficult to master, but by learning the basics, you have increased your chances of success in the street dramatically. Let us delve into some basic grappling techniques.

BALANCE DISRUPTION

Break the balance of an opponent by pushing, pulling, and foot sweeps. Gain the inside position by placing your hands on the insides of the attackers arms at the biceps. Pushing and pulling is best applied from this position.

Foot sweep: From the inside tie position described above, push with your right hand and pull with your left. This will cause your opponent to pick up their right foot and step forward. Knowing this, as you perform the pushing/pulling action, lift your left foot and sweep their right foot as it moves forward to regain their balance. Continue the push-pull until they fall. If they regain their balance, immediately perform this movement to the other side. This will generally cause them to fall.

Another simple sweep you should practice is to grab the opponent's wrist, pulling them toward you and across their body. Use the same side foot to hook behind their heel and kick the foot in the direction that their toes are facing. This may or may not knock them down, but you will have succeeded in disrupting their balance and opening them up for follow-up attacks.

Basic hip toss: The mother of all throws. Done correctly, you will be able to effectively throw an adversary twice your weight. Throws are dynamic, and there must be movement involved to execute a throw. It is also easier to relinquish your space than it is to throw someone to another spot. Foot placement, movement, and hip pop are crucial to performing a successful throw. Thread your left arm under their right arm and have your head on the same side as your arm. This is called an *underhook*. Slide your left hand across their back to their opposite trapezius. With your right hand, grab their left arm at their triceps. Next, step across with your right foot, and then your left will follow as you bring your hip in and your butt across. Make certain that your feet are close together. Having them too far apart is the practitioner's biggest mistake. Flex your knees, pull on their left arm with your right, "punch" with your left as you pivot your feet, and finish the throw. In combat situations, attempt to have your adversary land directly on the top of their head. This will immediately end most confrontations. If not, maintain control of their right arm when they hit the ground and apply a choke or pull up on their arm as you stomp their head with your right foot. It takes repeating a move 1,000 times to be able to execute it properly, and it requires 10,000 repetitions to master it.

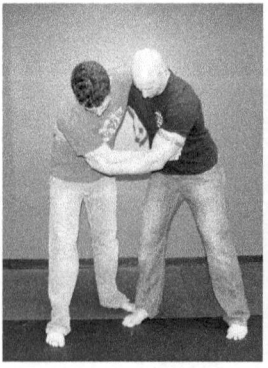

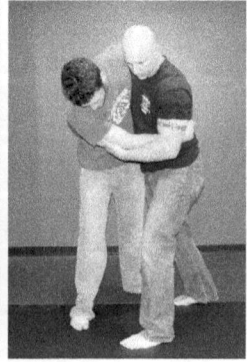

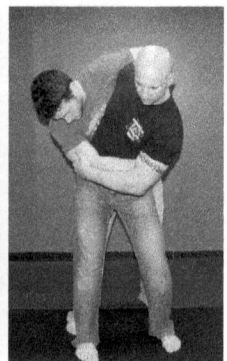

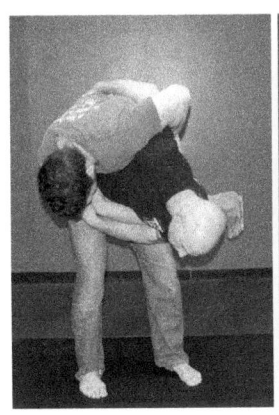

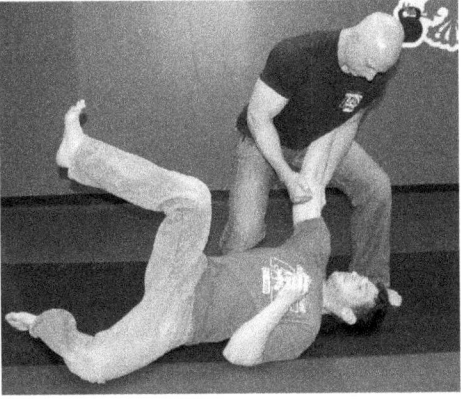

Sprawl: This one defensive maneuver is the single most important move to keep you on your feet when your legs get attacked for a takedown. When you are attacked with a double- or single-leg takedown, do not give your adversary both your hips. Drop your weight into your left hip as you drive your hip downward and throw your legs back. Take an *overhook*[35] with your left arm and loop it around his right arm as you are performing the sprawl. With your free hand, smash your arm across his face and turn his head away. Once you have secured this position and he can no longer take you down, strike him in the head with your free hand. You may also force him to the ground and spin behind him and take his back. Deliver your ground and pound from here, or apply a choke.

Spear double leg takedown: There are several immensely effective double-leg takedowns. I choose this one because you don't have to go to the ground and your head is in the middle, thus making it more difficult for your opponent to apply a choke on you. You need to be close enough to touch your opponent to be able to take them down. In the street or in an MMA cage, delivering a solid strike to their face prior to the shot is a very effective means to gain entry. As you prepare

---

[35] Overhook, also referred to as a whizzer, generally occurs when your opponent has an arm around your waist or when your leg is grabbed in a takedown situation. Loop your arm over theirs and bring your fist close to your own arm while you drop your hip into them.

to execute the takedown, lower your level by bending your knees as you *shoot your takedown.*[36]

Bull your neck and aim your head to his solar plexus as you grab behind both of his knees. Thrust your head into him, pull with your arms, and drive with your legs until they have hit the ground. It's very important to make certain that you don't reach with your arms or put your head down when you shoot. You must get your body onto theirs. Be cautious following them onto the ground. You may get rolled or injure yourself on the pavement. It's better to knock them down and administer kicks to them.

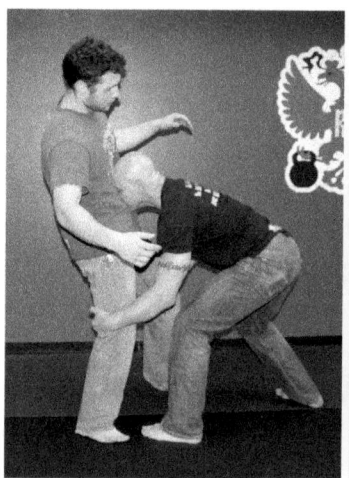

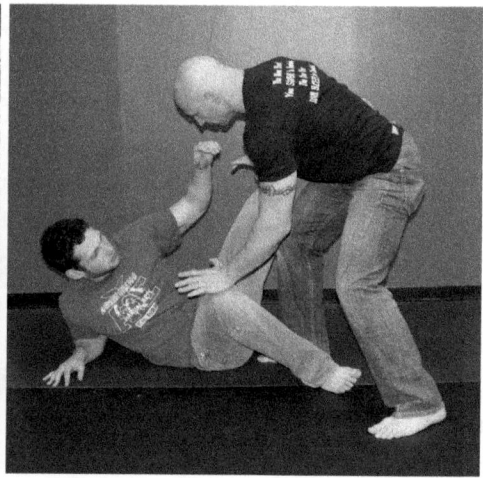

There are several extremely effective grappling systems: wrestling (collegiate, freestyle, Greco-Roman, submission, and catch), Brazilian jujitsu, judo, and sambo are the most effective for combat training. They are some of the most effective forms of unarmed combat available, but are the most difficult to master. Seeking professional instruction in one of these arts will teach you a great deal about your body and how to move.

---

[36] Shooting a takedown is the act of dropping your level and taking a penetration step into your opponent. Driving forward with your legs as you grab their legs with your hands. An unsophisticated shot resembles a tackle.

12
COMBINATIONS AND SERIES

The saying "One strike, one kill" is actually a misinterpretation of the Japanese saying regarding strikes. When karate started to become popular, people feared black belts. They knew the death touch, and they were trained to "kill you with one blow." This notion is nonsense and has since been debunked. The true saying was "To strike with killing intent." Is it possible to kill someone with one shot? Yes, but death usually occurs when someone gets knocked out on their feet and hits their head on the ground as they fall.

How do we use our strikes? Use combinations. I like to throw nothing less than three techniques. You need to consider percentages. If you consider the punch statistics of a professional boxer, most fall short of landing 50 percent of their strikes. These professionals throw thousands of punches any day, and most of them land only a little over a third of the punches thrown. This is one of the most important reasons for throwing multiples: you will most likely miss. Additionally, multiple strikes are generally required to neutralize an assailant.

Listed below are some very effective combinations to practice. These should be practiced in front of a mirror, on a heavy bag, and with a partner. Use the mirror to check your technique, the heavy bag to develop power, and your partner to work on distancing and timing.

Hand and Foot Combinations

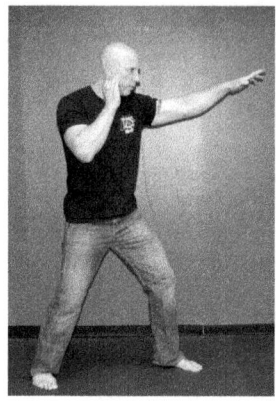

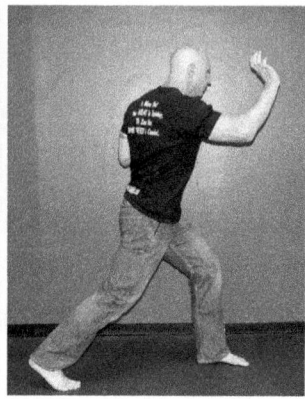

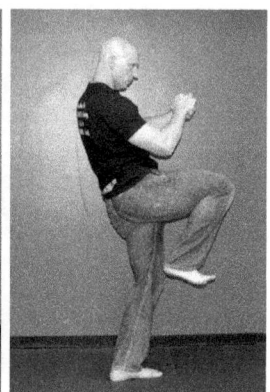

Short and long axehand

1,2, cut kick, chin jab and knee
Elbow across, elbow upward, straight knee and round knee
2 straight knees, downward elbows
Sidekick, backfist, hammerfist smash
Palm heel, elbow downward, knee drives
Lead-leg roundhouse kick, backfist, elbow smash
Elbow across, angle down, angle up, straight knee
Strike and subdue drills
Finger jab-chin jab-knee strike
Backhand slap – low side kick – elbow smash
Duck-side step-body shot-knee-hook-elbow
Lunge front kick (big boot) knees-redirect and/or smashes 14 (rear attack) Foot stomp, backward head butt, back elbow
Dual ear slap, eye gouge, springboard knee to groin
Parry, V-step, and clothesline
Head butt, tracheal choke, knees
Piet a te, back slap, knifehand chop to neck
Skipping side kick, knee drive, sweep
Sliding lead leg front kick, shin kicks and foot stomps, strikes

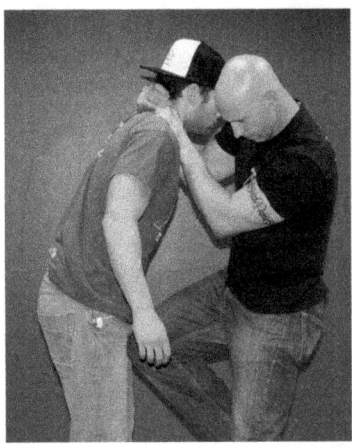

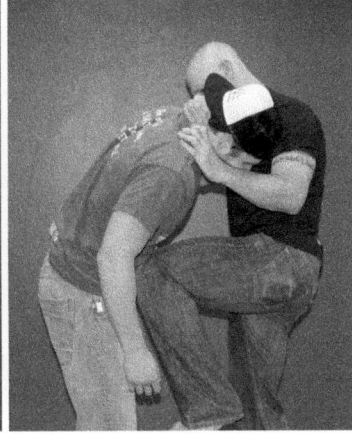

BLOCK AND ROCK

The complete block and rock series is counteroffensive. Step back and shift your weight onto your back foot. Once you engaged and deflected the attack, immediately fire back with a straight cross to your opponent.

High block and strike
Hammerfist block and strike
Outside middle block and strike
Knifehand front and side
Hammerfist, front and side

13
STREET APPLICATIONS AND TACTICS

Here's a real life story for the ladies. Most of the incidents that are recounted in this book have men depicted in various situations. There are quite a few women I have trained that defended themselves successfully in the street, but none as dramatic as the incident that I will relay now.

I was sitting at the desk of my martial arts studio back in December of 1995 when in walked the mother of one of my students who was away at college. She began to kiss and hug me, not that I minded it; but I asked her why. She told me that I saved her daughter's life. I replied, "How?"

Elizabeth had trained with me from the eighth grade through high school. She was 110 pounds, 5'4", and stunning, and just had finished her first semester as a college freshman. However, all during her time with me, she trained hard and was very serious about her martial arts. She was attending the American University in DC and left a party early to go home and study. She did break one of my rules—she was traveling alone at night, but she was wearing the proper attire. While walking across the campus, she was accosted by a large-knife-wielding assailant.

Her reactions, choice of kicks and strikes, and knowledge of distancing, zones, and movement all came into play. This was the first time she had ever been in a street situation. Prior to this incident, her only fighting experience was what we did in class and in tournaments.

Elizabeth launched an attack. She front-kicked him in the groin, applied a sidekick to his knee and then a roundhouse kick to the face when he hit the ground. She then booted the knife out of his hand and took off. All the kicks and movement she applied were all part of our daily basic training.

The result? He was arrested and hospitalized, with ruptured testicles, a dislocated knee, and a broken nose. When the DNA was taken, it matched the DNA present at four other rapes that occurred on campus. Her training saved her from becoming victim number 5.

There have always been debates about what *system* or *style* of fighting is best suited for the street. Martial arts can be broken down into three categories: self-perfection, sport combat, and self-preservation. Which works best for our purposes?

Self-perfection martial arts such as aikido, tai chi, many kung fu styles and any of the kata or forms-based karate styles. They are completely useless for street application. If people want to argue, fine. I'm judging this upon what I've seen work in the street and sound training principles. The aforementioned arts are fantastic for peace of mind, learning stances, developing discipline, and providing fitness as well as mobility, but knowing 57 different katas will not help you win a street fight. There is no need to discuss these arts any further.

Sport combat was created for practitioners to train against another human. This develops the reflexes and body awareness applicable for actual combat. There is nothing like drilling and training with a live person to develop your skills and a more usable type of strength for combat. The only drawback would be the rules applied to sport combat. The rules are implemented for the safety of the participants. Certain movements and target areas are disallowed. This, along with equipment, is geared toward the safety of the participants, and rightly so.

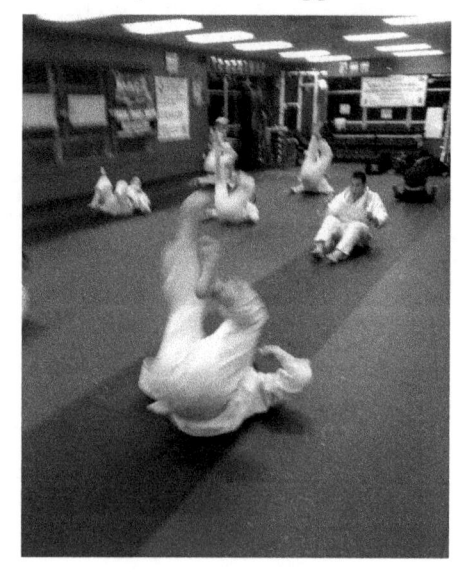

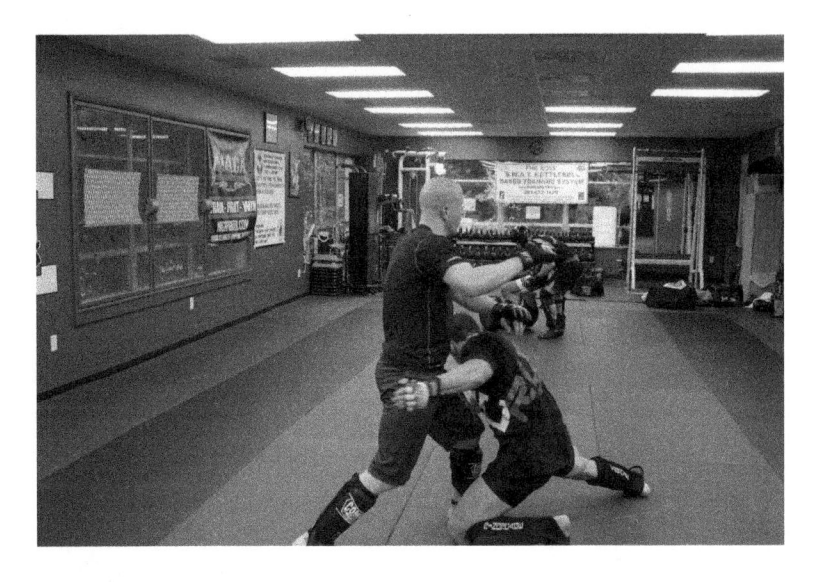

A number of years ago, I was training with the World Kickboxing champion, Carl Moffett. He was watching my guys and me using virtually no equipment and beating the crap out of each other. He thought that we were nuts (maybe he was right) for "conditioning" our bodies for combat in that manner. He advised us to lessen our injury occurrence by padding up and ramping up our body conditioning in methods other than full-contact, no-equipment sparring. Great advice. Combat is unpredictable. Take precautions while you are training.

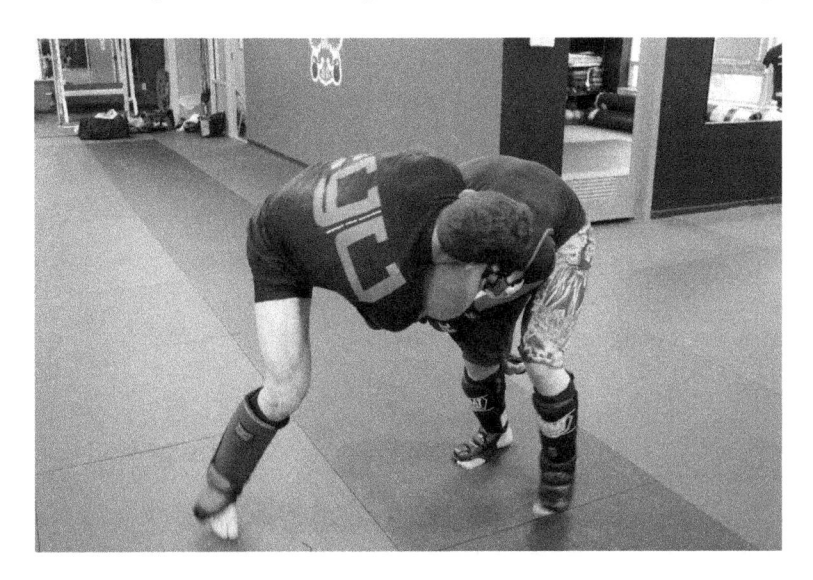

You may also consider which sport combat art is best. Each sport combat art has its drawbacks and limitations. On the onset, you may think that a mixed martial artist has the immediate advantage. Maybe, maybe not. Most street fights last only 10 seconds or less. Most fights start with the fighters standing up, and all are without a referee telling them when to start. Usually, the guy who lands the first shot wins. So a boxer or an accomplished striker would have an advantage over a grappler in this scenario.

If the fight does not end in the first few blows, it will ultimately go to the ground. What happens if it does go to the ground? You would think that an MMA fighter or a Brazilian jujitsu black belt has an advantage there. Not necessarily the case. In the street, generally, it's the guy who has the most friends who wins the ground fight. While you're attempting to apply an armbar, his buddies are kicking you in the head.

Even if you are in a one-on-one street fight, submissions may not be the best option. Look at the practicality: if someone tries to apply a triangle choke in the street and the other guy picks him up and slams his head off of the concrete sidewalk, now how practical are his ground fighting techniques? You would be better suited as a wrestler with a good ground-and-pound game. Take him down with a solid double-leg takedown and oil rig[37] his face with a barrage of punches, open-hand strikes, and elbows.

A fighter with a kicking-based art such as Taekwondo, Muay Thai, Savate, and various karate systems have their set of disadvantages as well. First of all, anytime you pick your foot up off of the ground, you just sacrificed 50 percent of your balance. This makes you easier to take down. What if the surface is slippery or unstable with gravel or loose footing? What if there is an obstacle, such as a pole or a chair? You would not be able to apply your kicking techniques. What if you are seated in a chair? Ask Jean Claude Van Damme what happened when he fought Chuck Zito[38].

---

[37] Oil rigging is the act of holding down an opponent with one hand and punching them, usually in the head, repeatedly with the other fist. Generally, the striking hand is your dominant side.

[38] It's an urban-legend fight between Chuck Zito and Jean Claude Van Damme. As legend goes, they got in a confrontation at a gentlemen's club in NYC, and Chuck

You may now be saying that boxing is the best. Maybe, maybe not. Most boxers train with gloves and wraps. The use of gloves was implemented for the protection of the boxer's hands, not to lessen the severity of a blow to the heads of the combatants. This method of fighting actually prolongs the combatants' exposure to mind-jarring blows. That being said, a boxer's hands are very quick and their movements good, but most of their hands are not conditioned for street combat. A closed fist, in order to resist injury, must be conditioned properly for bare-knuckle[39] fighting. If you punch someone in the head and don't hit them perfectly, your hand will break.

What if the boxer gets kneed in the groin? Or taken down to the ground or faced with a weapon? How about a kick to the knee? Most boxers are not trained to deal with such attacks. Even if they bob and weave out of the way of a strike, they may get cracked in the head with a knee as they move under the attack.

Wow! You're probably asking yourself, *How the heck am I going to be able to defend myself? Boxing, wrestling, BJJ, taekwondo? They all have such apparent weakness. What the heck do I do? How can I train to defend myself? Is this hopeless?*

Have patience. The answer will be coming. I'm just not ready to give it to you yet. Keep reading.

Self-preservation, or pure self-defense systems. Pressure point training, Krav Maga, Russian Systema, the various tactics practiced by our Special Forces, etc. Some of these systems are based on a great deal of reality and are excellent. Others leave a lot to be desired.

I cannot speak for all systems, nor can I earnestly speak for all instructors, but for a self-preservation or self-defense system to have validity, there

---

knocked Van Damme out cold with one punch. They were in punching range. So much for JCVD's kicks.

[39] Bare-knuckle fighting is fighting with no gloves or hand protection.

must be some type of actual sport combat training against another human. If an instructor states "We don't spar because we only practice death techniques and cannot spar in fear of the safety of our students and others that may come in," that's a load of crap! Many of these guys have never been hit in the face or kicked in the groin and would wet themselves if they ever got cracked. They hide behind their "death techniques" because they are pathetic fighters and are, rightfully so, very insecure about their ability to perform that they create a guise of unsubstantiated nonsense. They lull their students into adopting a false sense of security while setting them up for failure and lining their pockets with the hard-earned money of their pigeons.

There is only one other type of worse self-defense fear predator that I despise even more—the one that misleads the unwary on a grand scale: the Internet Video Huckster. These guys purport to have "secret techniques" that are "banned by the government." They flood the Internet with false advertising and promises of street invincibility with their secret arsenal. They claim that their programs are so complete, so devastating that simply by purchasing their DVDs and practicing the moves in your basement, you will be able to defeat an MMA fighter in mere seconds! That's like saying to someone, "Watch this video on swimming and you'll be able to beat Michael Phelps, without ever getting into a pool!"

Enough time spent on the phonies. I just wanted to give you a heads-up to what to watch out for. If it's too good to be true, it's too good to be true. Enough said. Let's get back to some useful material.

SO WHICH IS METHOD IS BEST?

"Now, some Special Forces guys become expert martial artists. And most of them will tell you that your particular style or discipline is as good as another, the thing that matters is the effort and heart you put into it. And they put as much time and effort as any other black belt in anything does, and they'll tell you they did it on their own time."[40]

---

[40] This is a quote fro the WeaponsMan blog, written by a former Special Forces member.

There is no one answer. What you need to do is train in our system or a system akin to it. You will need to be in shape and make your body as strong as possible. It is an imperative to engage in some sort of real sport combat practice. This would include training in all or a combination of boxing, kickboxing, Brazilian jujitsu, mixed martial arts, wrestling, sambo, judo, or other combat sports, where there is contact between you and your practice partner. You next must practice your defensive tactics with fluidity, purpose, and control. For the safety of your partner and yourself, one cannot practice these techniques with full force.

What type of training should I start with, and what do I need?

I am 100 percent honest with my students, and I have been 100 percent honest in this book. So, I will not stop now. To be able to handle yourself in the street, there are certain base arts that you need to train in. Simply said, they are the most practical and translatable to real combat.

I will tell you that the best two arts to learn first would be boxing and wrestling. Here's why: Most fights occur within the punching range, so learning how to box is very important. Wrestling is important because you *don't* want to get taken down in the street. Wrestlers are trained in how to resist being taken down and develop great balance. Both boxing and wrestling are tough methods of combat and require getting hit, slammed, and roughed up. The weight shifting, body conditioning, development of reflexes and footwork (movement) for both of these combat sports is unmatched. If you so choose, you may then add an art with practical kicks and then one with submissions and locks. I'm not trained in sambo specifically, but I worked with a bunch of sambo practitioners, and that's another solid base art. There are others, but make sure that there are real combat components to whatever you choose to train in.

Next, learn how to use weapons. The more you know about a weapon, the better you are able to defend yourself against it. It is important to know your own body and how to make it move *prior* to learning weapons training. So don't rush into using a weapon. If you're not good at it, you will most likely wind up getting the weapon taken away from you and the assailant using your weapon on you! Be cautious. We will discuss practical weapons in chapter 16.

I come from a wrestling and boxing background. Most of my street fights started with me throwing punches and then landing a takedown. When I learned karate, I would kick, punch, and then land a takedown. As far as submissions, I would primarily use wrist locks and choke holds when I was working as the situation dictated that I subdue someone.

Real-Life Example

In the 1980s, I worked as a bouncer in several establishments. It was 1983, and there were three of us working as security at a bar called Quincy's in Greenbelt, Maryland. The bar was formerly a "biker bar" called Jimmy Comer's, and we were part of the crew that converted it from a bike bar to a dance/sports bar and restaurant. The three bouncers on that night were Kirk, Percy (wrote a passage for this book), and me. It was Beat the Clock, night, so patrons were encouraged to drink early and a lot! So now you have the background on the evening.

Most bar fights start for very stupid reasons, and this incident was no exception. Kirk was about 6'4", but thin and wiry. He wound up getting into an argument with a patron about the video game Ms. Pac-Man. Yes, that's right, Ms. Pac-Man—not even the original Pac-Man, but Ms. Pac-Man! There were three of them, and they were big. One was about 6'5", 270 pounds. The others were 6'2" and 6'3" and approximately 30 to 40 pounds lighter. The argument ensued, so Percy and I walked over. Now Percy was only about 5'11", but he was tipping the scales at 250 pounds, and his barrel chest arrived 5 minutes before he did. At the time, I was 5'10" and around 195. As we stood there, Kirk and the big guy decided that they were going to have their fight outside so they would not mess up the bar. We tried to keep the fights outside to minimize damage to the bar and not incite more patrons.

Kirk made a crucial mistake: he turned his back on the foe to walk outside. The guy cracked him in the jaw. Kirk did not fall to the ground, but his body bent at the waist, and he fell backward. By the time he regained his balance, I had the guy who hit him on the ground, and Percy had dropped one of the other guys by slamming him into the brick wall. The third guy put his hands up, stating, "He was cool and wasn't going to make trouble."

So how did this transpire? After the big guy hit Kirk, I ducked under his punch and hit him with a right hook (body shot), and then I got behind him, reached between his legs, and suplayed[41] him backward. Once on the ground, I quickly scrambled to the top position with him stunned and on his back. I applied the python lock, securing one of his arms and my other hand wrapped around his windpipe. (I saw Percy's feet on either side of his head. His legs were shaking due to the adrenaline dump.) I then told the big guy I had on the ground to relax or I was going to bite his nose off. He relaxed fairly quickly, and then I informed him I was going to let him up. I also advised him to not look back, say a word, or do anything but walk out. He complied.

Why this story? Well, a few reasons. One, I used boxing and wrestling to take out a much larger adversary. I was able to use the submission hold only after strikes, and after I secured the position. Also, my coworker Kirk made a tragic mistake by turning his back on a guy he was going to fight.

WHAT ARE THE MOST IMPORTANT STRIKES AND KICKS TO LEARN?

I fear not the man who has practiced 10,000 kicks once, but I fear the man who has practiced one kick 10,000 times.

—Bruce Lee proverb

---

[41] *Suplay* is a wrestling move used most often in freestyle and Greco-Roman wrestling. Often confused with the *suplex*, which is a move from "fake" or "pro wrestling." Once you are behind your adversary, lock your arms around their waist, pop your hips in, and lift them as you bridge backward. If you keep the bridge, they will land on their head or the back of their neck. If you turn at the last moment, you will land on top of them, and they'll be prone.

There are dozens and dozens of striking techniques. How do we choose what ones to use? What are the most effective? Refer to the list of single techniques in chapter 9 for the complete list of recommended kicks and strikes in our system.

In chapter 1, we spoke about the magic number 7, +/- 2. In a stressful situation, the brain is able to respond to the immediate external stimulus with anywhere from five to nine movements. You may now be asking yourself, why learn all of these movements? I can only use 9 moves at the most. Isn't training with those other movements a waste of time? No, it's not. Here's why.

First of all, you have a different set of responses for different stimuli. A set for grabs, strikes, different weapons, etc. So you must develop those series sets of movements. You wouldn't perform a double-leg takedown on someone with a gun to your head, but you'd shoot a double if you just slipped a punch.

Secondly, how do you know which movements work best for you without having tried them? This is very akin to the little kid that only wants to eat macaroni and cheese and chicken nuggets. If you don't try the other foods, how are you going to know what suits you best? Unless you try a variety of movements, you'll never know which ones work best for you and your students.

Another point is that the better you know a technique, the better able you are to defend against it. If you want to effectively defend a punch, you had better know the mechanics involved in throwing a punch. The same holds true for kicks, grappling, and especially for weapons. It's beneficial to become well versed in various movements and strategies. Know thy enemy.

As stated before, the basic movements work best. You will use your basics 90 percent of the time. Once you have honed in on the basic set of movements that works for you, the other 10 percent of the movements may work specifically for you. Here are some examples: Let us suppose that you have a fighter. Most of his scoring techniques are his basics—front, round and side kicks, jab, cross, and hook. However, he has a great jump-back kick. Let's consider a grappler: Most of his submissions may come from the rear naked choke or the armbar, but he happens to have a nasty Peruvian necktie. In these instances, theses fighters have their basics, but a small percentage of their repertoires come from techniques that work well for them specifically.

One final word on this: even though I never recommend throwing a jump spinning kick in the street, it's beneficial for coordination, balance, and development of stabilizers and intrinsic muscles to increase the performance of your technique set. You will most likely never use a spearhand technique, but the practice of it increases the range of motion and strength of your hands.

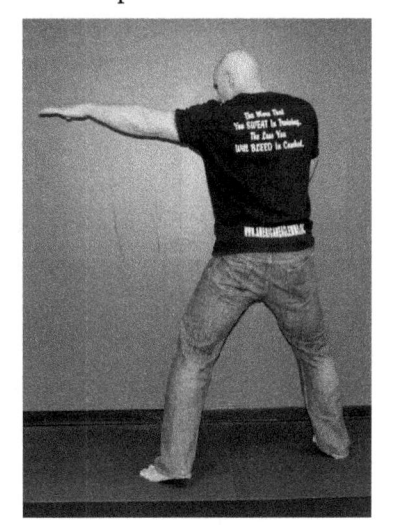

Basic Techniques

Hands: Closed fist, punches 1–6. Open-hand strikes such as the axehands, slaps, and palm heel strikes are the most effective.

Elbows: Elbows can be delivered up, down, across, back, and on angles. The general targets are the temple, jaw, groin, solar plexus, ribs, and spine.

Knees: Straight knees delivered to the groin and bladder work best. Roundhouse knees directed to the sciatic nerve, quads, and hamstrings are most effective.

The **Fabulous Four Kicks** are as follows:

Roundhouse. An extremely quick, powerful and versatile technique used to cause damage on many parts of the body. The Roundhouse family of kicks also includes cut kicks and shin kicks.

Side kick. This thrusting technique may be used with equal effectiveness either defensively or offensively. Striking with your heel to the knee or body of your opponent. The Side kick variations include stepping, skipping, and kicks off the back side of your body as in the back kick or mule kick.

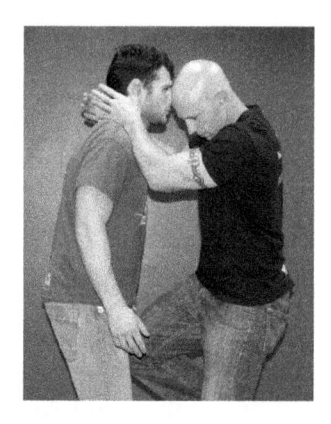

Front kick. Virtually any area of the body may be attacked, either with the ball of the foot, full bottom of the foot or the heel. Groin, shin, solar plexus, ribs, etc…This kick may be used as a push to drive an opponent backward as well.

Stomps. Foot stomps, parachute stomps, heel stomps directed to the top of the foot, shin or to any accessible target on a downed opponent.

So what do we do?

The most important component is your mind-set and willingness to win—even more important, *your hatred of losing.* If you ever had witnessed me win anything, I never demonstrated excitement more than a smile. When I'm in a competition or a "situation," I am supposed to win. That's what I'm there for. I *expect* to win. So when I win, I'm simply doing what I should do. I hate to lose, more than anything. Show me a "good loser" and I'll show you a loser.

Maybe you couldn't see that I'm disappointed or mad, but I don't take losses lightly.

Three weeks after I earned my black belt, I entered a professional karate tournament. My first fight was against the #3 ranked fighter in the world, Larry Kelly. I will tell you that he surreptitiously spanked me. I couldn't lay a glove on him. He didn't hurt me, but damn, he embarrassed the hell out of me! He avoided all of my attacks and simply hit me when I missed. After the bout, I didn't speak with anyone. I was an amateur champion, and I expected to win at my first pro event. When I got home that night, I ran five miles and then went into my basement and hit the heavy bag so long and so hard that I was completely exhausted and both my hands were bleeding. I really didn't care; I was extremely pissed off at my performance. It was the last time I was ever embarrassed. I made sure it never happened again.

WHAT TO DO WHEN THE PROVERBIAL S———T HITS THE FAN?

Five-time UFC World Champion Frank Shamrock was posed the question, "What's the best advice anyone has given you about fighting?" He stated that the best advice he was ever given was, "Keep your hands up." That's some great advice. When you are in a fracas, get your hands up by your head! As I tell my students, you can do push-ups to strengthen your upper body, you can do sit-ups to make your abdominals strong, but there is no such thing as "face–ups," so you better protect you face and head by keeping your hands up!

I would also advise you to move. Simply start moving, but not backward. Move your head around and circle. Change directions. A moving target is much more difficult to hit than a stationary one. So *keep your hands up and move.*

WHAT'S A GOOD BASIC PHILOSOPHY TO ADOPT?

The element of surprise is an element that is especially beneficial to smaller and female practitioners. In most self-defense situations, the assailant is looking to impose their will on someone that they believe that they can subdue with minimal effective resistance. Use this opportunity to launch your counterattack. Quick, repeated, and powerful strikes in resistance are all that you may need to afford yourself the time to escape with minimal injury.

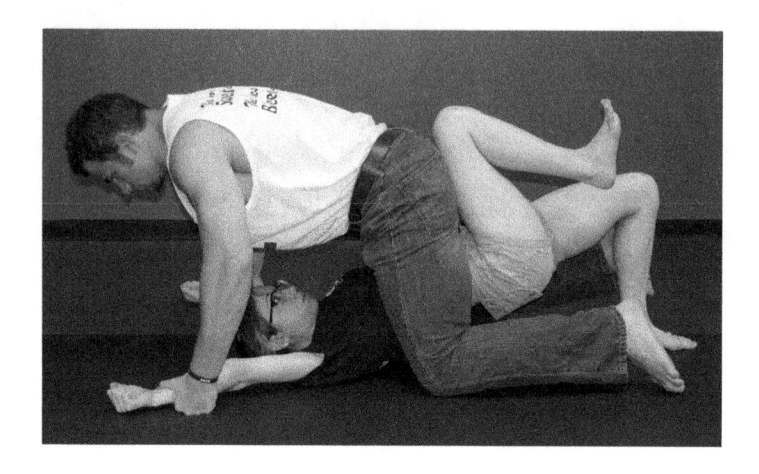

As far as actual movement and fighting strategies are concerned, a good premise to use as your base is what I refer to as *the Xs and Os principle*. Think of it as the *X*s and *O*s in football, where the *X*s represent the defense and the *O*s represent the offense.

When defending, your movements should contain *X*s, and when attacking (or counterattacking), use *O*s, otherwise known as circle striking. If you consider many martial arts movements where the arms cross in front of the body and move to another counteroffensive position. This X in defending principle applies to ground fighting, stand-up, and weapons. Some examples would be as follows:

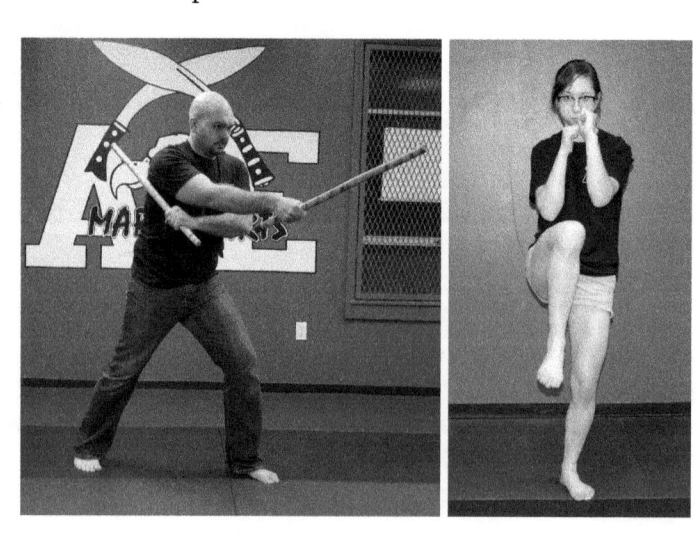

The *O*s is for offensive circles of striking combinations. My preference for attacking and counterattacking is in a circle. An example of a circle or O combination would be a left round.

Roundhouse kick to the body, left jab, right cross, and right cut kick. You start at the midsection, move up and then across and down to the opposite side from where you started, thus making a complete circle. I will say that there are certain circumstances when I employ an *X* for striking, but as a general rule, I utilize a circle, or *O*.

HOW SHOULD WE TRAIN?

There is a false opinion espoused by some so-called experts that all you need to do is to practice your self-defense and death techniques. *(Chuckles.)* Others claim that if you are used to "pulling," or controlling your strikes, you will do so in the street.

Well, both are incorrect. Consider this: if you didn't pull your techniques or exhibit control while sparring, everyone would be banged up and unable to compete or train. My training partners and I have had plenty of knockouts and submissions in competition, so that theory is out the window. When you are in a situation, treat it like a training session that you don't have to hold back in. If you don't roll or spar live, you'll never be able to develop the kinesthetic awareness of movement with and against another human being. This is also why live drilling is tantamount to your training. You need to practice your real sport combat *and* your defensive tactics, plus strength and conditioning, as well as your body toughening techniques. Don't neglect any of these areas.

I have never had an issue making the transition from my training in the studio to application in the street. Neither have any of my friends, students, or my training partners. When I've been squared up with someone in the street, I treated the situation like I was sparring - except more emotion, adrenaline, and knowing that I *didn't* have to hold back! It was go time! Those who disagree with this either never have been in a fight or have been trained in an inferior system. The sparring and reaction to human movement, getting hit yourself and seeing how you react, plus practicing your defensive tactics is a great place to start when preparing yourself for a street encounter.

You need to train so that your defensive maneuvers are purely reflexive. Once you have this, IT takes over. You have now developed instinctive technique. The body and the mind are in such sync with each other and you are so attuned to them that you will respond properly. Here's an example of what I'm referring to: I had graduated college a year or so before, and I was in a bar in NYC with a group of friends. As we were making our way through the crowded, dark, and very loud club, I felt someone grab me by my traps from behind. I immediately turned and captured both of the assailant's arms with one of mine and readied my fist to smash into his face. Luckily for him, I recognized him. He was a buddy from college. I pulled the punch before I hit him in the face and let go of him. I said, "Greg, what are you doing!"

He said, "You are crazy!"

I replied, "Me? You know me and ought to know better than to grab me from behind!"

IT took over. IT responded. IT did what I had trained IT to do. Protect me. IT did its job. As IT had many times before and after.

Listed below are specific responses to specific attacks. It is impossible to train for every potential situation. However, the concepts of the responses are universal and applicable to multiple attacks and scenarios. The attacks addressed are some of the more prevalent. The defensive tactics employed are the most universal. This meaning that most people will be able to perform these movements against most assailants.

All self-defense techniques have three components (or ingredients, as I often refer to them): *distraction*, *release*, and *finish*.

The distraction is in the form of a stomp, smash, or a strike to the vital and semivital areas. The release occurs when you free yourself from their grasp or hold. The finish takes place once you are free and need to temporarily (or permanently) disable the assailant while securing your safe escape. At worst case, once you are grabbed or attacked, immediately strike back.

Listed below are over 50 prescribed self-defense techniques. It would be an arduous, if not impossible, task to teach, train, and practice every possible defensive tactic maneuver. Not to mention developing the muscle memory required to execute the techniques under duress. Instead of focusing specifically on the techniques, we focus on the principles of responses to attacks.

So why do we even practice techniques? There are several reasons. We need to know how to move with another person and how a body will react when both being attacked and attacking. These are some well-known, prevalent attacks. Preparing oneself for these instances is practicing due diligence. The main reason is teaching your body how to apply the principles of human movement. Thus developing the IT, or instinctive technique, necessary to effectively protect yourself.

REAL-LIFE EXAMPLE

It was May 1984, and I had just finished my finals at the University of Maryland. It was a long day of celebration, and the night had wound down. It was around 2:00 a.m., and there was a group of us hanging out in my apartment eating pizza and such. Only the screen door was closed, and suddenly, there was a knock at the door. I could see the door from where I was sitting, clad in only a pair of shorts. I got up and went to the door. There was a guy there, approximately six feet tall and 210 pounds. He was covered in blood, said that he had been in an accident, and asked if he could use the phone to call his brother. I said OK.

Well, as he was on the phone, I noticed something propping up his shirt in the back. I was getting a strange feeling, so I followed him out of the door and looked around as he started walking off to the right. I looked to the left and saw a guy lying on the ground bleeding about a half of a block away. I yelled to the guy who just left my house. He took off. Game on!

I took off after him and caught up with him at the end of the street. He turned and faced me with the knife in his hand. I open-hand–slapped his knife hand, hitting the back of his wrist with the heel of my palm, and the knife flew about twenty feet or so and landed in a gully. I moved to the side and hit him in the back of his neck, then I foot-swept him and took him to the ground in a prone position.

Pushing his face into the dirt with one hand, I jacked his hand up behind his back with the other while jamming my knee into his tailbone. In the interim, the police arrived in full force! There were a dozen cops surrounding the action, lights and sirens blaring, with their guns drawn on the two of us. Quickly, I looked up and said, "Don't worry, boys, I got him!" By some miracle, the victim lived. He had survived eight stab wounds, one of them puncturing his lung. I wound up being the recipient of two letters of commendation from the Prince George's County chief of police and the county executive. If you look at what I did, there was nothing fancy about it—just concise, powerful movements and quick action.

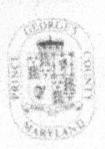

OFFICE OF THE COUNTY EXECUTIVE

PARRIS N. GLENDENING
COUNTY EXECUTIVE

June 19, 1984

Mr. Phillip Gerard Ross
4212 B Guilford Road
College Park, Maryland 20740

Dear Mr. Ross:

    The Prince George's County Chief of Police has brought to my attention an event occurring on May 20, 1984 during which you made possible the apprehension of an individual who had committed a serious crime. Your assistance to the police in this matter, while you knew the culprit was armed with a knife and was dangerous, was a display of unusual courage and indomitability.

    The action you took as a citizen without laboring on the hazards involved is heartening to governing officials, such as myself, and I speak for the whole County when I tell you your action was truly commendable. When citizens take alert action that reflects respect and consideration for the personal and property rights of others an attitude of uprightness and fairness is shown that is a lasting credit to such a person.

    Again thanking you for your action, it is my hope that you will maintain this attitude of helpfulness. If I may be of assistance to you in the future, please feel free to call.

                        Sincerely,

                         Parris N. Glendening

Common Attacks

The defenses listed to the following attacks may be performed with either side of the body. For simplicity's sake, we will discuss only one side per attack. However, be certain to practice both sides, you never know what circumstances will dictate. You may have an injury, or your dominant side may be otherwise occupied.

We describe initial responses to attacks. If executed with intensity, precision, and power, the prescribed techniques will resolve the situation. However, things don't always go as planned. So you will need to be prepared to improvise. I call this "catch as catch can." Whatever comes up, hit it. Adhere to the principles of movement, and you will tilt the scales in your favor.

There are many bonafide self-defense techniques. The responses listed are the ones that I have found to work the best for the largest majority of people. Most of these techniques have been done personally by me in a real-life situation, or someone I trained with had performed them in a similar situation. After years of practice, you may discover variations that better suit you. If so, perfect! Good for you, use them. We're simply giving you a point to start at or a different perspective if you are already trained.

Chokes

Front choke, two hands: This is the "stereotypical" front choke attack when someone reaches out with both hands and attempts to strangle you with their hands. Bring your shoulders up with a shrugging motion as you bring your chin down, just as if you were a turtle going into his shell. As you are doing this, strike your opponent in the nose with a palm heel strike with you right hand. Next, you will simultaneously step back with your right foot as your left hand comes over with a slap to the assailant's ear. These combined motions will free you from their grasp. Plant your right foot firmly on the ground and deliver a side kick to the attacker's knee. On a side note, if you have fingernails (one for the ladies), you can scratch their face with your open-hand slap and leave identifying marks.

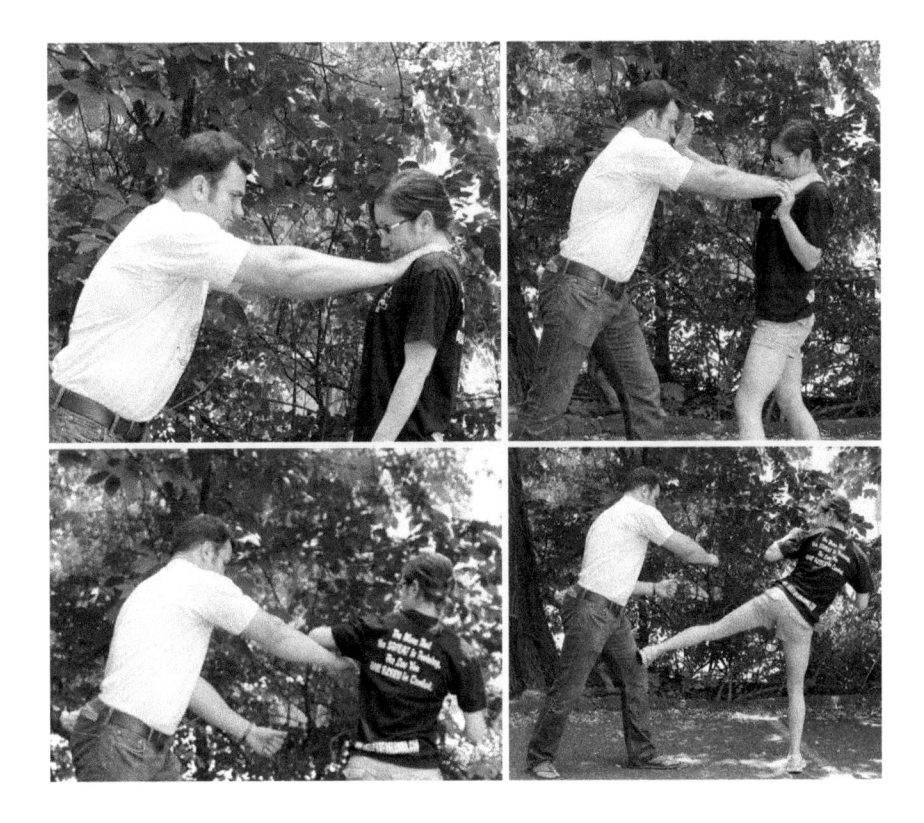

Front choke, one hand: There are two basic methods that you can defend yourself with in this situation. One is to the inside, and the other to the outside. The latter is the preferable method, but you are not always afforded that luxury.

Outside: When you get attacked with one hand, the hand will most likely be used to punch you in the face. This is why moving to the outside of the opponent is preferable. If the assailant grabs you with their left hand, you grab their wrist with your left hand and place your elbow up so that it is covering your face. Step with your right foot, making sure their left arm is straight as you deliver a hammerfist strike to the extended arm at the elbow. As you finish that blow, immediately strike their face with a side hammer smash.

Inside: There may be the occasion that you are unable to take the outside path and you need to be aware that you could be stepping into a punch. If the perpetrator grabs your throat with their right hand, secure his wrist with your left. As you step in, make certain that your right hand is up. We do this for two reasons: one, as a means to protect your face when you move in, and, two, so that your hand is in a position to deliver the knifehand chop to the biceps insertion. This is located above the bend in the elbow. Bounce your strike from the biceps and drive an elbow into your assailant's face. Your fist will be clenched and your palm facing downward. Capture your opponent's neck with your right hand and deliver upward knee strikes to the groin, head, or bladder.

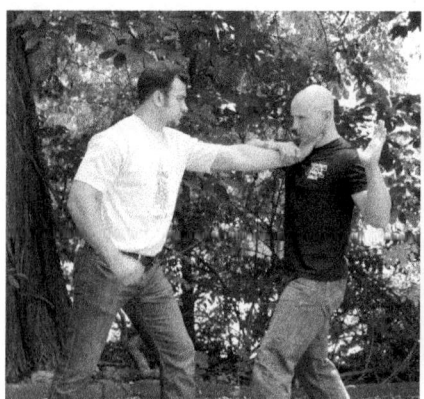

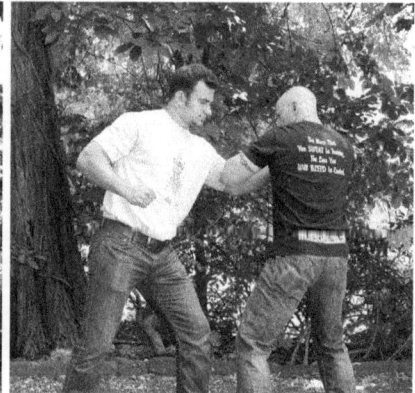

Rear chokes: There is a common thread with all choke defenses. You need to make space and do it quickly. If the assailant knows what he's doing, you'll be unconscious in 3 seconds or less. When you have an arm around your neck, you'll need to bring your shoulder up, tuck your neck in, and take your middle finger and your ring finger, insert them into the crook of the attacker's elbow, and pull down.

You will now need to turn so that your chin is placed in the crook of the elbow. You have now bought yourself some time to escape.

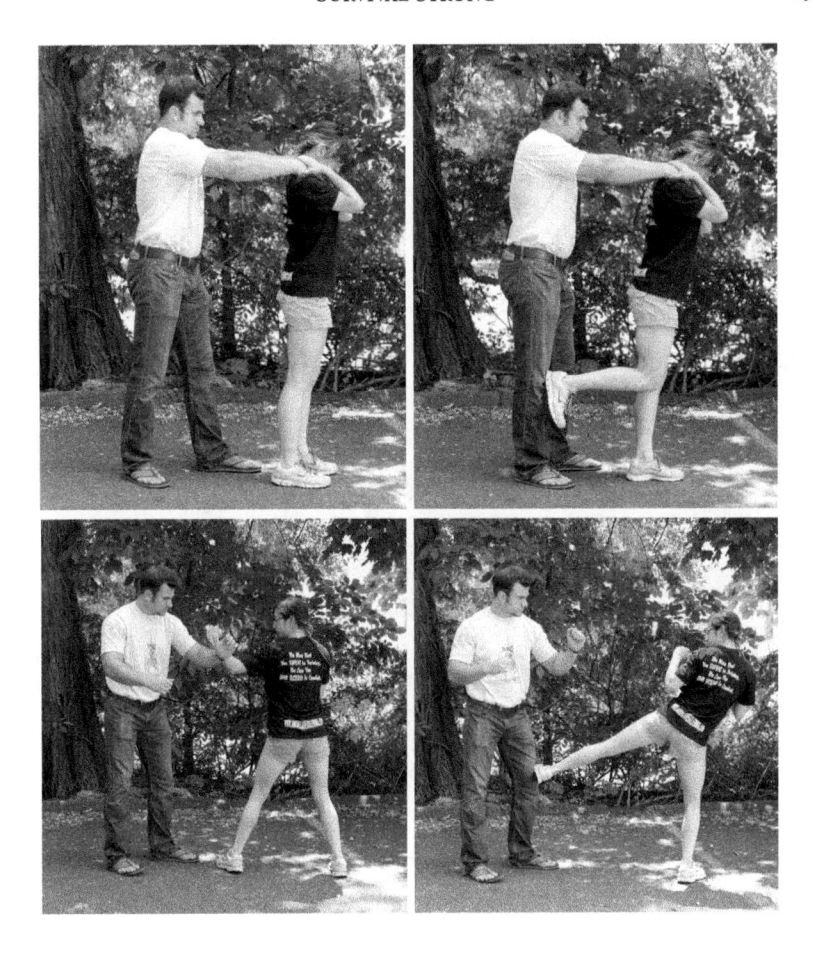

Rear choke with arm bar: This is a very commonplace restraining attack. The assailant will wrap their right arm around your neck and force your left hand up high by grabbing your wrist and driving it up. Lower your weight, stomp their toes and kick their shins, drive your head backward into their face, and then perform the sequence of movements described above.

Once you have loosened the grip and applied your distraction techniques, take your left foot and step behind your right foot as you bend your waist and duck out. This motion frees the arm that they are jacking up your back. As you turn and move, keep the grip on the arm that was once around your neck with your right hand and your newly freed left one. You will wind up on the side of your opponent. Drive your right shoulder into their arm as you sidestep and drag the opponent by the arm in the direction of their hand.

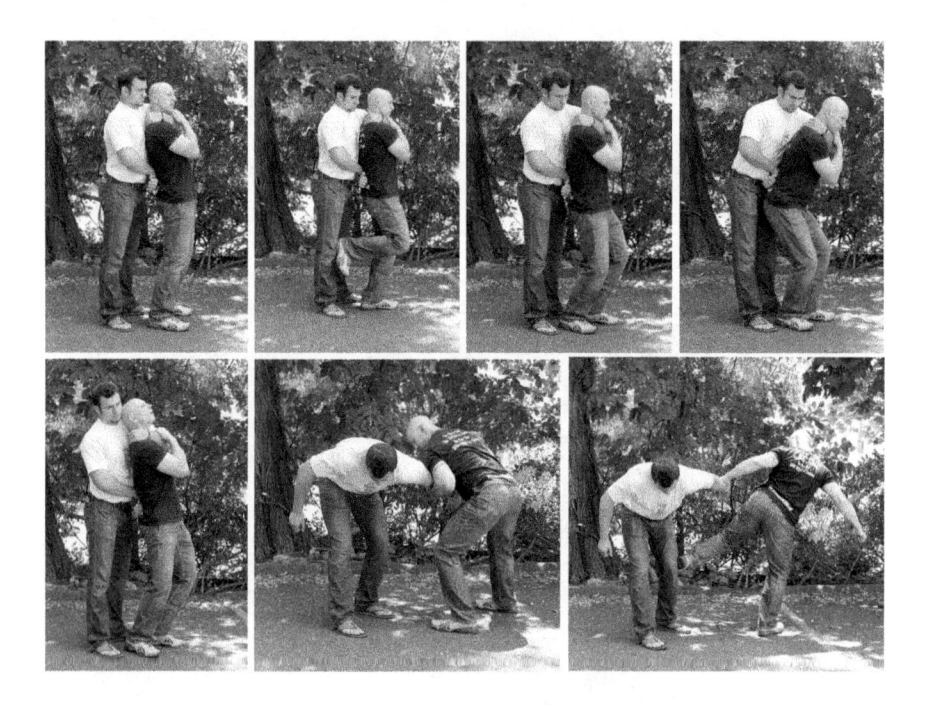

Rear naked chokes: There are more people practicing martial arts nowadays than ever before. Additionally, most thugs get their techniques from television, hence the gun being held sideways. There is no shooting advantage to holding your weapon in this position. That being said, a great deal of these guys see MMA fighters putting rear naked chokes (RNCs) on their opponent's in combat. It's only natural that they will try them on you. So it's best to be cognizant of this fact and prepare yourselves.

Standing: If attacked in this method, you would follow the same movement pattern as you would if attacked with the rear choke and armbar. However, you may not be able to throw the backward Head Butt; the lock may be too tight. You will most likely be able to back into the attacker as you deliver a barrage of kicks and stomps to the feet and shins. Repeat the same steps used in the Rear Choke with the Armbar.

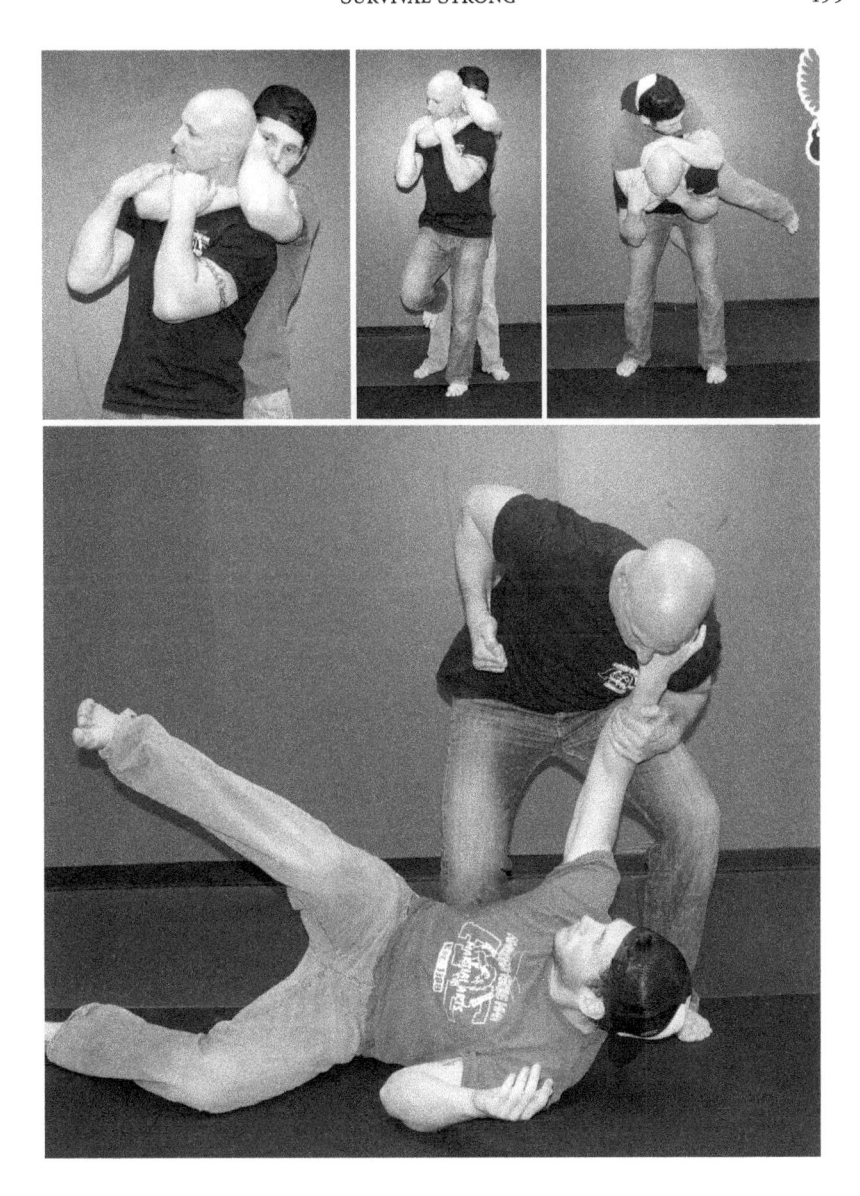

On the ground: This position is a little more dangerous, unless you have friends with you to kick and stomp the attacker. If not, here's what you'll need to do. First of all, he will most likely have his hooks[42] in on

---

[42] Hooks in: This is a term used in MMA and BJJ to describe the position when one person is directly behind the other and he hooks his legs inside the opponent's inner thighs. This position may be achieved while both are sitting on their buttocks or with both people prone.

both of your legs. Some people like to escape to the choking side arm; others like to get to the free arm side. You may not have a choice, so practice your escapes to both sides. Let's consider escaping to the choking arm side. Follow all the steps to relieve the pressure on your throat as you slide your body down toward his feet as you put your butt on his thigh. Eventually you will slide yourself downward and get your butt on the outside of his leg. You are now able to cut your hips and flip over so that you are belly down and scramble[43] to a side mount, full mount, or to your feet. After you get here, it's catch as catch can. I got you this far—you're training takes over here.

Wrist Grabs

When someone grabs your wrist, at least one of their hands are compromised. They are as tied up as you are—for the time being, anyway. You need to take advantage of this before they realize that they do not have the advantage. They are also vulnerable to strikes, having one half of their defense compromised. It's important to keep in mind that you are always most vulnerable while attacking. You will also always want to twist your wrist so the edge of the wrist on the side of your thumb is lined up where there thumb and finger come together. There are many controlling techniques that you can

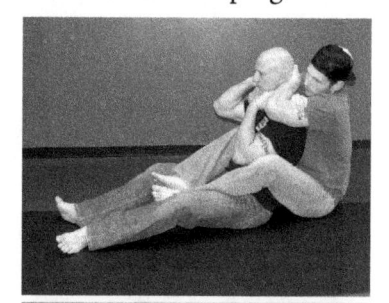

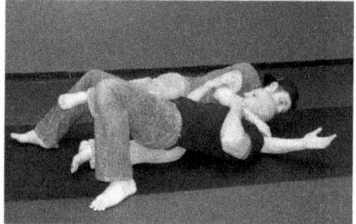

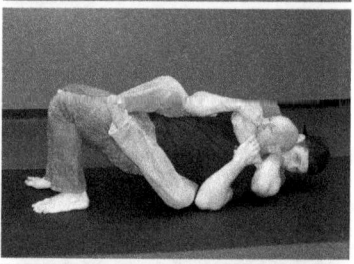

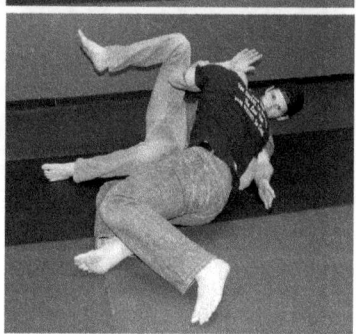

---

[43] Scramble occurs when you have freed yourself from a position and you employ perpetual motion to move to an advantageous position or escape.

use when your wrist gets grabbed, but they are reserved for situations that dictate control and non-lethal responses. We will not address these here. Controlling techniques are only recommended for those working in security or law enforcement. You have to be extremely proficient to subdue another human being without inflicting pain or damage.

One-on-one (single) wrist grab: Let us suppose that your left wrist is grabbed. The attacker will not simply stand there holding your wrist. They are either going to pull you, try to punch you, or a combination thereof. Step into the assailant with your right foot as you deliver an axehand with your right hand to their head. Now, as you twist your left wrist as described above, execute a downward chop on their wrist. Bounce that hand off of their wrist and strike them in the side of the neck as you grab their neck. Thread your left hand under their right arm and onto their back. Stomp the ground with your left foot and perform the springboard knee with your right knee, striking the groin, bladder, or head. Repeat the strikes until they drop. Whether you are attacked with the same side wrist or the assailant grabs the cross wrist, the defense remains consistent.

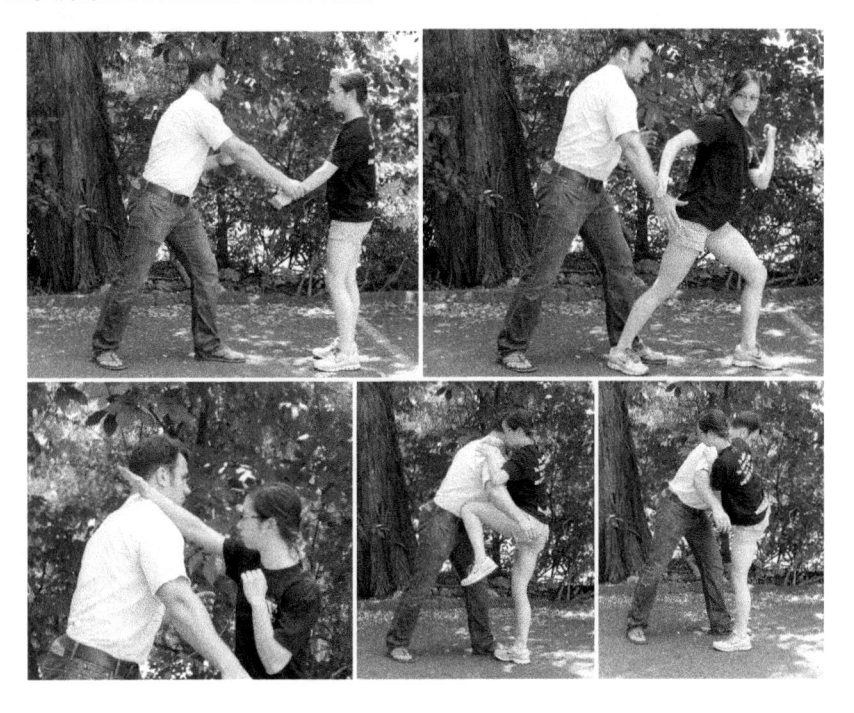

Two-on-one wrist grab: The assailant grabs your wrist with two hands. Deliver a palm heel strike to their face, aiming for the nose. Reach between their arms and "shake hands" with yourself and step back with the opposite foot of the hand that is being grabbed. So if your right hand was grabbed, step back with your left foot as you pull your hand free. The opponent steps toward you, delivers a side elbow to their face. If he steps away or remains stationary, administer a side kick to their knee.

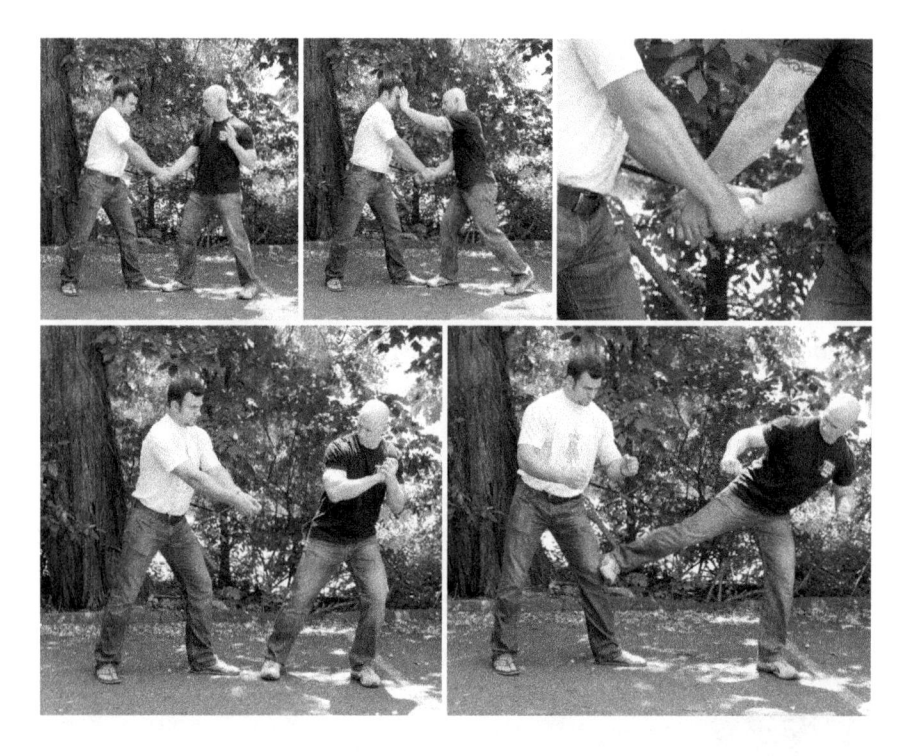

Two-on-two wrist grab: One of the easiest and most effective manners to free yourself from a two-on-two wrist attack is to force your hands in and, as they pull your hands outward, to counter what you have done, deliver a front knee strike to the groin. Repeat this until they fall. If they don't pull your hands apart, punch your left hand downward and grab their right wrist with your right as you deliver a kick to their left shin with your right foot. Stomp the ground and move to your left and kick their right knee, step to your left and side-kick their right knee as you free your hand.

Two-on-two wrist grab, control: If the situation arises where you need to control the attacker and both of your wrists are grabbed, first, kick to their talus or shin. Next, turn both palms up, right hand positioned over the left, and grab their left hand with the fingers of your left hand on the thumb portion of their palm. Your thumb will be up as you pull your fingers toward you, push your thumb toward them as you shove their hand toward them and downward to the outside as you deliver a palm heel to the side of their head.

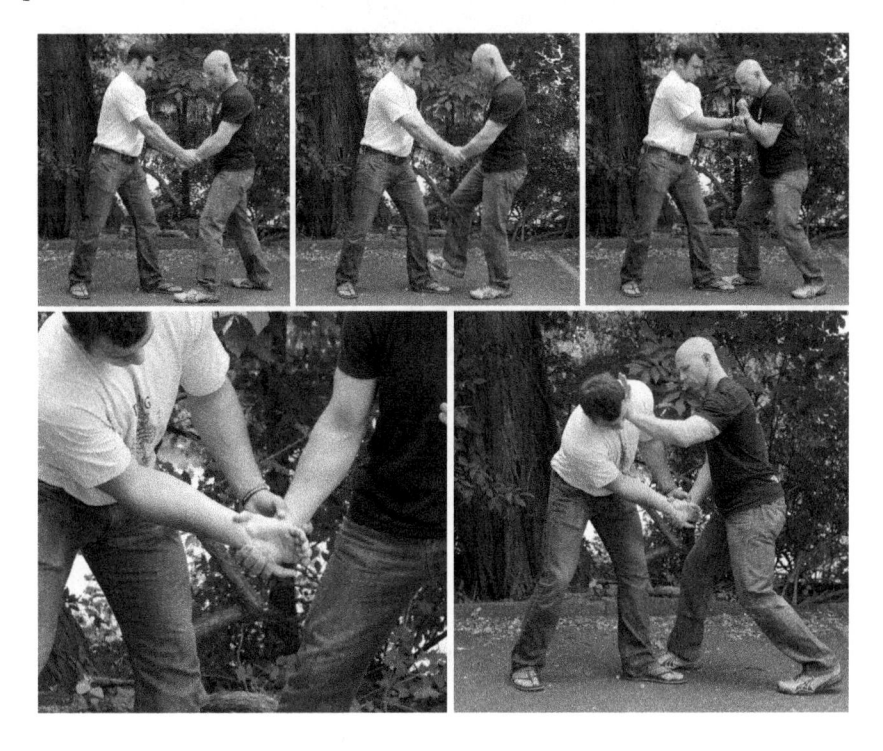

Two hands on one arm from behind (arm behind back): If your right arm is grabbed and controlled by your assailant's hands and your arm is placed behind your back, first stomp his feet, and kick backward into his knees as a distraction. Next, bend at the waist and step across with your left foot and pivot 180 degrees. You will now be facing your attacker, but off to their right side. Free your hand, either by utilizing a small circle with your wrist or by attacking with chops to his wrist. Employ a finishing technique.

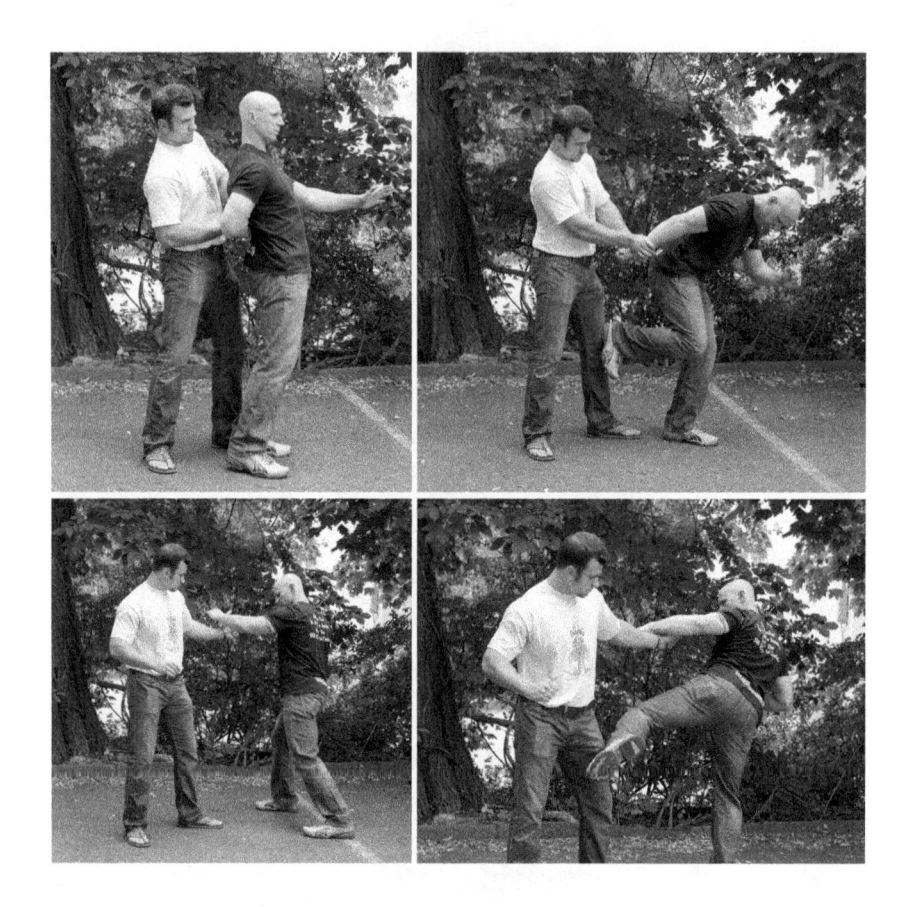

Two-on-one arm from behind (around waist): Suppose you have been grabbed from behind and your attacker grabs your left wrist with his right hand and grabs your right forearm with his left hand. This is generally referred to as a two-on-one wrist control position. If they position themselves properly, their face and groin will be obscured. You'll only be able to use foot stomps and shin kicks as distraction techniques.

To free yourself from this, thread your right hand under their right hand as you grab their left wrist. Bring your right elbow up high as you "pop" his right hand off of your wrist and then drive your left hand straight downward. You will now be free to unleash your barrage of counterattacks.

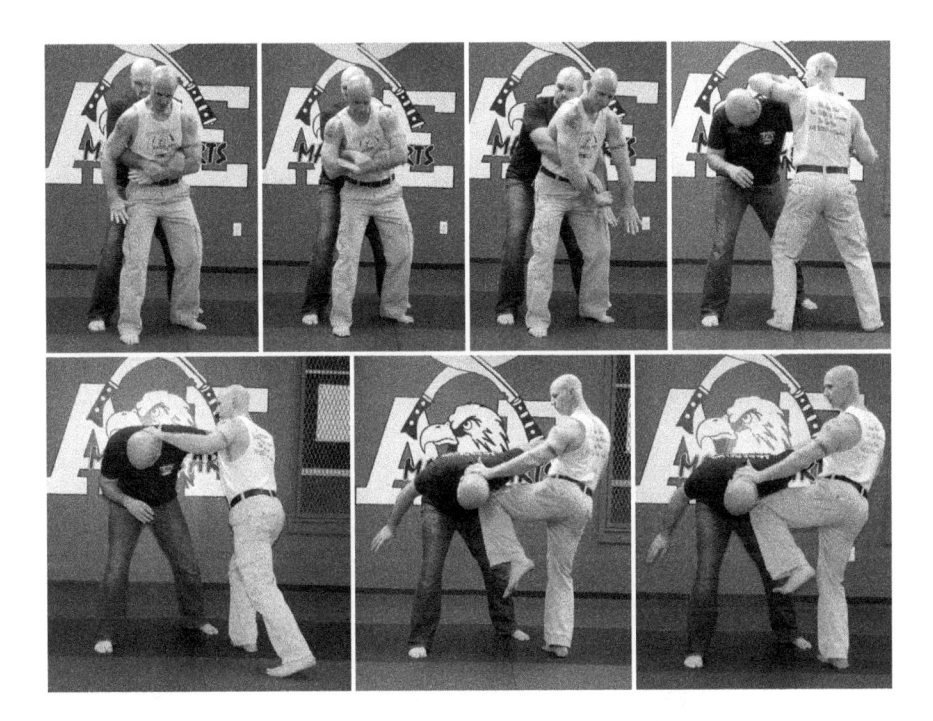

Punches

It's very humorous to me to watch movies and see these action stars catch someone's fist in mid-punch and then proceed to flip them through a wall. This will not happen in real life. We need to concentrate on the fact that all punches begin at the hip and then come from the shoulder. Stopping the punch at its origin is the only chance that you'll have. You'll never catch their fist, so it's a waste of time to even think about it. Parries, movement, and stopping the punch at its origin are the strategies that work best.

Single straight punch: If you are attacked with a straight punch, the person throwing probably has some idea of how to throw a good punch and most likely has had some training. This person is more dangerous and will leave fewer openings.

Let us assume that you have your hands up and that the attacker is throwing a straight right hand at you. Move to your left and toward them with a 6 step (pie stepping in chapter 10), parry their strike with your left hand anywhere between their fist and elbow as you deliver a strike to their abdomen with your right hand. Next, slide your right hand up to capture their extended right arm and deliver an elbow strike with your left to their head.

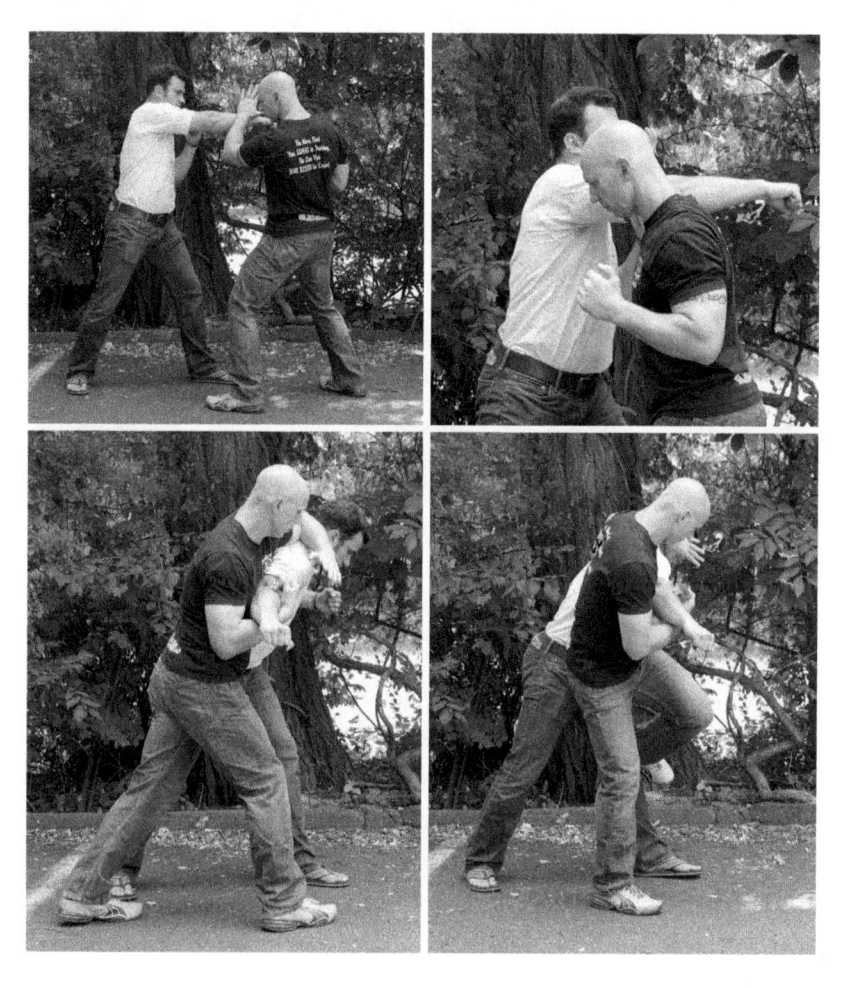

Two straight punches: This defense is identical to the single straight punch, except there are two parries due to the two punches, and we'll finish with a knee drive to the groin and a downward elbow smash to the back of the head of the doubled-over attacker.

Grab and punch: If someone grabs your lapel, you can bet that there will be a punch sailing to your head shortly thereafter. If they grab you with their left hand, cover it with your right and immediately direct a palm heel strike to their right shoulder with your left hand. We strike the shoulder because every punch, whether a straight, hook, or uppercut, emanates from the shoulder. Stop the punch at its source. Back to the defensive maneuver: keep your assailant's left hand secured to your chest and after you have struck his shoulder with your right, execute a chin jab, then an elbow strike across his chin from right to left.

Next, perform an axehand strike from left to right and then grasp their neck with your right hand as you slide your left hand under their arm and across their back. Now you deliver knee strikes to the groin, solar plexus, and bladder until you determine it's time to implement your redirect throw.

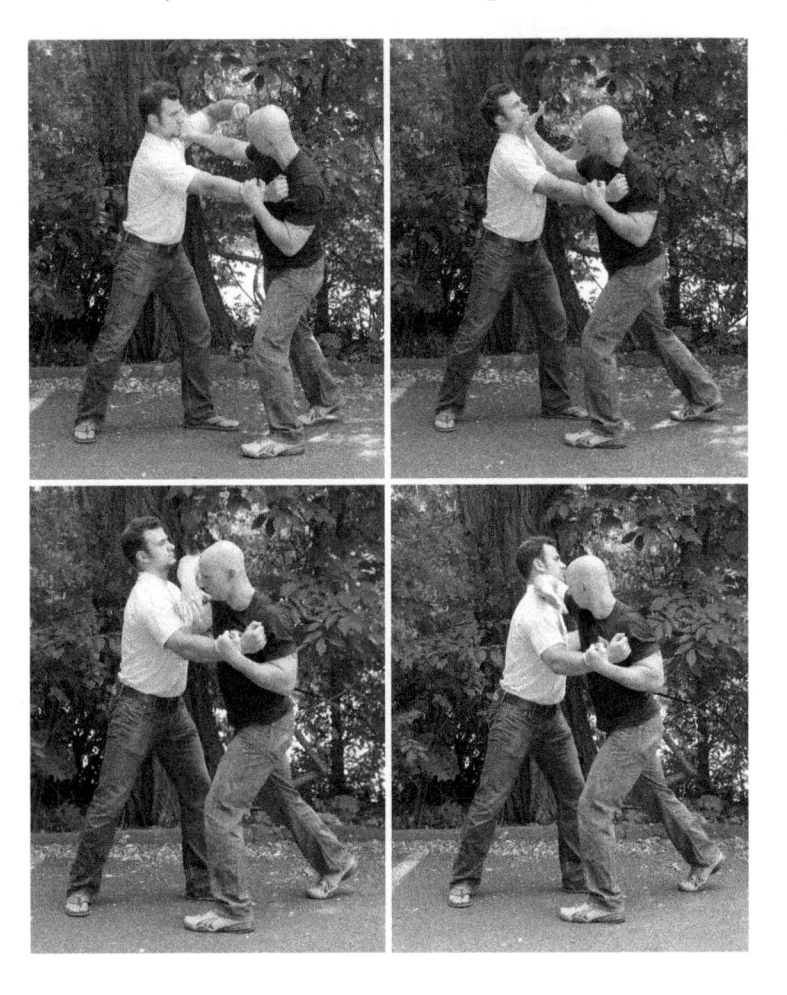

Double punch (haymaker): This defense is against an attacker throwing haymaker punches at you. As the looping punch comes in, perform knifehand chops to the biceps of the assailant. Once you have blocked, immediately counterattack with a knifehand chop to the neck, grabbing behind his head with the same hand and then delivering an Elbow Smash to the face. Now repeat the position and the finishing as we had done in the grab-and-punch attack.

We use this finish on many attacks.

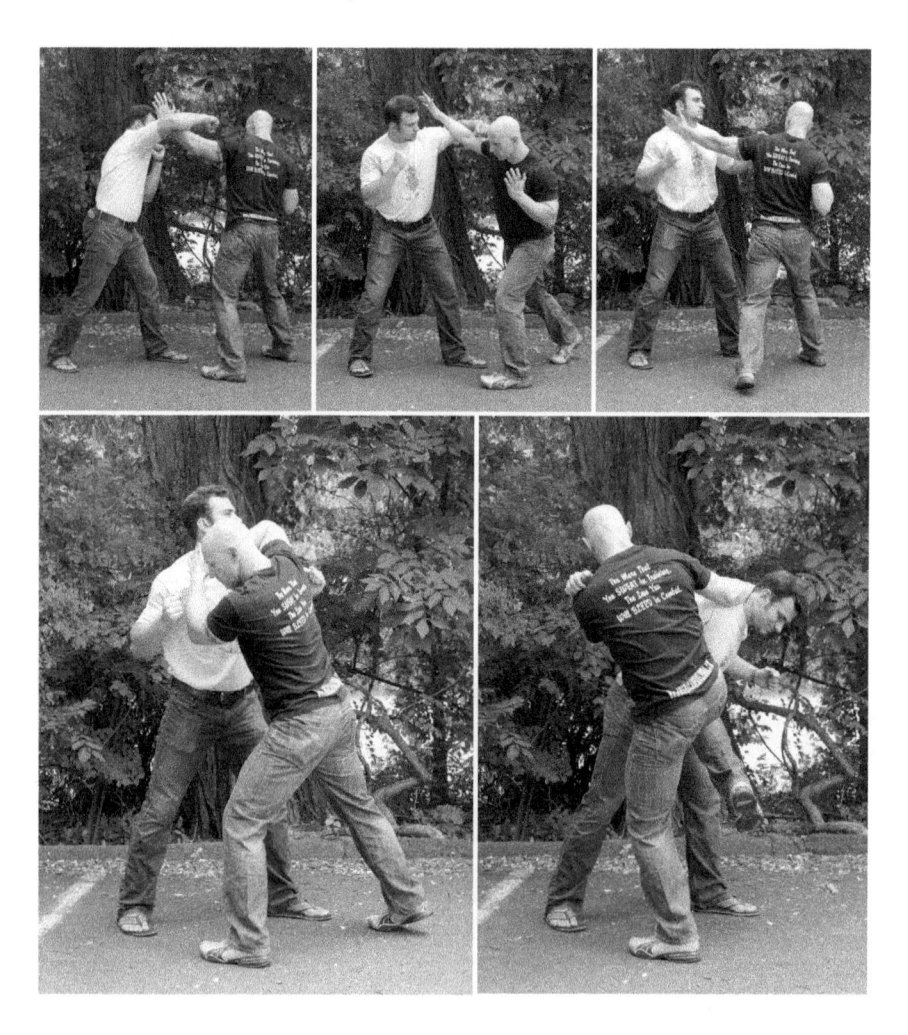

BEAR HUGS

Let's consider who will be attacking you. The chances are that you will be attacked in this manner by a larger, stronger individual who feels that they can overpower you. Just think about it: if you are 6'2" and 225 pounds, it's highly unlikely that a 5'1", 123-pound assailant will attack you in this fashion.

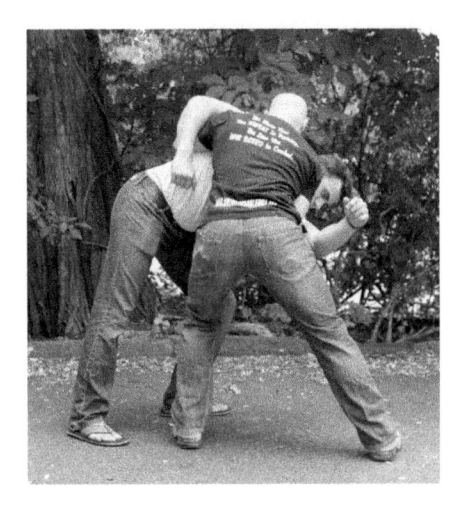

Front bear hug: There are three different situations with the front bear hug attack—entering arms trapped, locked in with the arms trapped, and arms free.

Entering, arms trapped: An assailant steps in to grab you and wraps their arms around you. Step back into a front stance with one leg straight and locked out and the other knee bent as you drive your palms into their hips. Make sure that your thumbs are pressed against your hand so your hands form "flippers." When the attacker pulls you into them harder, go with it and deliver Knee Drives to his/her groin and/or bladder until you are able to free yourself or they fall the ground. You may now execute kicks or a parachute stomp to the downed perpetrator.

Front bear hug, arms free: Both of your hands and your arms are free. You have most likely been lifted off the ground, so you can't use the ground to aid you in your power. No worries, you won't need it to administer a head butt and then cup your hands, clap their ears, and gouge their eyes with your thumbs. As described beforehand, take your thumbs, start at the bridge of the nose, dig your thumbs in and scoop to the outside.

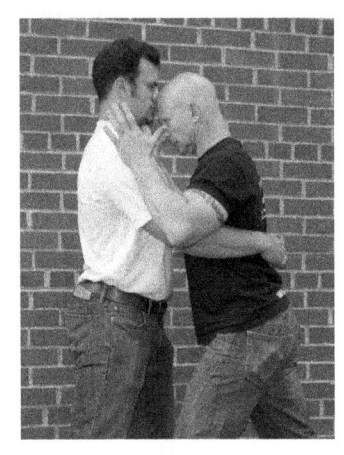

Front Bear hug, arms trapped and tight to you: You may have been caught completely off-guard and your assailant secured a tight Bear Hug over the arms on you and they are crushing you. Begin with a head butt to the nose as you make your hands into fists and press them together, lower your weight, pull your hips back and drive your thumbs into their bladder or groin. If the attacker is a male, grab, twist and pull the groin. If they are a female, strike to the groin and then gain enough space to deliver Knee Drives.

Side bear Scramble: Occurs when you have freed yourself from a position and you employ perpetual motion to move to an advantageous position or escape.

Hug: You get attacked from the side and your arms are trapped. Lower your weight by bending your knees and keeping your back straight. Capture their hands with your hands and stomp their foot, do a side head butt and then a hammerfist Strike to their groin with your hand closest to him. Step behind your outside foot with the foot closest to him and drive your outside arm up into the air as you make a 180-degree pivot with your feet. Maintain a grip on his wrist and kick his knee with a lead leg side kick.

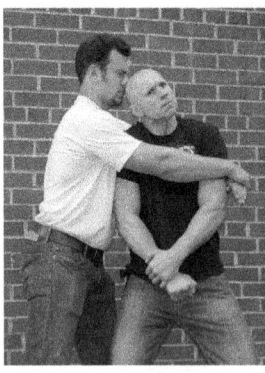

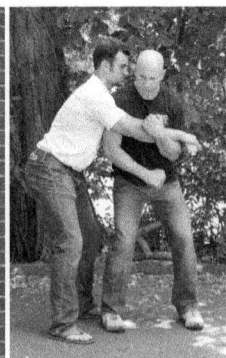

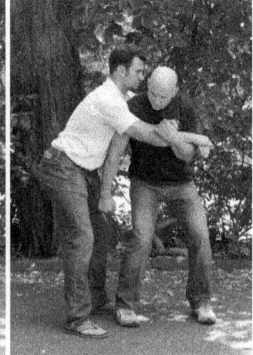

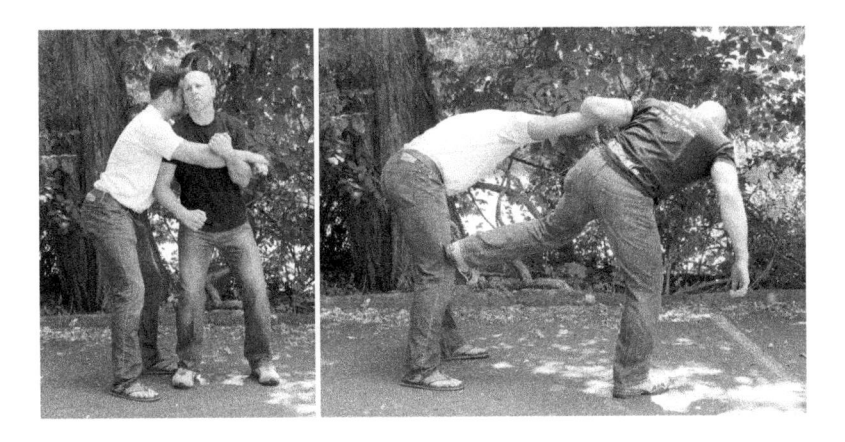

Rear bear hug: You will either be attacked with your arms trapped or free. The Arms free is an easier attack to defend.

Rear bear hug, arms trapped: The defense for this attack is virtually identical to the side bear hug attack, except adding the application of a "butt butt into their groin as part of the loosening-up sequence. The butt butt technique is exactly as it sounds. You drive your butt into their groin.

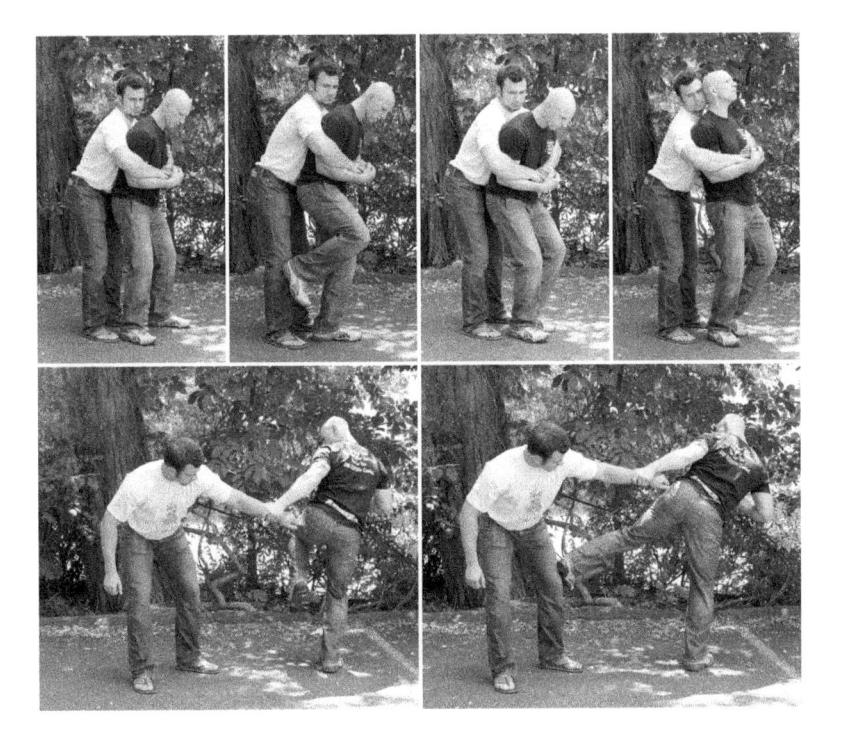

When your arms are free, drop one leg back and deliver one, or a combination of, the following, and double ear slap, cupping your hands as you force the air into their ear canal. Then move to an eye gouge, knees to the groin, or any of the many other finishing techniques. When grabbed, you may also attack their *episternal notch*—the little "hole" at the base of the throat above the collarbone. I like to brace with one hand behind their neck and drive my thumb in and downward. If you simply go straight in, you will not shift the throat cartilage to the side, thus enabling your thumb (or fingers) to get at the sensitive throat. If you have smaller hands, use two fingers to jab the area. My favorite to do is the *thumbs to the carotid*. Grab their neck and place your two thumbs on their carotid artery and jam them into the area with great force. This will send a *shock* through the assailant's body and enable you to deliver kicks, knees, or other strikes to finish them off, affording you your escape.

Kicks

If you are being attacked with kicks by someone who throws them with proficiency, the attacker has probably had some training. Also, a kick, even from an untrained person, is more powerful than a punch. Your legs are much stronger than your arms. This is fact.

Also remember that your movement and blocking drills will come in handy when facing a kick attack.

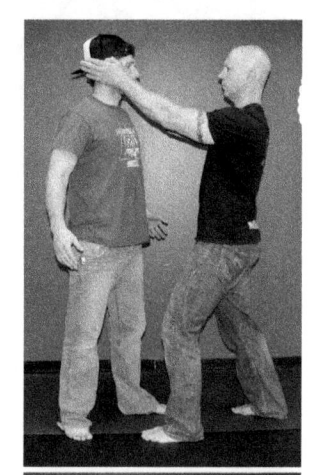

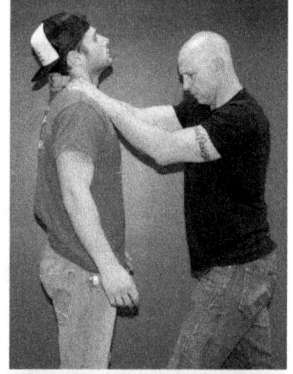

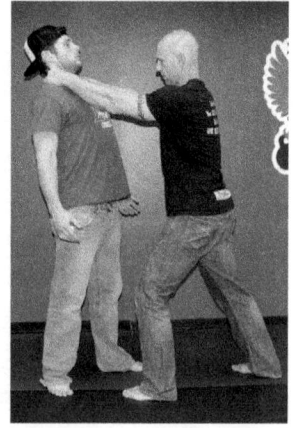

Front kick attack: If you are attacked with a front kick, you will either have a lot of room or very little. For example, a lot of room would be in a parking lot. A little room would be in a parking lot between two cars.

Front kick, a lot of room: Use your box step and deliver a side kick to the back of their knee with your right foot and then cut-kick their same leg with your left. Next, side-kick their other leg with your left foot before placing it down. Now, either deliver elbow strikes to their head or apply a standing rear naked choke.

Front kick, no room: You will need to parry their foot to the side with your hands. We normally don't drop our hands this far down, but in some instances, you will need to take chances to neutralize the most imminent attack. All else is identical to the aforementioned defense, minus the first kick.

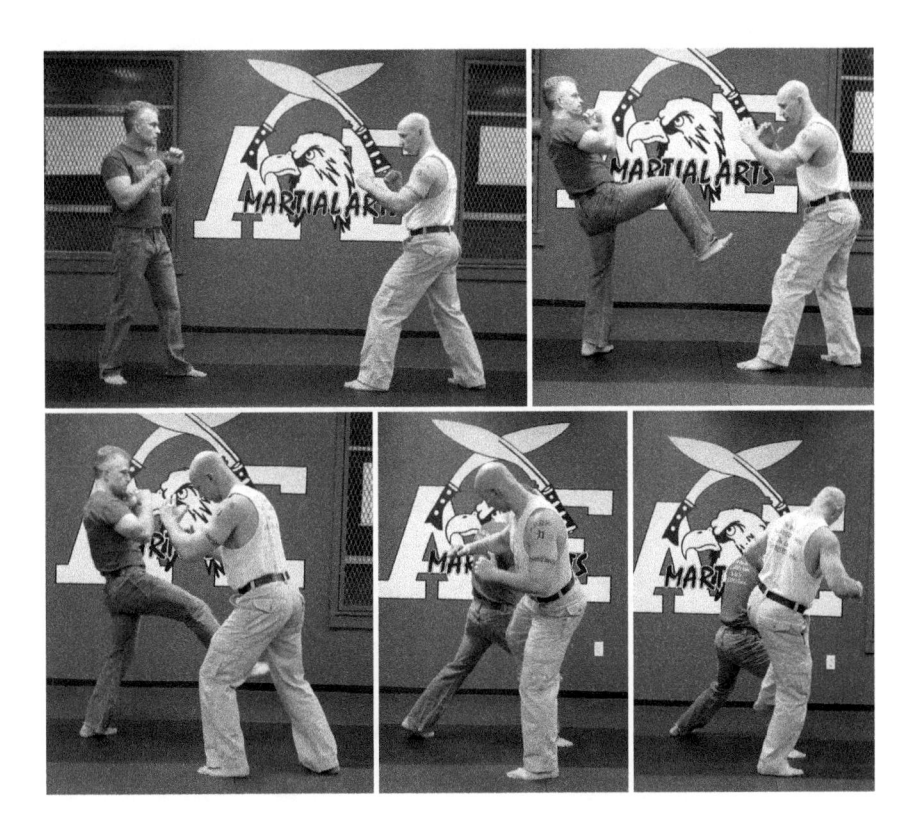

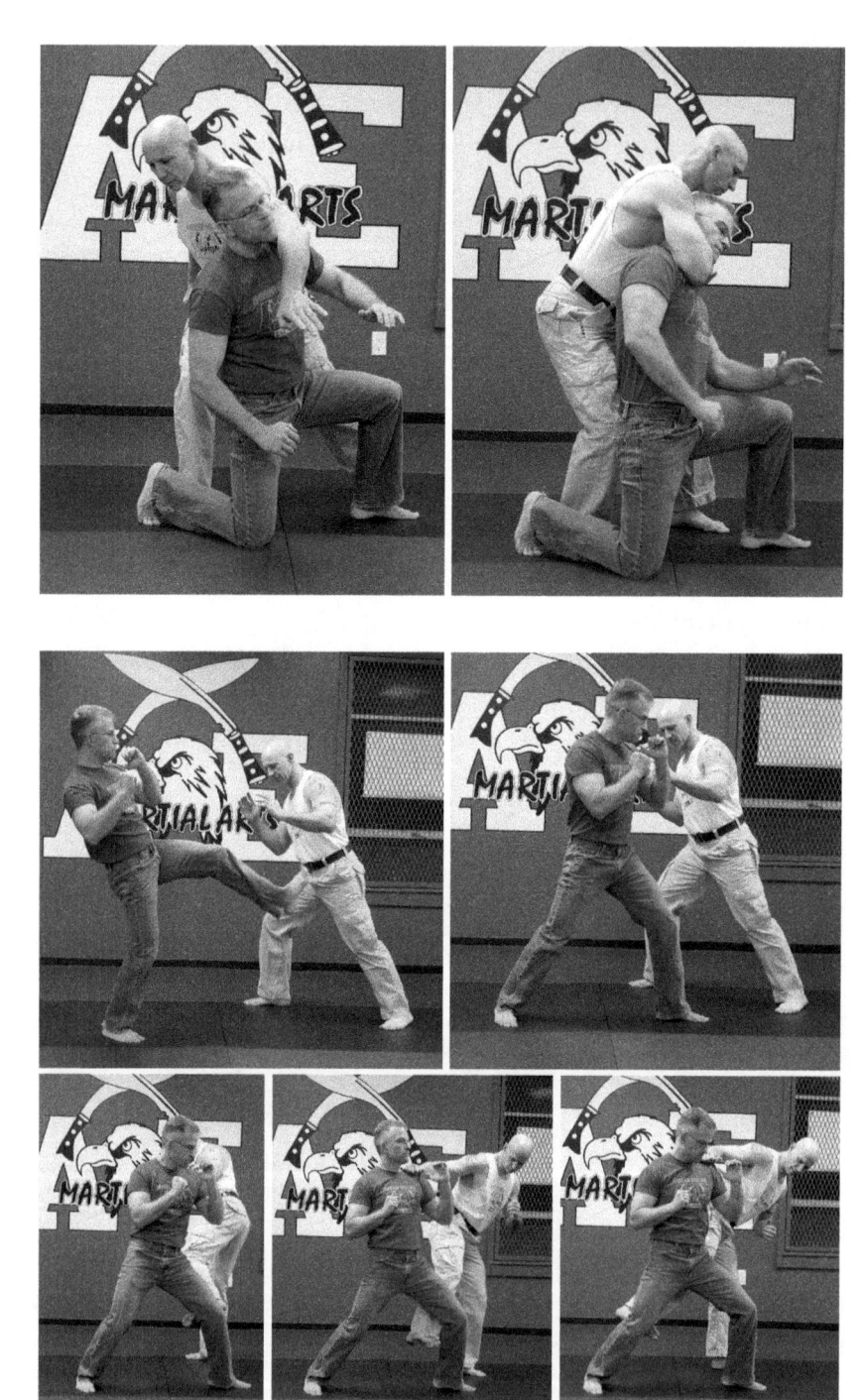

Roundhouse kick attack: The most dangerous part of this kick is the foot. A well-placed roundhouse kick is like a powerful whip. If you get hit in the head, groin, or ribs, the results can be devastating. It's important to get inside the kick and cut the power off at the knee. Step in with your hands up, elbows directed into their leg as you perform a combination block/strike. Next, you will grab their leg and secure the python lock (figure 4) on their leg, kick them in the groin, and take them down by lifting the captured leg and sweeping the remaining leg. Maintaining your hold on their leg, it's now time to employ the Italian gas pedal. [44]

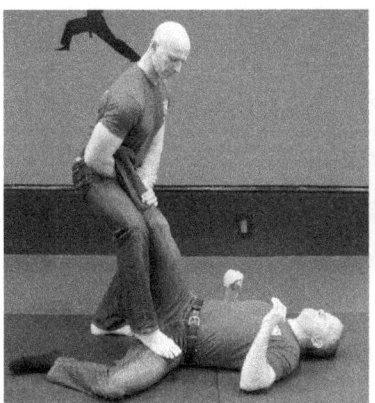

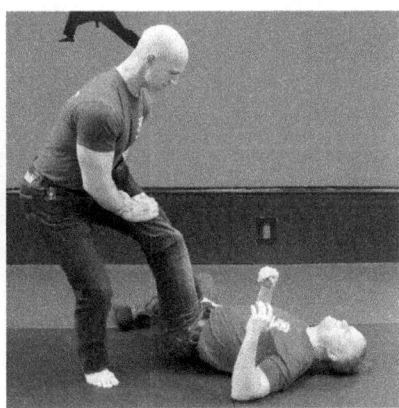

Cut kick attack: As we are aware from our training, a cut kick is a particularly devastating kick. Following are some of the most effective streetwise methods to defend yourself from this attack.

Kick stop: If you are being attacked by the right leg, pick up your left foot and push-kick the attacker anywhere between the knee and the hip.

Quick kick: Once their attack is thrown with the right leg, quickly switch your hips, bringing your left leg to the back. Immediately "bounce" your foot off of the floor and deliver a counterkick to the back of theirs.

---

[44] Italian gas pedal; While your opponent is supine and you are standing above them with one of their legs in a python (figure 4). Grip, take your foot closest to their groin and stomp down on it as you pull up on their leg.

Leg check: As the right kick comes at you, lift your lead leg and angle your knee or upper shin toward the oncoming kick. You want to have your knee slightly pointed toward the outside of your foot on approximately a 15- to 20- degree angle. Step inside and implement your counterattack.

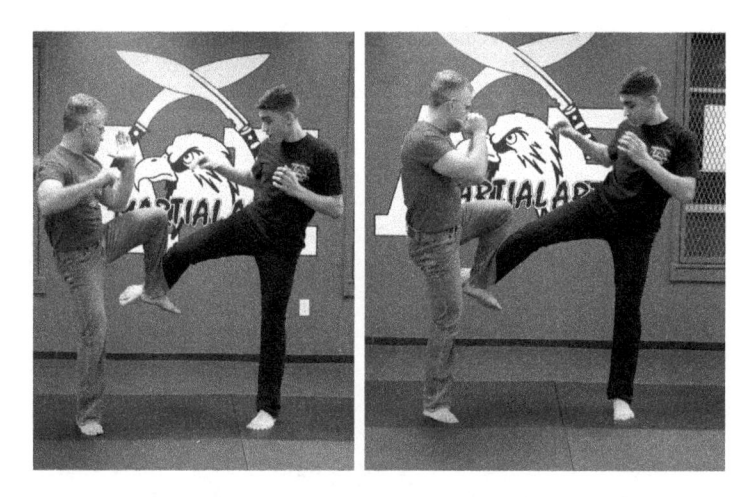

Kick stop: Since we know that all techniques start at the hip, we will focus our attack here. If the opponent starts to throw a kick, or if you believe that they are, bring your corresponding leg up quickly with your leg straight and "shove" your foot into any spot from the top of their knee to their hip. Stopping the kick at its origin. Move forward with your counterattack.

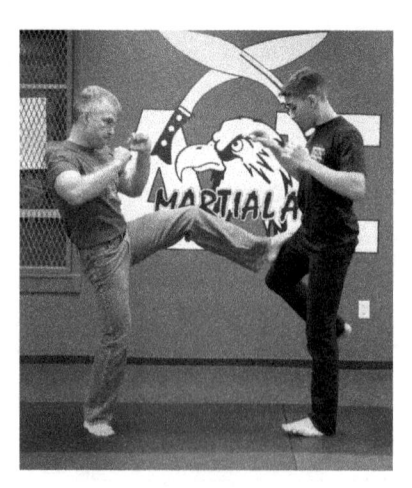

Grabbed leg: So you now have become an accomplished kicker and you train to throw your kicks in a confrontation. Fine, but what do you do if your leg gets grabbed? Sprawling is one excellent option, but what if your leg is up too high? What can we do first? If your leg gets grabbed, you opponent's both hands will be occupied, leaving his face and head open for a counterattack. Instead of moving away from him, launch yourself toward him and grab the back of his neck with one hand while delivering elbows to their face and head. Once you have loosened them up, drive your knees into their groin and bladder until you are free or they are incapacitated.

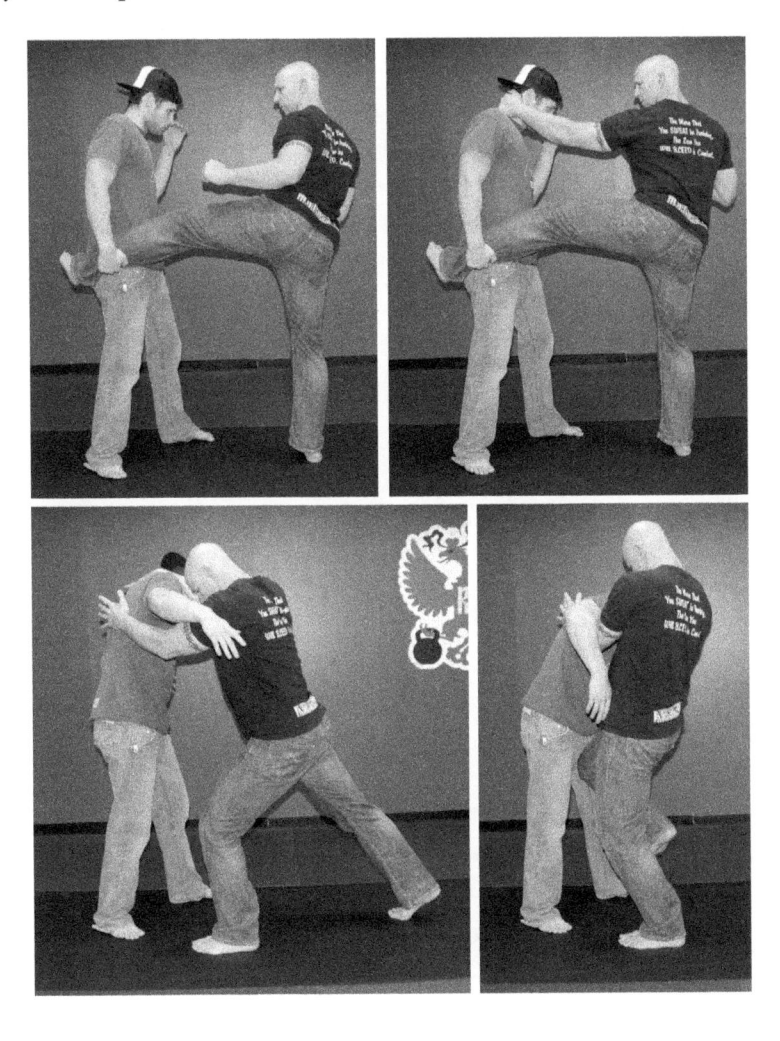

Ground Pins

Before we discuss ground techniques, you must consider how you got there. Were you taken or knocked down? Were you hit with a strike that caused you to fall? Were you simply lying there and got caught by surprise? You may need some recovery time to gather your wits. This may entail hugging the attacker until your head clears. We will focus on the worst of the scenarios: your assailant has you in a full mount with either your arms pinned or choking you.

Arms pinned: You are in the full mount, and your assailant has your wrists both pinned against the floor. There are several movements that must be done simultaneously to be successful. Shoot your hands off to the side as a bridge toward the ceiling and drive your right knee into their coccyx bone. Trap their left arm with your right, bridge again, and roll to your right while pushing on their ribs with your left hand to add power to your move. It is time to finish the maneuver. You will be in their guard, or at least between their legs and on top of them. Place your forearms on their abdomen and levy punches to their chin and elbows and their thighs until their legs open. Now you smash the groin.

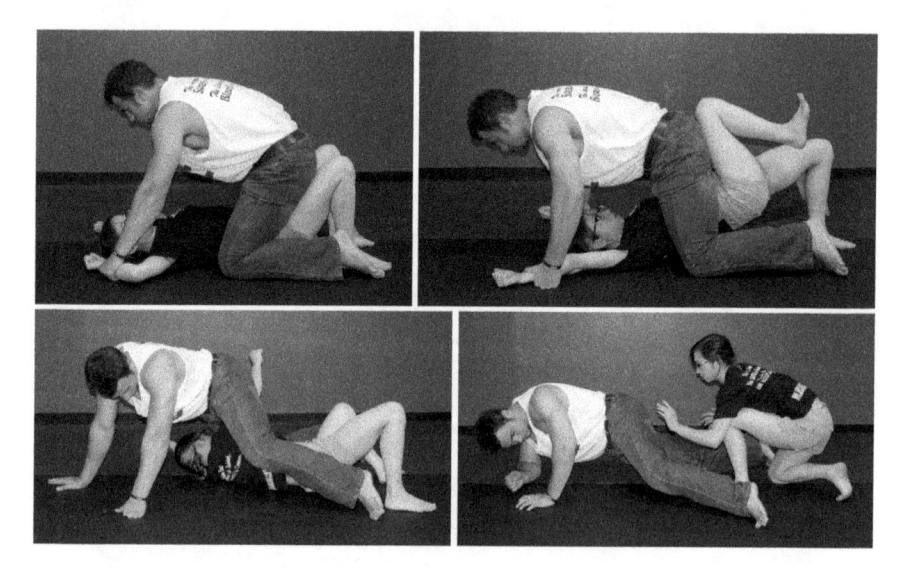

Choking: You are in the same position as you were in the previous move, except that the attacker is choking you while sitting on your chest. You do not have much time. The first action will be to punch your attacker's ribs and then finger-jab them in the eyes. This is followed by a double knifehand chop directed to the assailant's elbow pits. After the chop, clamp their left hand to your chest with your right hand. Strike them in the throat with a left-hand scissor punch as you perform a bridge pop and roll to your right. Do the same finish technique as you did for the arms-pinned defense.

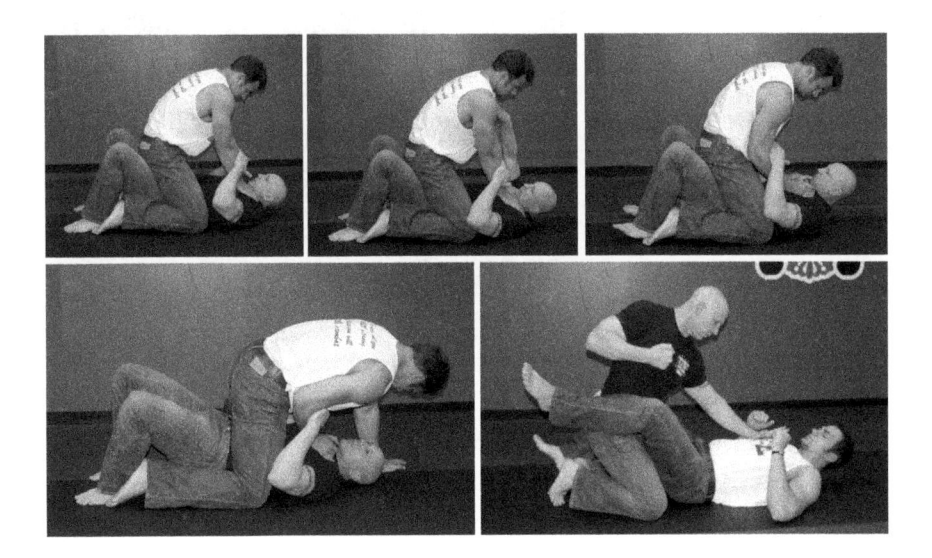

Hair Grab

I personally have the world's best defense for the hair grab: my head is completely shaved. So unless you are sporting the same hairstyle, you'll need to learn a defense for this attack. Another important tidbit to note: rapists love ponytails. Rapists consider them handles and use them to grab and control women.

Front hair grab: The assailant facing you grabs a fistful of hair with their left hand. They will tend to grab and twist, yielding a tighter grip and then pulling you forward and down. Place both your hands on top their left hand and step into them. As you step in with your left foot, deliver a knifehand chop to their biceps insertion with your left hand while maintaining the grip on the hand on your head with your right. After the chop, smash them in the face with your elbow as you pull their hand in the opposite direction. Think of the movement as if you were yawning and stretching, making your chest big—only, doing this very quickly. Grab them by the back of the neck, thread your hand under their arm, and give them knee drives until they drop, just as we have done to finish several other defensive tactics.

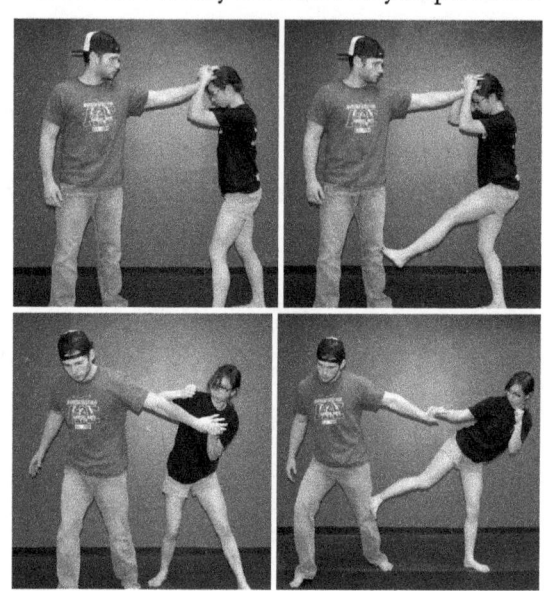

Rear hair grab: Once you are attacked from behind with a hair grab, place both of your hands on their grabbing hand and move backward quickly into them as they pull. They will be expecting you to pull away, so this will disrupt their balance and buy you some time. As you are moving backward, kick and stomp their shins and feet. This may free you. If not, suppose that they have grabbed you with their right hand, step with your left backward, and bend at the waste as you snap their hand down. Once they are bent over, pretend as if it is fourth and long and deliver a punt to their face. For you non-football fans, simply kick them in the face with an upward front snap kick.

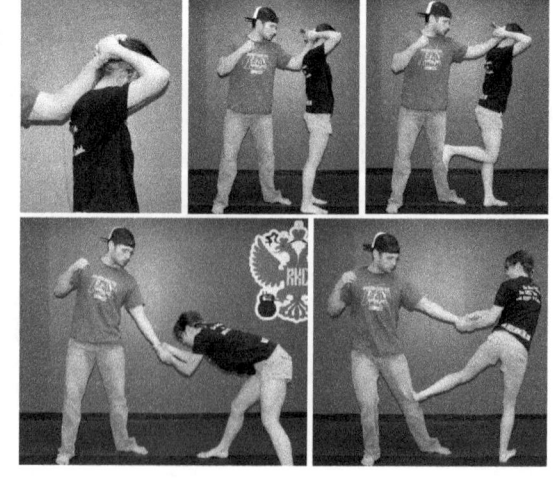

Double Lapel Grab

On this attack, it's important to note that both of your attacker's hands are compromised. He probably thinks that you won't resist, and he wants something from you. This is an advantage for you. A disadvantage in this situation is if there are multiple attackers—one grabbing you and the other committing some other sort of act against you. We'll address the single attacker defenses here and the multiple attackers at the end of this chapter.

Chop defense: Once your lapels have been grabbed, palm-heel-strike the assailant in the nose, double-clap their ears, rise up on your toes, and drop your weight as you do a double-knifehand chop downward on the bend in their elbows. Finish them with a head butt to the nose and knee drives to their groin and bladder. Push them away and front-kick them in the nearest, most vulnerable available target.

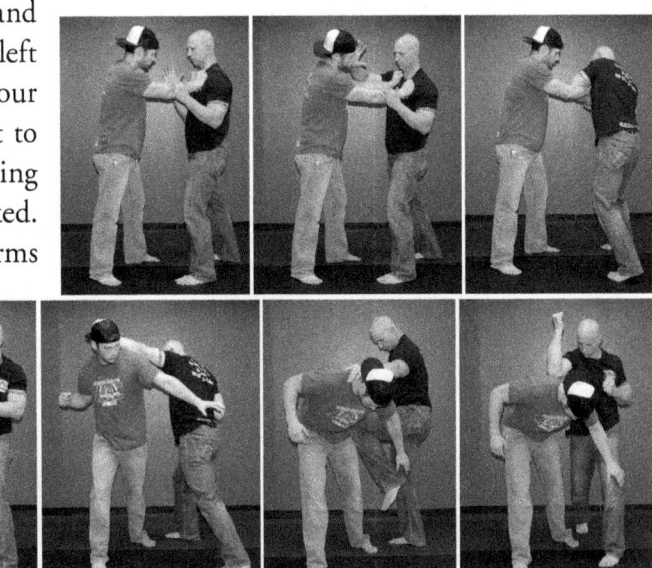

Thread defense: Begin your defense again with the palm heel strike to the nose. If you strike with your right hand, thread your left under their wrist. Pressure down on their right wrist with your left elbow and position your left hand so that your fingers are facing upward and the back of your hand is against their left wrist. Twist your hips from right to left while keeping your arms locked. Trap both his arms with one hand. This position is transitory, so start to strike immediately, directing your blows to their temple, floating ribs, and peroneal nerve.

Tackle

A tackle is generally a rage attack, and the attacker is filled with fury as they rush you. The negative for you is they are committed to the move and the direction, and they are coming at you hard.

This is also to your advantage; they are unable to change directions easily when attacking in this fashion. There are three basic options for defense: the Front kick, knee drive, or a redirect.

Front kick: You need to be very confident and possess a very powerful and quick front kick to pull this one off. As they charge, stand your ground and time your full front kick (off of the back leg) to land as they get into range. It's risky, but if you're good at the front kick, your results will be favorable, and the damage that you cause is debilitating.

Knee drive with side step: When they are charging at you, wait until the last possible second and hop to the side and deliver a round knee to their midsection and a knifehand chop to their neck.

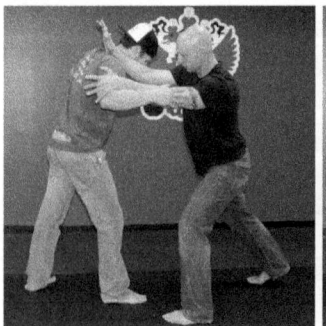

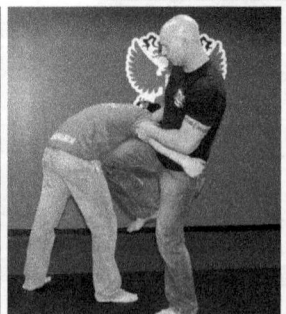

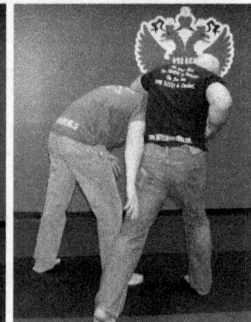

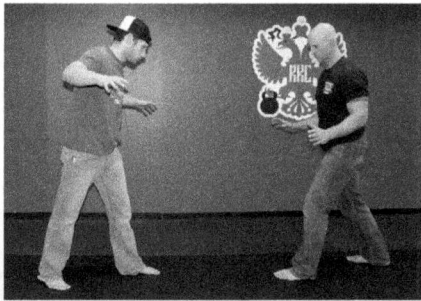

Redirect: This is another timing-based defense. Just before they reach you, axehand-strike them to the side of the neck or head with your right hand and thread under their outstretched left arm. Perform a 180-degree step with your right foot as you redirect their head downward and toward their right knee as you lift up your left arm, thus turning them so they fall onto their back where you were previously standing. Do what is necessary to finish them. Kicks to their head and body, or use your parachute stomp to end it.

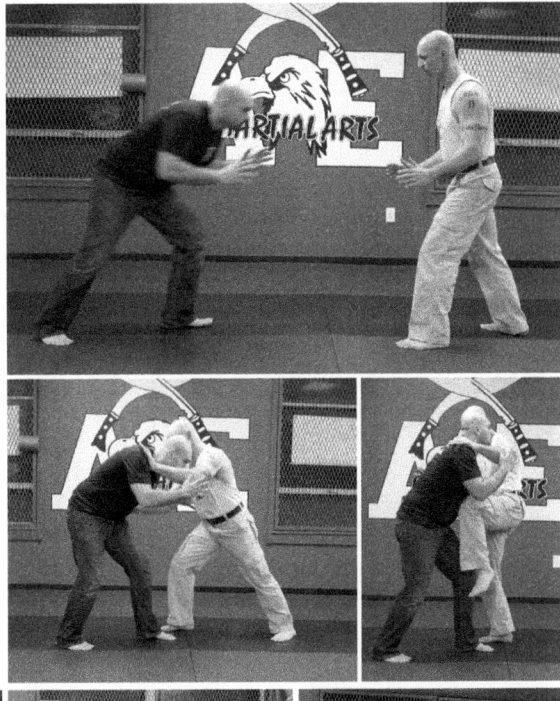

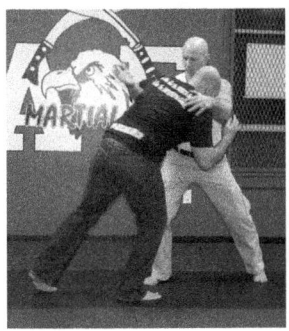

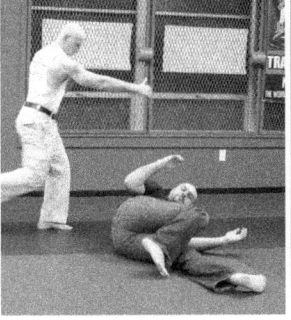

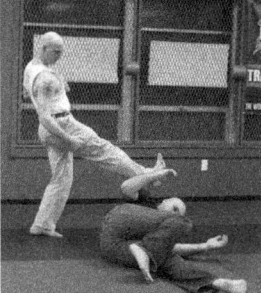

From the Ground (Knocked Down)

If you fall or get knocked to the ground, assume the side position where up on your elbow with only one side on the ground, not lying on your back. This position has great advantages for fighting, other than the fact that you are on the ground and could easily sustain an injury from broken glass, nails, sticks, etc., that may be on the ground. However, if you are here, you need to be able to defend and move from this position. I generally mix the following defenses together, changing from one defense to another. I change sides and circle to throw off the attacker.

Upkicks: This was seen a great deal in MMA. I would not rely on this for the street, though: your groin is open. In MMA, the groin is an illegal target area. In the street, there is no such thing. Knowing this, upkicks are still acceptable to mix into your defenses, provided you deliver a side kick the perpetrator's face as you rise up on the non-kicking foot and balance yourself on your elbow and the hand of the side of the kicking foot.

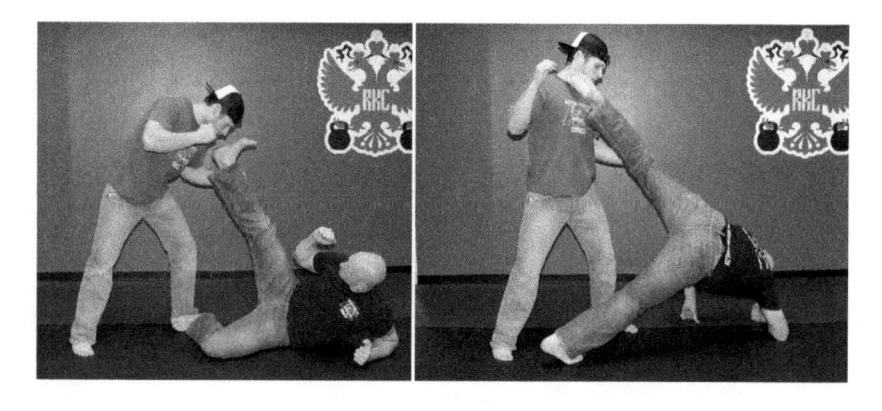

Circle and kick: While propped up on your elbow and on your side, rotate and follow your attacker as they try to circle to your back. You may also flip to your other side by switching which hip is on the ground. As you implement a barrage of kicks to their knees, move into them and "chase" them down kicking and launching yourself aggressively at them.

Circle and scissors sweep takedown: You are on the ground and on your side, you're kicking away at his legs, and either he manages to step in, or you close the distance. If his left leg is forward, place your right foot on top of his left and your left foot behind his left knee. Use your hips, not your legs, to turn toward him rotating 180 degrees. This will knock him to the ground facefirst. To keep things simple, roll on top of him and take his back or stand up and kick his ribs and head.

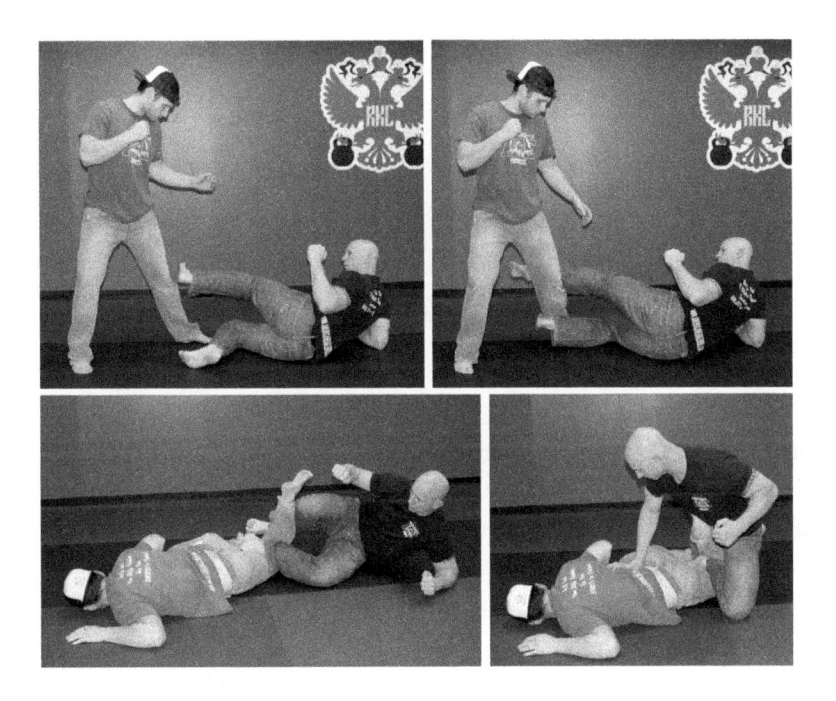

Multiple Attackers

There is an infinite number of possible multiple-attacker situations that you may be faced with. It would be virtually impossible to even attempt to address them all. As with all the other described maneuvers, focus on the principles and apply them to the situation at hand.

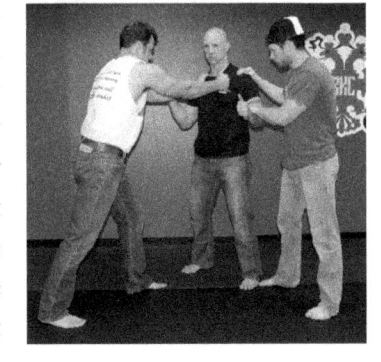

One in the front and the other on the side: If you are confronted with one assailant grabbing you in a double-lapel attack and the other on your right, grabbing you by the back of your shoulder and chest from the side, direct a side elbow with your right to the face of the attacker on the side. With the same hand, smash the other opponent in the face and then strike them with your right knee to the groin; and without placing your foot down, direct a stomp to the side attacker's inside knee with the same foot. It's catch as catch can at this point. Move and do whatever is necessary to provide yourself an escape.

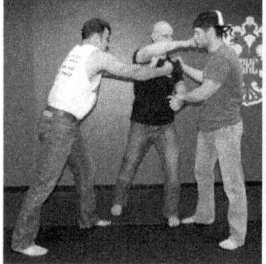

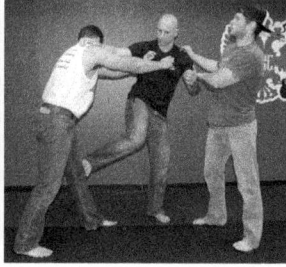

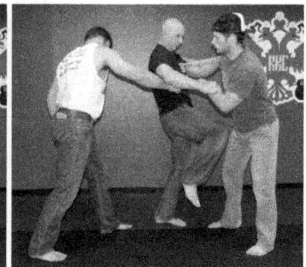

One assailant on either side: Two guys grab you, one on each arm, and they are trying to take you someplace against your will. Resist at first for a short time and then go with it, but running ahead of them. As they strive to catch up to you, jam on the brakes and stop dead in your tracks and you punch both fists straight down. This will cause their grips to release you. It's now time to unleash a hellish onslaught of kicks, stomps and strikes and make your escape.

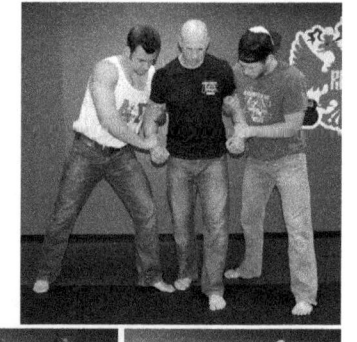

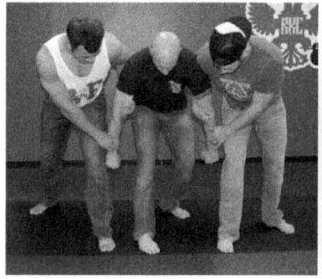

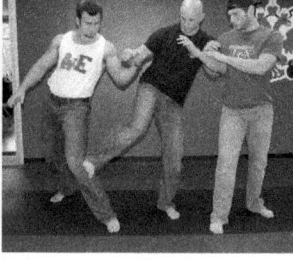

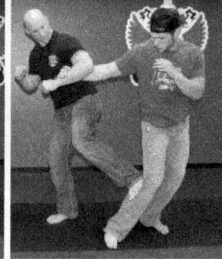

BASEBALL BAT AND CLUB

Blunt, accessible, and extremely lethal, the ends of a bat or club are the business parts. There are techniques using other sections of these weapons, but for the most part, you will be faced with an instrument being swung at you, even if the assailant has been trained. Back in the 1980s and 1990s, police were issued and trained in the use of the PR24, which is essentially a Tonfa. This was a club with a handle on it that was supposed to revolutionize policing and crowd control. All the departments were issued the PR24 (Tonfas), their billy clubs discarded, they were trained for hours on end on how to swing and block with them.

Well, after a few years, it was soon discovered that the police were simply flipping the PR24 over and either using the handle like you would a hammer head or simply using it like a regular club. Bottom line: no more PR24's. Man, I wish I had that contract for the furnishing of the PR24's and the administration of the training. I'd be retired! So the point that I'm trying to get across is that under stress, people will only effectively use gross motor movements. Swinging a bat or a club is a gross motor movement. Fancy movements are not. As a general rule, you will be attacked with either a side-to-side, an overhead (downward strike), or an attack somewhere in between.

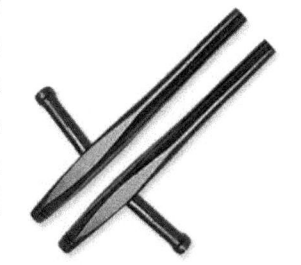

Side to side: If the attacker swings a bat with two hands as if they are Derek Jeter, you need to avoid the business end. If you get hit with any part of the bat from the sweet spot[45] to the end of the barrel, you will sustain damage. You have two choices here, either move in quickly with a lunge step as the bat is drawn back or fade back out of the way and lunge in after the barrel has passed the center of your body. Once it has passed, the dangerous part will not be a danger until a backswing is performed. So, to do the aggressive step in defense, lunge at the opponent with both hands up at a 90-degree angle with your fingertips facing up.

---

[45] The sweet spot of a bat is the area located approximately 5 to 7 inches from the end of the barrel.

Smash into him with both of your arms and grab the bat by lopping one arm over it as you axehand his head with the other and executing knee drives. For the fade back and then attack, do as described above, and once the tip of the barrel is past your midline, lunge at him, and do the same finishing technique as before.

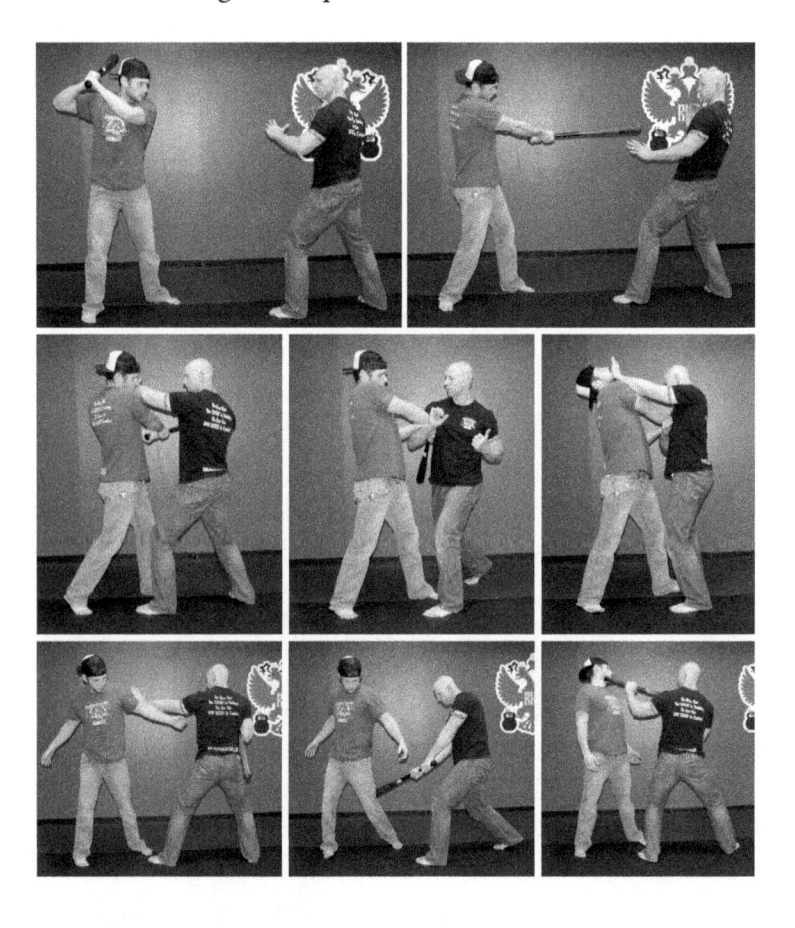

Overhead: Pick a side and use lateral movement and parry with the inside hand as you step. Take that same hand and wrap up your arm around both of his as you palm-heel-strike him in the face with the other hand. Kick, knee, and stomp and deliver more palm heel strikes until you are able to secure the weapon and incapacitate the attacker. If you are being attacked on an angle, step to the side that the attack emanates from, not where it's going.

If it's a one-armed attack with a club, either move to the outside or the inside. As a general rule it's always better to move to the outside: it gives you a better position, and your opponent less options for counterattack. However, you are not always afforded that luxury, and you may be forced to step inside due to the environment, or maybe a person you are with is in the way.

Outside step: If you are attacked with a right overhead or angled-downward attack, step inward on a forty-five-degree angle with your left, perform a high block with your right and your wrist meeting his.

With your left hand, do a downward chop (thumb first) at the bend in the assailant's elbow. Shoot your left hand across, locking your left hand onto your right forearm, thus creating a figure four lock. Continue the step inward with your right foot and bow in a semicircle to your left. This will put a great deal of stress on their shoulder and elbow and cause them to fall to the ground. Disarm them and render them helpless with kicks and stomps.

Inside step: If the attack is with the right hand, step in with your left foot and execute a left high block. Do a thumb-down knifehand chop with your right hand and thread your right hand through to your left forearm, locking in a figure 4. Step with right foot and pivot toward your left bowing in that same direction, taking them to the ground. Finish them as detailed above.

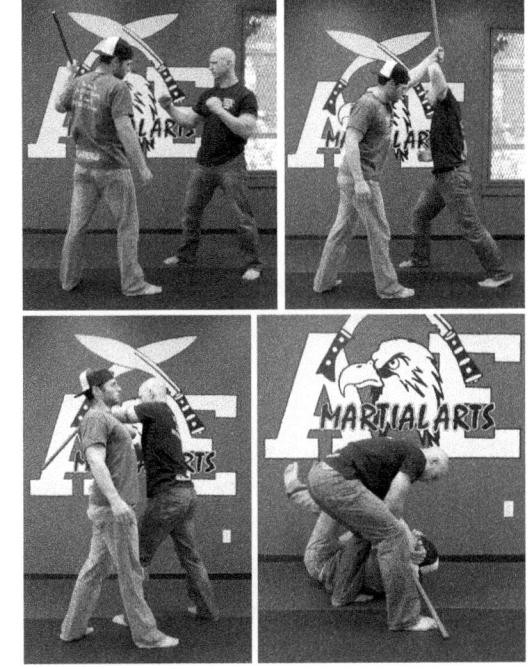

Knife

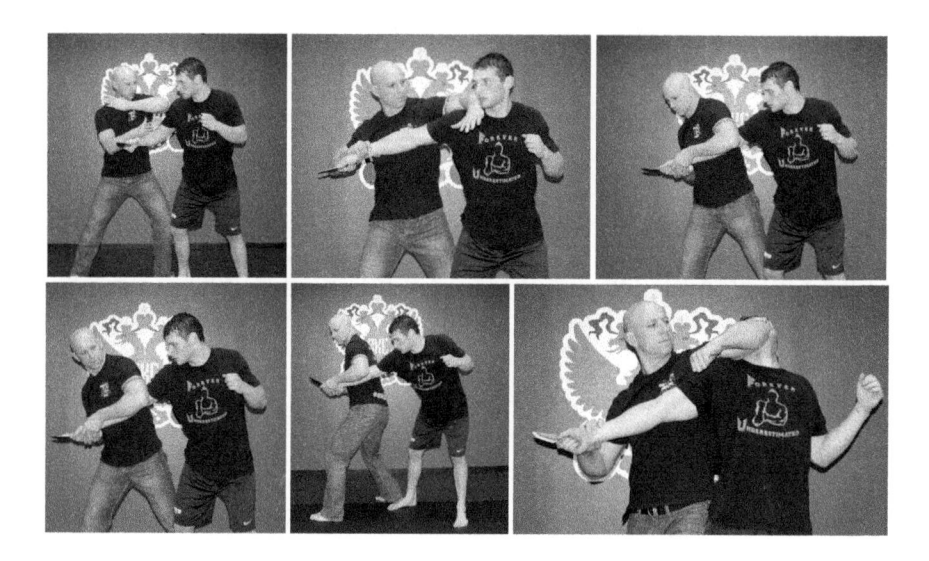

Know this: If you are attacked with a knife, you will be cut. Knives are very accessible, everyone has them. Heck, you used to get a free set of steak knives when you filled your tank with gas back in the day! Statistics demonstrate that the percentages are higher from deaths by stabbing than deaths shooting. Imagine that! You have a better chance surviving a gun attack than you do a knife attack. So, not only are knives more accessible than guns, but they are more lethal. You had better know your way around a knife.

Throat: If you find yourself with a knife to your throat, consider yourself dead and every second that you are breathing is extra time on earth. On the good side, if they wanted you dead, you would be dead already. Lucky for you they want something from you first. Once they have that, though, you are done. You had better act quickly. Get space between your throat and the blade; this may entail sustaining a cut on your hand, but that's quite a bit better than getting one on your throat!

Front of the throat: Let's presume that the attacker has the knife up against your throat, and the knife is in their right hand with the knife point facing toward your left. Put your hands up in the air, placing your right hand slightly higher, and shake them. This will draw their attention to the right hand and away from the left. This is important because you will grab his knife hand with your left. This is the gutsy part: you don't pull away from the blade on your throat. It's against all your natural instincts, but if you shy away from the blade, you'll rob yourself of much-needed room when you need to execute your defense. You need to perform several motions simultaneously. Rip your head backward and turn your right shoulder forward and you grab his blade hand with your left hand.

You may have to grab the knife, not just the hand. As you do these movements, slap the assailant with your right hand and then with the back hammerfist, smash them in the face. Take control of his knife hand with both of your hands, placing your thumbs on the back of the hand and grabbing their hand with your fingers, thus placing them in a wrist lock. Step forward with your right foot and snap their arm to the left over your right hip and kick their knee with a mule kick. Secure the weapon and finish them with any of the variety of methods.

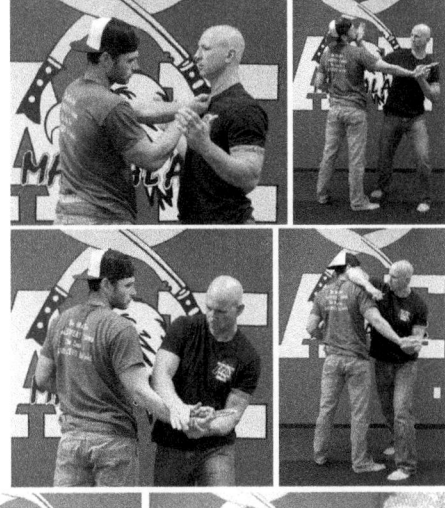

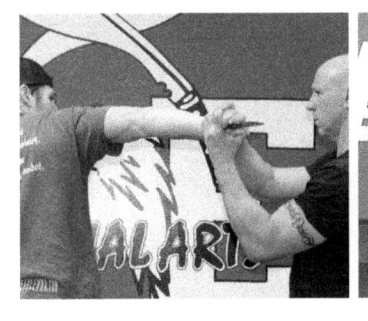

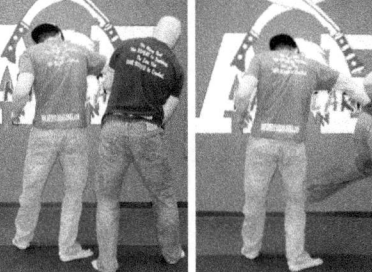

Knife on the throat from behind: You have a knife to your throat with the attacker behind you. Let's make it even more interesting: he has your arm jacked up behind you. His right hand has the knife, and his left hand is controlling your left. Rip your head backward as hard and fast are you as able as you grab his knife hand with your right. Step behind your right foot with your left and direct his knife into his chest or abdomen. Do what is necessary to secure your escape.

Menacing: If you are approached by a knife-wielding attacker, it will be in one of two manners. They will be moving a little or moving a lot. It makes no difference what the attack is, and overhead, a thrust, a slash—it simply doesn't matter; only the movement matters. Look, this is *not* the movies. You are not going to simply grab the knife, flip the guy around, and throw him through a wall. It won't happen like that.

Here's how it will really go down. The rule of thumb here is, if they move a little, you move a lot. If they move a lot, you move a little. Abide by this axiom, and you will prevail. When it comes to fighting an attacker with a knife, boot him. Read on to see how...

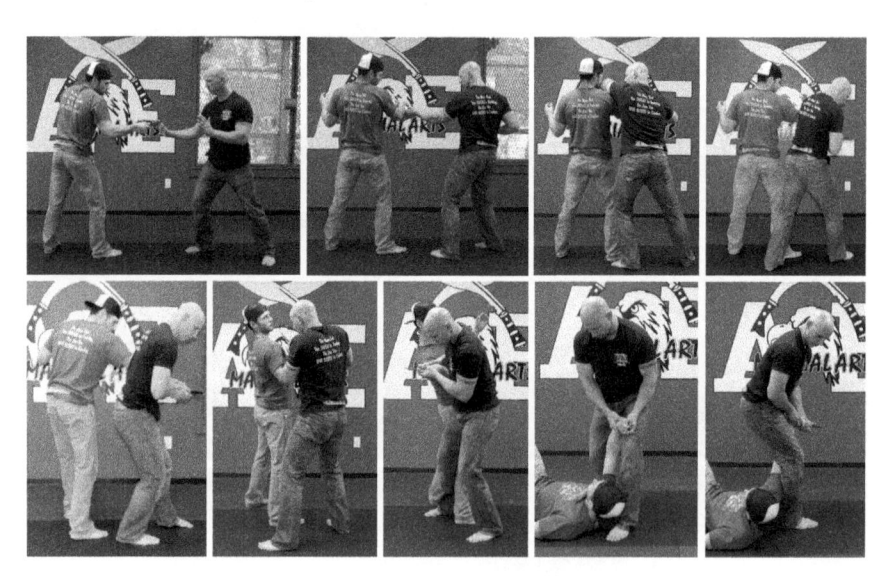

Moving a little: Suppose your attacker is only moving a little. Meaning they are standing between you and your escape, menacing, and preventing you from leaving. As the rule goes, you need to move a lot. So launch your attack with the big boot (lunging front kick) directed toward their center mass. Generally, they will be holding the knife out in front and somewhere in the center of their body. The chances are good that if your kick is directed to the center, you will kick the knife. Whether or not you kick the knife is inconsequential, because you will drive them back and levy axehand chops to the arm and wrist of their knife hand. You will next secure the knife hand and deliver an elbow smash to their face as you pull on the knife arm extending them and adding additional power to your strike. If the weapon hasn't flown out of their hand at this point, it's now time to secure the knife and administer any of a number of finishing sequences.

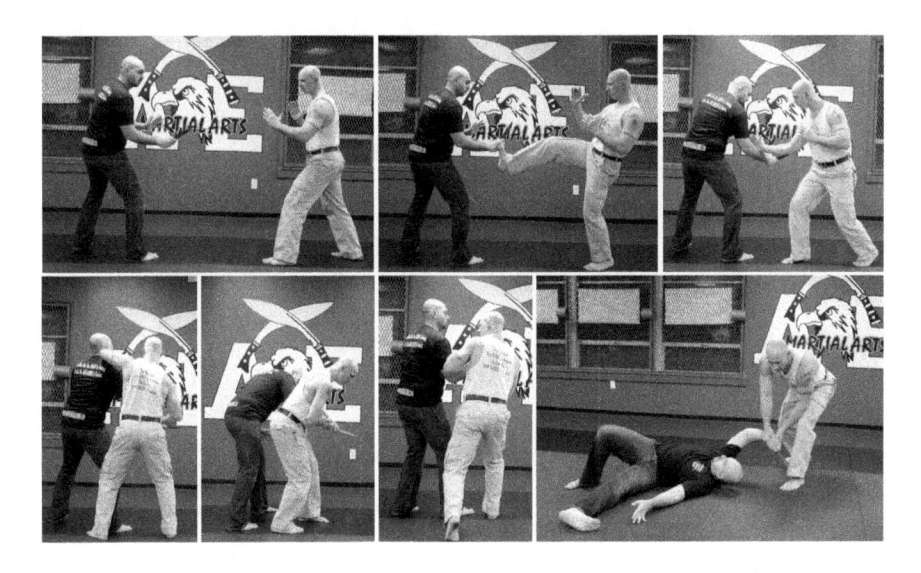

Moving a lot: You are faced with an aggressive assailant who is coming at you fast, thus moving a lot, you will need to move very little and employ impeccable timing. As with the moving a little attack, the type of attack with the knife does not matter—overhead, thrusting, slashing or flicking. When you are charged, jump to the side at the last possible moment and deliver a side kick to their knee, driving it to the floor and forcing them to collapse to the ground. Follow this move by hacking their knife arm with downward axehand chops. If these movements do not cause the knife to be dropped, grab the knife hand and perform any of a number of wrist locks, securing the weapon and incapacitating the attacker. Finish with kicks, stomps, and/or the parachute stomp. It's important not to stop until you are sure that he is incapacitated. He may have another weapon on him. Don't leave that to chance.

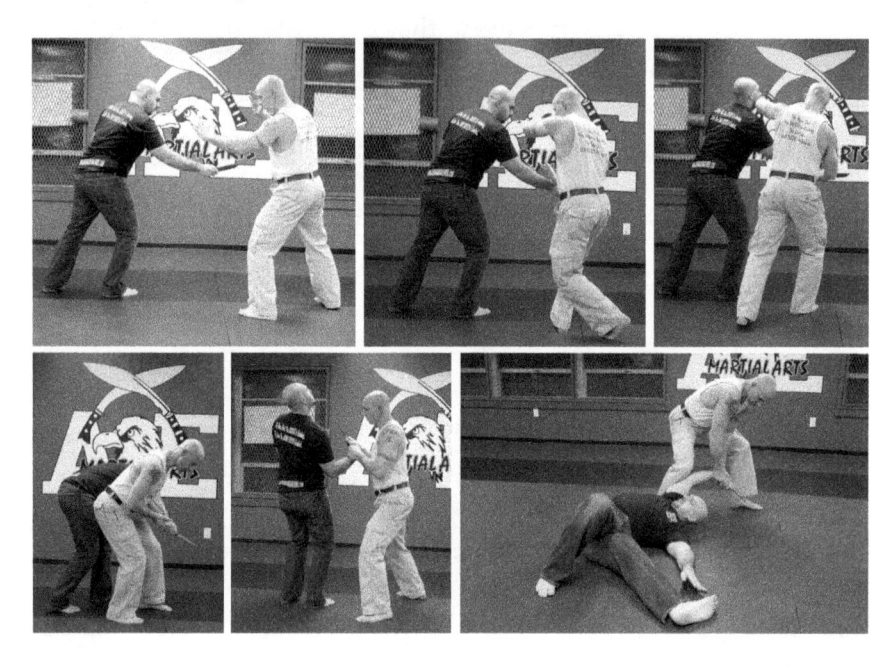

Gun

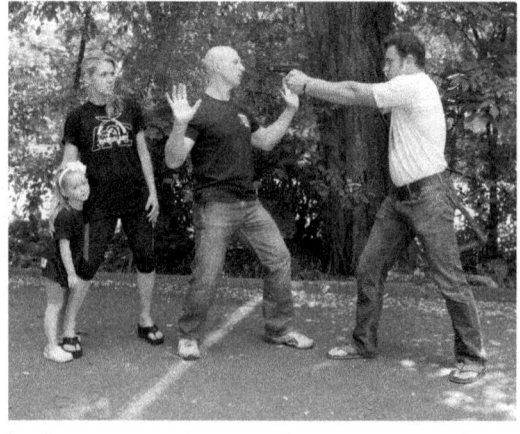

There are many things to consider when being on the wrong end of a gun. Both a fool and a coward can pull a trigger, so there is not much skill needed at the point blank range—just a willingness to harm. If an assailant is 5 to 10 feet away from you with their gun pointed at you, it's a tough call; you'll be better suited to get them to come closer to you. As with the knife, consider yourself dead and living on borrowed time when staring down the barrel of a gun. You have to understand the mind-set of the gun-wielding assailant. They feel in control and are empowered by having this gun in their hand. They are in charge. They are the aggressor.

To draw them in, put your hands up and take small steps backward, many times, this will prompt them to move toward you, generally with larger, more aggressive steps. This will bring them closer to you and within a better striking range. If none of this works, you will need to move. Move to the side and in toward them. If you have to take a chance, so be it. Many times you can get them to miss or their gun may misfire. Guns take care to maintain good working condition. Most thugs don't spend the time to clean and make sure their weapon is in good repair.

Remember who you are dealing with. They are most likely not going to be a professional hit man. If they are, you did something to someone that you shouldn't have. If a true professional wants you dead, you won't even know it happened.

If you are attacked by a sideways gun-holding moron, they have no idea what they are doing and have learned their gunmanship from TV. If you hold an autoloader (semiautomatic)[46] gun sideway and fire it, the chances of it jamming are very good.

Listed below are some of the more prevalent manners that you may be attacked with. There are others, but the principles that you apply here will transcend to the other situations you may face.

Gun to the head: The two basic attacks that a gun-brandishing attacker will employ will be either to the front or the back. Most thugs do not want to be seen, so they will generally be close to you. The good news is that if they wanted you dead, you would be already. They want

---

[46] Autoloader: Many antigun people have no clue as to what they are speaking about. They speak of automatic weapons and really are referring to auto-loaders or semiautomatic firearms. Auto-Loaders simply slide another round into chamber after the previous one was fired. One finger pull, one shot fired. An automatic weapon fires rounds as long as the trigger is depressed.

something from you first. The bad news is that once they have gotten what they want, there is no guarantee that they will not shoot you. If you are alive, you can act. Use your opportunity while it's still there. There are other very good methods that I like, but as with most of these techniques, the listed group is the most universal.

Front: If you have a gun to your head, put your hands up as you did during the knife-to-the-throat attack. Drop straight down by. Many anti-gun people have no clue as to what they are speaking about. They speak of "automatic weapons" and really are referring to auto-loaders or semiautomatic firearms. Auto-loaders simply slide another round into chamber after the previous one was fired. One finger pull, one shot fired. An automatic weapon fires rounds as long as the trigger is depressed. These weapons are considered "machine guns" and have been illegal for most civilians to purchase or own in the US since 1986. Bending your knees and drive your hands directly upward, forming your thumbs into a "V" as you pop the barrel of the gun first upward and then grab the gun with both hands. Snap the gun downward while pointing the barrel upward and toward the attacker. Straighten your knees and resume the standing position, pointing the gun at the assailant. Do whatever you deem necessary at this point.

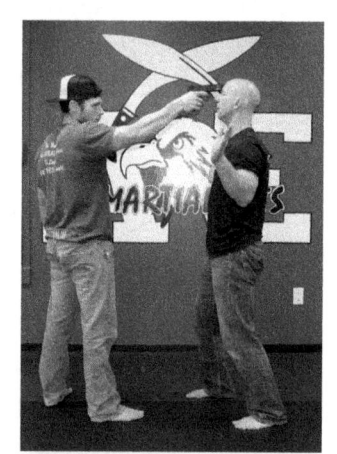

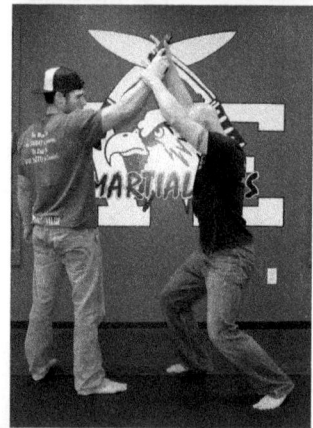

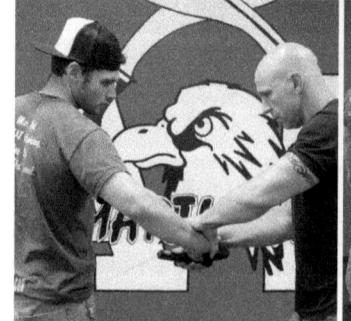

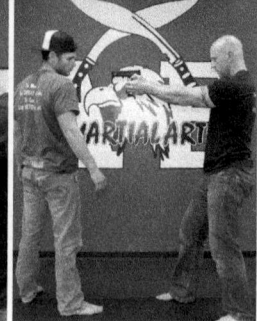

Back: A gun to the back of the head poses several problems. First, you have a gun pointed to the back of your head, which is never a good thing. Second, you don't know which hand the perpetrator has the gun in. It is always preferable to work toward the outside of the gun hand. If, while you have your hands in the air, are able to determine which hand he has the gun in, great, work to the outside. If not, no worries, the initial movements will be the same; just the finishing will be different. Let us assume that the attacker has the gun in his right hand. If you are able to determine which the arm side is, you will step with your left foot so it crosses your right as your hands hit his arm. Let you right hand slide down his arm, secure the hand at the wrist, and then hit his extended arm at the elbow with a left hammerfist as you pull on the arm.

Suppose that we launch or counterattack only to discover that the opposite hand has the gun. Since you are moving, keep going in that direction. Your left hand will along the inside of his arm and makes its way to his right hand, securing a grip at the spot where the wrist and the hand meet. As this is happening, your right will deliver an elbow smash to his face.

Next, perform a knee to the groin and then place both of your hands on his gun hand and mule-kick his right knee.

Stomach: Again, we will operate on the assumption that the gun is in the right hand. However, be certain to practice being attacked with either hand holding the gun. If your hands are down and you find yourself with a gun pressed into your stomach, turn quickly toward your right and smash the back of your left forearm into his right hand. As the barrel of the gun moves away from you and is past your body, slide your right hand, thumb facing upward, down to the wrist and hand of the assailant's gun hand. As you extend their arm, strike their head with a side elbow strike and then secure the gun with both your hands. As you do so, direct a sidekick/stomp with your left foot to their right knee and cause them to collapse to the floor. Turn the gun back toward them as you bend their wrist inward and remove the gun. Finish as necessary.

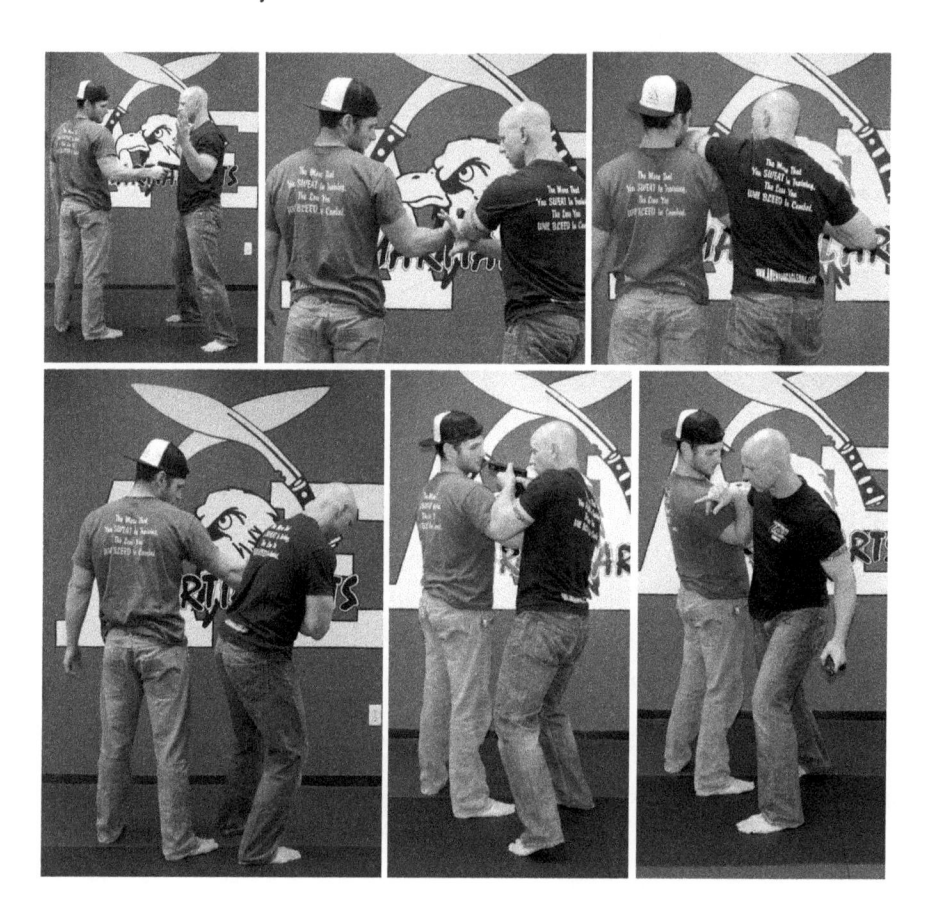

Back: We addressed the gun to the back of the head; the defense for the gun to the back is not much different. After you put your hands up, step with your left foot crossing in front of your right. This will also put you off-line from the barrel of the gun. Turn, and as your arms come in contact with theirs and slide your right hand, fingers up, down to their wrist and implement a left elbow strike to their head. Pivot your right hand on theirs so that your thumb is now upward and slide your left hand down placing both hands on their gun hand. Step forward with your left foot and snap their elbow against your hip by driving your hip into their extended elbow and yank their hand to the right using your hip as a fulcrum. Deliver Mule Kicks to their right need and complete the encounter.

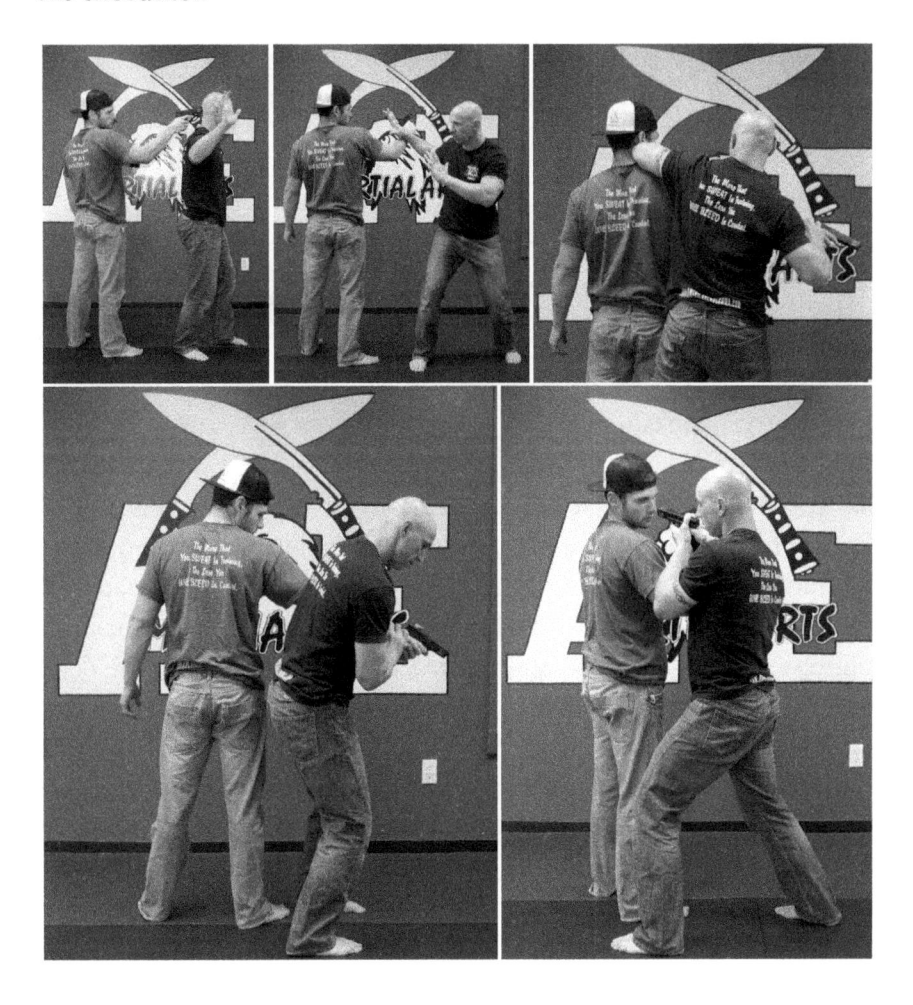

Execution style: If you find yourself on your knees with the attacker standing in front of you with a gun shoved in your face, here's what you do: Put your hands up and start begging for your life, shift your head to the left, and drop your head down, and to the left, as you grab the gun with both hands. Your right hand will have your thumb facing upward and your left hand will come over the back end of the gun. Push with your right and pull with your left and swivel your hips as you land on the ground putting you on your right hip. You will now be pointing the gun at your attacker with the newly secured weapon on your left hip. Finish the encounter as you deem the situation dictates.

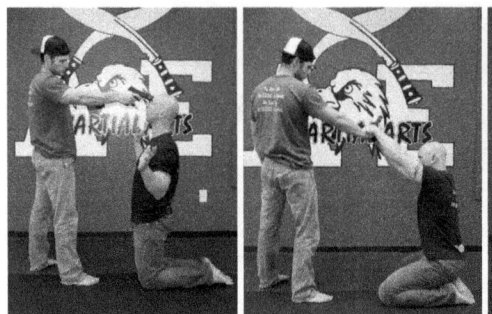

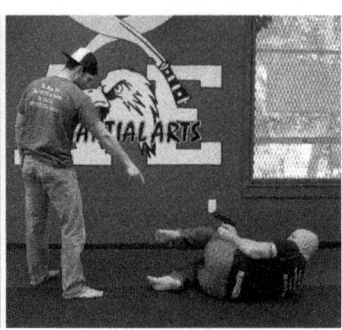

LAST RESORT MEASURES

We live in a different world now and any of us, at anytime may be faced with a seemingly insurmountable situation. These may be in the form of a hostage, terrorist, psychotic shooter, or a kidnapping. Let us consider the scenarios with the "best", if any of these situations can be deemed such, chances in degrading order. But before we delve into the situations, we must be prepared to adhere to the tenets that we have espoused throughout this book. Cooler heads prevail and the "all or nothing" principle. We must also realize that if faced with a dire situation and we find ourselves outnumbered and on the wrong end of a weapon, that every second we are alive is a gift. We need to make the best of it.

Now, it's a virtual impossibility to address every single potential situation, but principals are universal. Make sure that you have practiced your situational awareness and have put SIPDE, (Scan, Identify, Predict, Decide, and Execute) into play. Don't bring attention to yourself. When you have the opportunity, act swiftly and decisively.

Here's the situation, you're in a crowded area. This could be a restaurant, a concert hall, stadium, shopping mall, park, college campus or just about any other place where large groups of people congregate. Do not immediately flee, hit the deck and get a visual on the situation and make an educated move. Keep your cool! The perpetrators are counting on you to panic. They want to inspire mass hysteria, and you may run from the frying pan and right into the fire. Stick with the protocol. Remember that you can't count on anyone else. You have to have the mind-set of "Do something or perish." Yes, there is an element of bravery involved here. Recall the three Americans on the train in France. While others ran and hid, they attacked and subdued the terrorist and saved countless lives. God gives you one shot, take it. The second chance may never come.

In the event that you are too far away to mount a counteroffensive, stay low and keep calm. If you see a clear path toward an escape route, take it. If not, you may have to play dead or wait until help comes. Try to become as invisible as possible. The good thing for you is that not everyone will buy this book, so a great deal of them will be panicking, thus drawing attention toward them and away from you.

If you are fortunate enough to have a legal carry permit, good for you! You live in a region that respects the rights of the law abiding citizenry. This being the case, your best bet is to drop to the ground and find some cover. Assess how many assailants are involved. This may or may not be 100 percent apparent at first, but you have limited time to react, so you have to work with what you are presented with.

We will make the assumption that you are very familiar with your weapon and shooting abilities. The chances of the criminal having a bulletproof vest are pretty high, so a head shot would be best. If you are not an expert marksman, it would be best to aim your first shot relatively high on the chest and make your other shots moving up the body and toward the head. I will also recommend that you get some professional shooting instruction. There are many components to becoming a great shooter and they must be addressed if you are to be successful in a stressful situation. There are tactical shooting instructors that have skills superior to mine. I know what works best for me, but I strongly recommend that you get the training to make you a proficient shooter.

There are several general scenarios that we will address. These tactics are effective when you are unarmed or equipped with a knife. I do recommend that you carry a knife with you at all times, whenever possible. An assailant will either be drawing their weapon or reloading it, and you will be positioned either in front of them or behind them. There will also be times when they are simply looking around for more targets. If you are too far from them and have no escape route, it may be best to play dead until your opportunity arises. The most important physical aspect of this training, is how quickly you are able to cover what distance. How far away can you be from the assailant and still reach him (or her) without being shot? How can you make them miss? What obstacles are in your way? What is available in the environment as an unconventional weapon? Are there chairs, tables or garbage cans? Can you throw a salt shaker or can of beans at them?

Drawing Weapon

If you are faced with someone and you observe them drawing a weapon and you are within your practiced distance from them, rush them! Address the weapon with your thumb up and fingers down as you shove the weapon into them and downward. With your free hand, strike them to the face or neck and then place your full attention to the weapon. Secure the weapon with both hands as you stomp and kick the assailant's feet and shins as you disarm them. Always keep the barrel of the gun pointed away from you and toward them, if possible. Place one hand on the barrel and the other on the pistol grip for a handgun and barrel and the stock of a longarm. If you left hand in on the barrel, step with your left foot in the direction of the barrel as pull in on the grip (or stock) toward you so that your hip becomes a fulcrum with their arm on your hip as you apply force against the elbow joint with the goal of snapping it against your hip. The disarm is consistent for most of the standing disarms for this scenario.

As mentioned previously, know the distance that you will able to cover while the gunman is drawing their weapon. Practice these tactics with obstacles as well. Something lying on the floor, a table or chairs that you must negotiate. Know your capabilities.

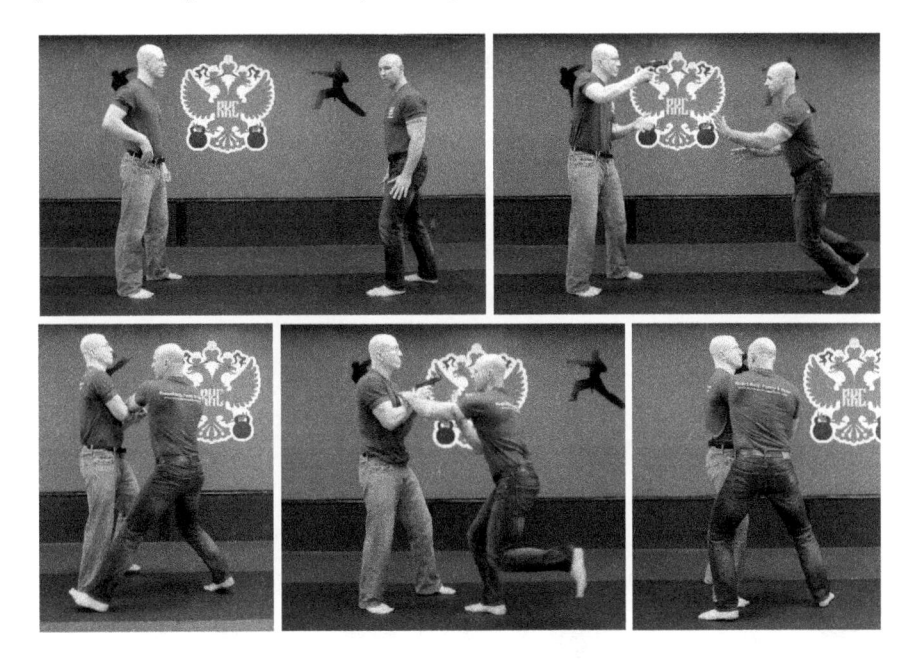

Reloading Weapon

The shooter is vulnerable for a brief time when they are reloading. If there are multiple shooters, you'll have to bear in mind your proximity to the one(s) not directly in front of you. Let us operate on the assumption that the other shooter(s) are preoccupied wreaking havoc in their particular area. At this point, you have determined your distance from the shooter, and it's one that you are confident you can cover before they are able to reload, aim, and commence with firing again. It's time to make your move! If there's a small table or chair that you can pick up en route to strike the shooter with, do so. If you are unable, utilize the same tactics to disarm the assailant as you would do if they are drawing a weapon.

From Behind

On the surface, one may think that this is the best scenario to be faced with because you are behind the shooter. However, if they are actively firing, they may turn and face you at any time and *best* becomes *worst* very quickly.

Take advantage of the fact that you are not in the direct line of sight and move quickly. Again, use your environment, if there is an object to strike with, pick it up. It may also act as a shield and help to deflect an attempted shot. If you are completely unarmed and void of any unconventional weapons, there are a few tactics that work best. If you are reasonably big (at least larger than the shooter), tackle him. This will knock him to the ground and stop him from shooting others. Immediately secure a grip on the gun and shove the barrel into the shooter. If the gun goes off, he will shoot himself. If you are smaller, the tackle may still work, but you will need to generate enough force to knock them down. If you have any hesitation or aren't confident that you will be able to knock them down, you will need to kick them in the back of the knee and deliver strikes to the back of the neck, occipital region, and trapezius. Next, secure the weapon. It won't be pretty, but it will nonetheless be effective.

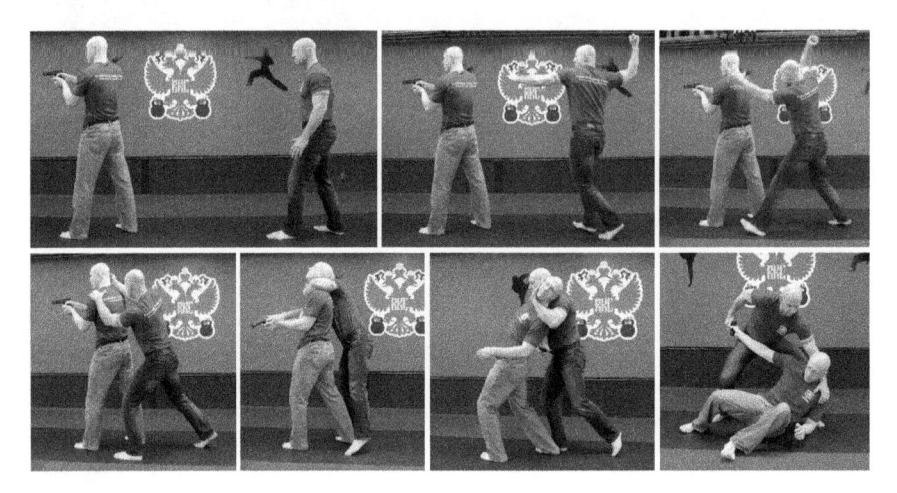

FROM THE FRONT, FIRING

The worst possible scenario is to be directly in front of a shooter while they are firing at you. It is an obvious overstatement to say that you need to work extremely quickly. You also have to be a moving target and make yourself as small as possible.

There are two basic tactics to employ. Distance and environment play a factor in which of these methods you decide to use.

Tactic 1. Execute a forward roll so that you end up rolling right into their legs. If possible, kick them in the groin on your way into them. Immediately work your way up the body and gain control of the weapon. Unleash hell, raining elbows down upon their head as you secure the weapon. Neutralize the threat, commandeer the weapon, and search for other assailants or exit the area quickly.

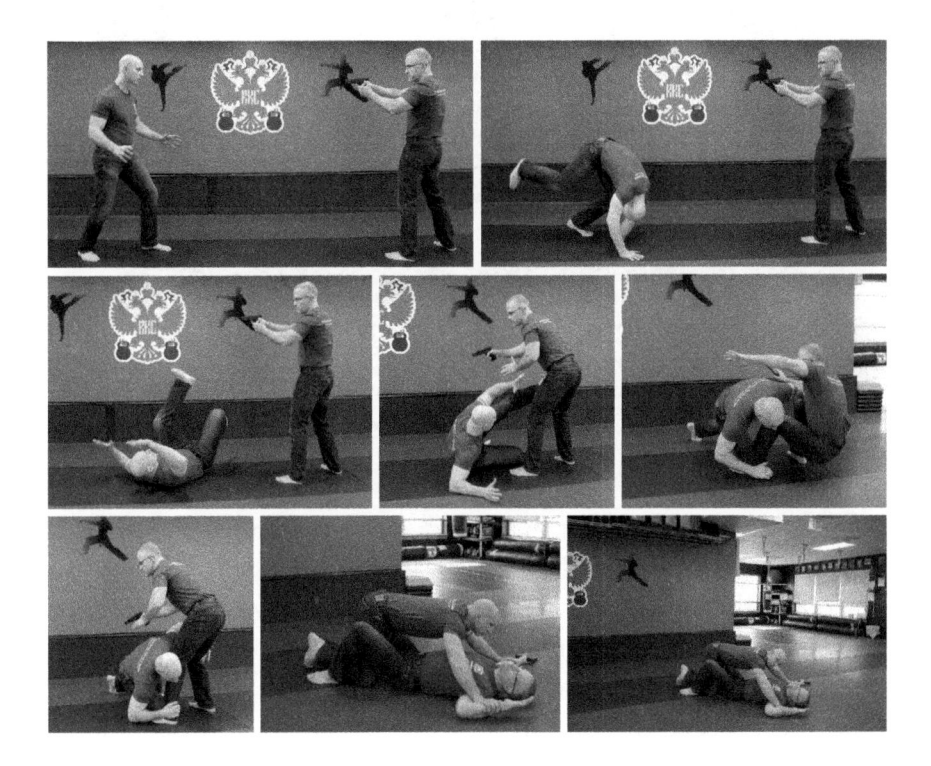

Tactic 2. Drop low and quickly "bear-crawl" toward the shooter. Drive your shoulder into their knees as you cup the back of their heels with your hands. As you drive your shoulders into their knees, pull their heels toward you with all your strength. As with tactic 1, work your way up the body and finish the process.

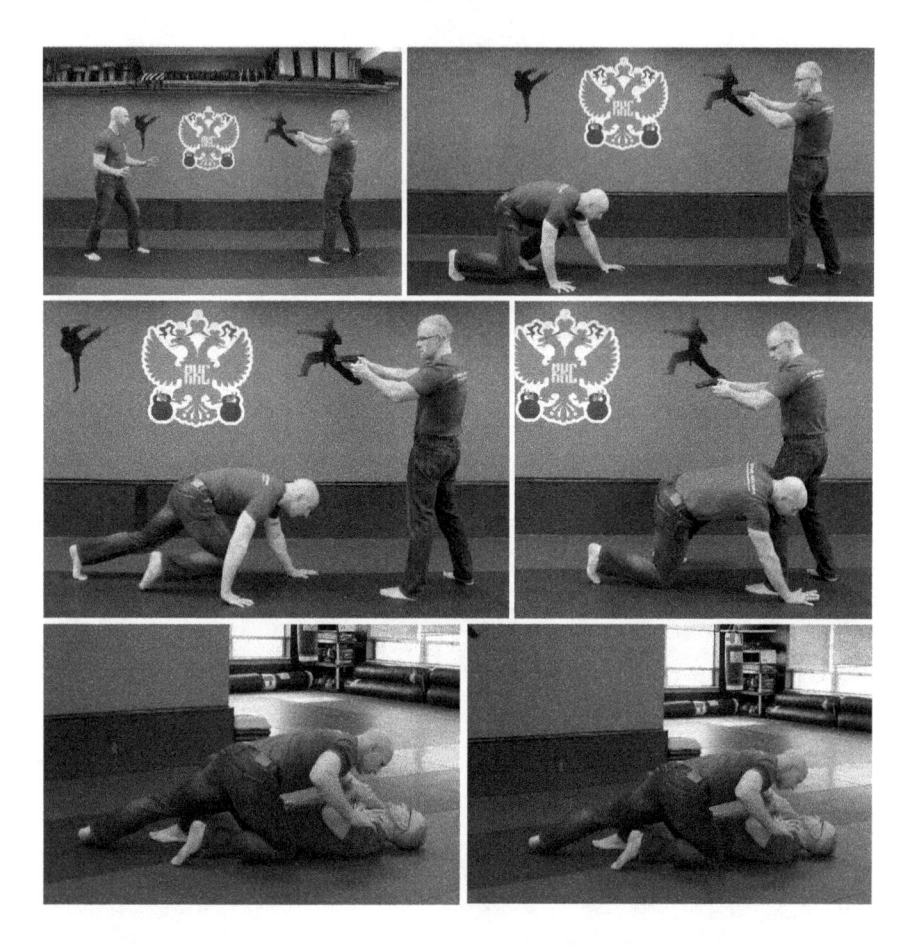

Again, folks, these are last-resort measures. Your dedication to the practice of the movements, conditioning of your body, and willingness to perform these acts under duress will determine your success. When facing a weapon, you are dead. Every breath that you have is on borrowed time, every second that you are alive is a gift, use them wisely and do anything you can to save your life and the lives of others.

14
PRACTICE AND TRAINING ROUTINES

MAN-TO-MAN STRENGTH

One quality of strength that is absolutely imperative for a fight situation is Man-to-Man strength. There is a dynamic and chaotic nature to grappling, boxing and kickboxing that is impossible to perfectly prepare for without actual fighting or grappling. Therefore it is important to not only improve your overall strength through proper training, but to also make sure that you spend some time with a bona fide "opponent." Below are a collection of drills to help you develop strength, balance, and reactions to aid you in fighting. These drills should be incorporated as part of your regular practice.

MAN-MAN DRILLS

Push-pull: Stand facing your partner with the same foot forward. Press the outside of your foot against your partner's and lock arms, hand to forearm. Push and pull each other in an attempt to disrupt your partner's balance. Practice this on both sides.

Pummeling: Stand chest to chest with your partner, and each of you has one arm under and the other over. One person moves forward as the other goes back, continually switching the under and overhooks, smashing your posterior deltoids into each other as you move. Once you get to the end of the mat, go back in the other direction so that you have switched who is moving forward and who is moving back.

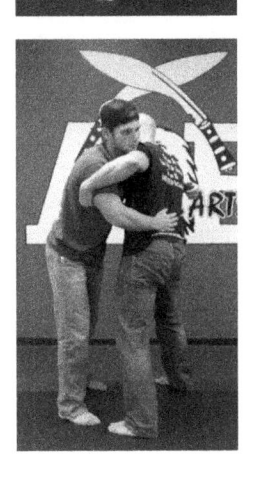

Inside control balance drill: Inside control is essential to grappling success, especially on your feet. Assume the inside position with your hands on the inside of your partner's biceps and push and pull them in different directions—back, forward, and side to side. Switch partners and then battle with each other for the inside control position.

Sweeps and disruptions: If you are wearing a Kimono or a jacket, you may grab on to the sleeves and lapels. If not, start from the inside control position and employ the movement practiced in the previous drill with the addition of tapping their feet with yours. Use the bottom of your foot to make contact with theirs. Use anticipatory movement knowing that if you pull them toward you, their foot will have to land for them to maintain their balance. Put your foot where their foot is heading. If they do not fall, immediately go in the other direction. This action will result in them falling or at least causing them to lose their balance, enabling you to secure a takedown or another advantageous position.

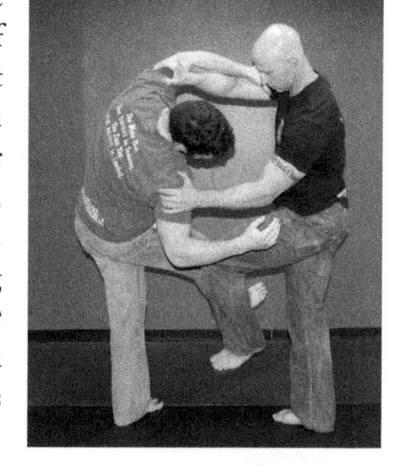

Throws: Practice all the throws that you know. Practice them slowly for technique and then work them hard. Do a "throw-around" by setting the timer for two to five minutes and going back and forth with your partner practicing your throws. Use pushing, pulling, and movement. Remember that throws are dynamic and require movement to be executed.

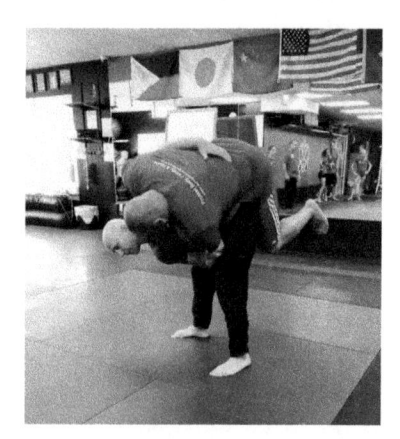

Ducks, slips, parries, and weaves: Have your partner wear focus mitts or simply use each other's boxing gloves as targets. If you don't have gloves, use open palms and slaps. Have your partner throw strikes at you as you practice moving out of the way and positioning yourself to counterstrike. You should barely get out of the way of the strikes so that you are closer, thus affording you a better opportunity to deliver your counterstrikes.

Partner carries: These drills can be used in a beginning of a workout as a means to warm up or at the end as an overload. Pick up your partner and carry them as you move quickly across the room. There are many different carries to use, here are a few. Double-leg, fireman's carry, marriage carry, piggyback and dog stance lifts. On the last one, your partner is on all fours and you are both facing the same direction. Wrap your arms around their waist, lift them and move them forward. They won't move too far, but it's a heck of a strength developing drill.

Stick grappling: One person holds the staff vertically and has their feet shoulder width apart, knees slightly bent and hands approximately a foot apart. The other person grabs the staff outside the stationary partner's hands and moves around them pulling and yanking on the pole and the stationary partner tries to maintain their position. Don't twist the staff, this does not help the drill, plus you may hit your partner or injure their wrists. Do this drill in spurts of 15 seconds on, 15 seconds rest and 15 seconds for the other partner. Repeat so that each person gets two to three rounds in as a warm up drill.

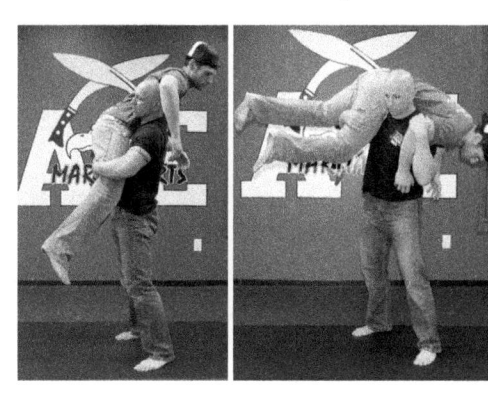

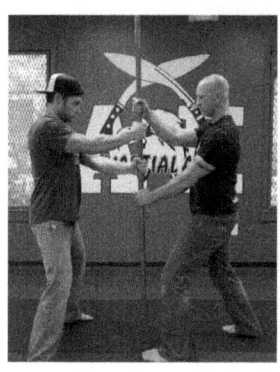

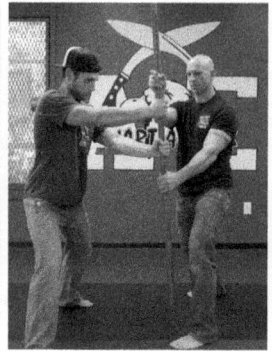

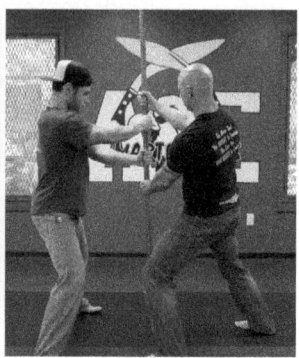

Wall drill (slaps):
One partner starts in a very negative position with their knees bent and their back against the wall. The other partner starts slowly and then builds to striking faster, trying to land slaps on their head, face, and body. Closed fists to the body are acceptable, and even help to condition their bodies. Don't try to smash your partner too hard, though. This is a reaction-developing drill.

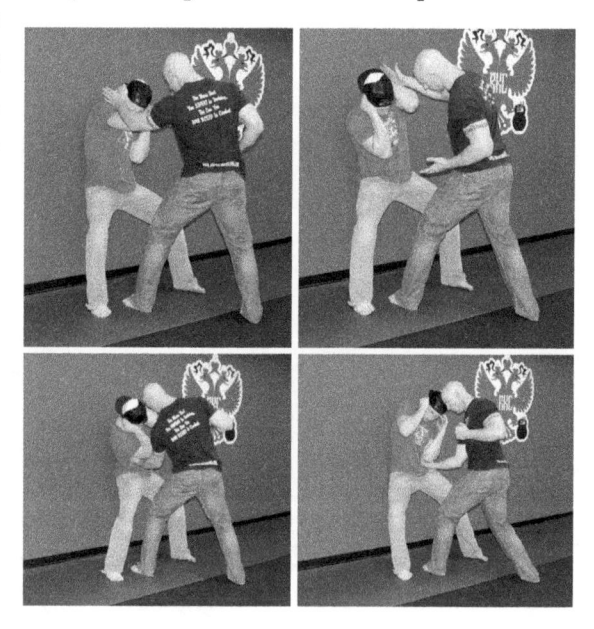

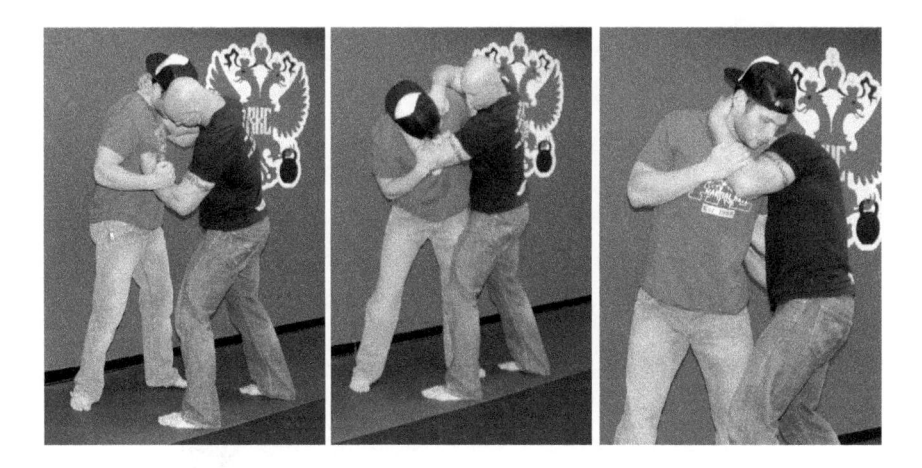

Defensive boxing drill into dirty boxing: One partner throws punches, and the other takes an angle, gets inside, and drives he other back onto their heels with strike and shoves. Grab the back of the neck or their arm and deliver strikes.

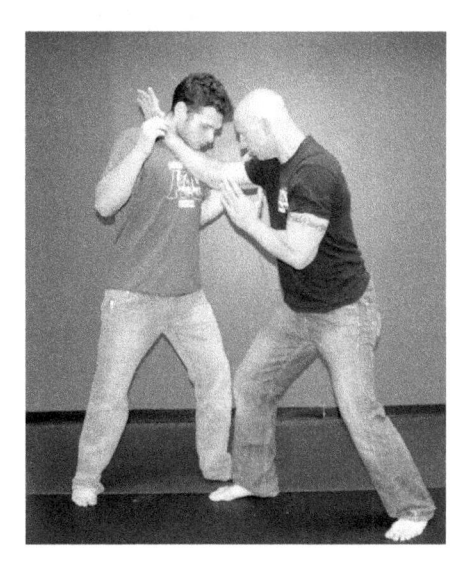

Drop out (balance disruption game): Both partners are on the floor facing each other in a push-up position. Using one hand (obviously), try to grab each other's hand and knock the others off balance. If you fall or your knee hits the ground, you lose.

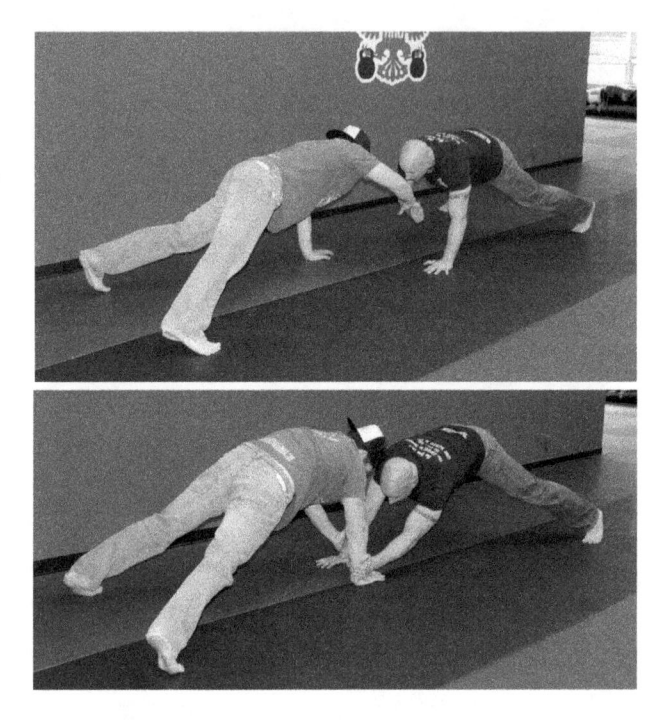

Pop shots: Both partners' face each other in a good grappling stance. Take both hand and pop your partner's shoulders as you lower your level, shoot a Double Leg Takedown and lift them into the air. Put them down without completing the takedown, so that they land on their feet. Repeat this move in sets of 10 repetitions for each partner.

Body lifts: Assume the Over/Underhook position and slide yourself to the side of the overhooked as you trap his far arm, lock your hands around the waist and press the side of your head against his chest. You are now in a Single Arm Bear Hug. Pinch his leg between your knees, pop your hips and lift your partner. Repeat this move in sets of 10 repetitions for each partner.

Bridge backs: Be very careful when practicing this drill. This should be used only by the more experienced and conditioned practitioners. Have your partner stand at your side, grab hands, and then he should use his other hand to support your elbow.

Bridge back as far as you are able to go. If you can touch the mat with your head, great, but I do not recommend that you start off this way. Once your bridge backward as far as you can safely go, come back up. Your partner should assist you as much as needed on the way down and on the way up. Start with 5 repetitions per set and increase to 10.

Sticky hands: This is yet another great training technique advocated by Bruce Lee. The goal of this drill is to develop sensitivity and awareness of your opponent's movement. Stand in front of your partner with one palm up and one palm down. Place the inside of your wrists in contact with your partner's. Now begin to move in small horizontal circles and gradually make them larger and "flow" to the back of the arm while shifting your weight. Do not force any movement, go with the flow of energy as you shift your weight and slide your arms against your partner's while moving and attempting to maintain contact throughout the drill. This is a fun drill and even though your goal is not to "win" per se, but to learn how to follow the movements of your partner. It is fun, though, to wind up tying your partner's arms up as they try to follow you!

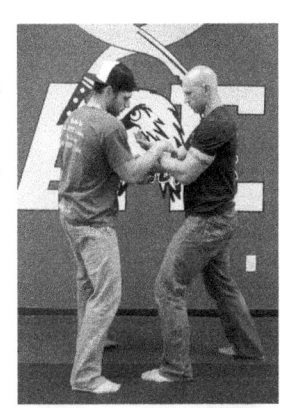

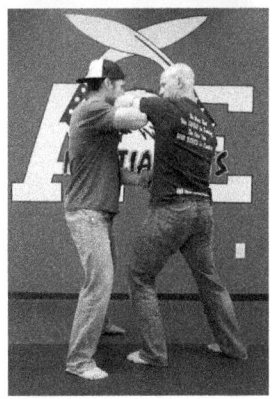

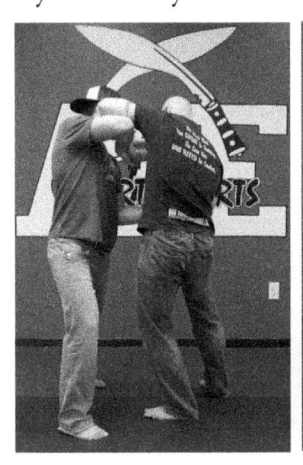

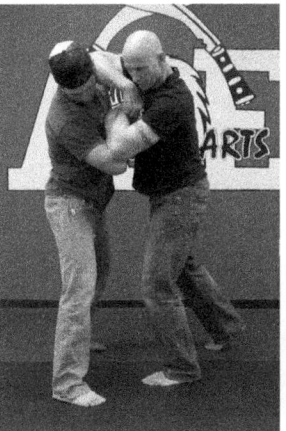

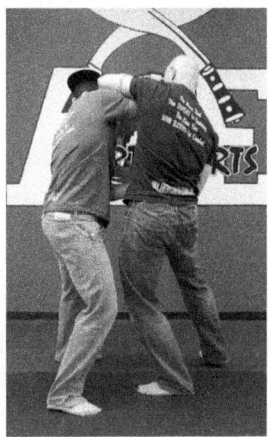

Punches: 1 thru 6 Combinations

Muscle memory is essential to be able to successfully throw combination in a stressful situation such as a confrontation. Practice these combinations in a mirror, on focus mitts, or a heavy back. Also, be sure to incorporate your bobs, weaves, slips, and general movement when striking. Always try to make it real.

1) 1, 2
2) 1, 3, 2
3) 2,3
4) 1,4,3
5) 3, 6
6) 6, 3
7) 2, 3, 2
8) 1, 6, 3
9) 1, 1, 2
10) 1, 2, 1

Endurance Punching Sequence

20 repetitions each sequence. Do both sides (right and left stance)

1) 1,2
2) 2,3
3) 3,4
4) 4,5
5) 5,6
6) 6,1

Bag Work

There are many people who hang a heavy bag, turn on the theme to *Rocky*, and start wailing away on the bag as the tempo to "Gonna Fly Now" picks up. Are they getting some cardio and developing some muscle? Possibly. Are they tired at the end? Most likely. Have they developed their striking skills and created some useful muscle memory? Probably not.

When you hit the heavy bag, you want to make the best use of your time. You need to hit the bag with purpose. You should hit the bag while utilizing movement, just as if you were fighting. Practice moving in and out, slips, ducks, bobbing, and weaving. Always either bring your hand to your head or your head to your hand. Develop *proper* muscle memory.

When you begin your training, you may be tempted to start with 10 rounds. I will not suggest that. Depending upon your fitness level, start with 3 to 5 two-minute rounds and then build from there. Be sure to keep a straight wrist and tight fist while punching and a flexed foot while kicking.

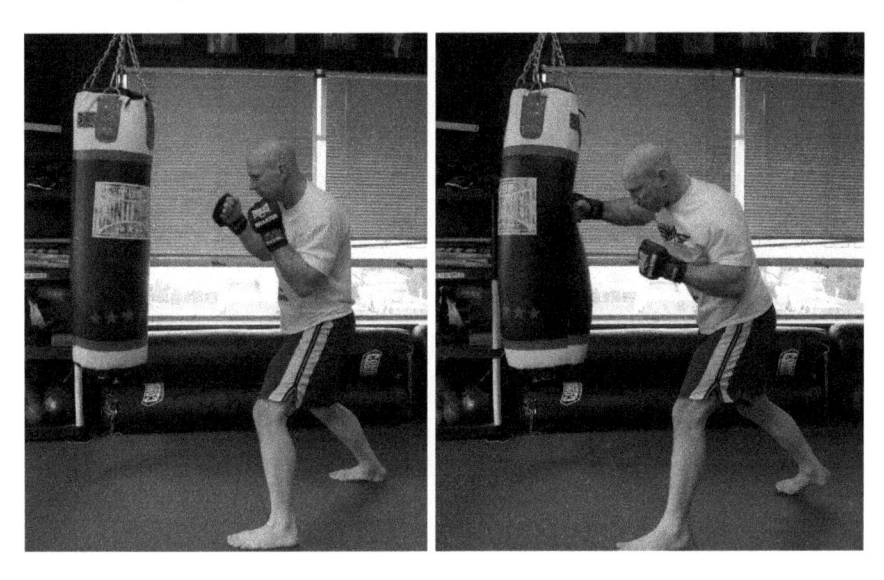

Ground and pound: There may come a time when you get someone on the ground and you have mounted them. It's time to unleash hell! However, be smart and don't simply throw punches at the downed assailant. Choose your strikes in a strategic manner and practice on a heavy bag.

Place your heavy bag on the floor and straddle it so that your knees are on the floor to either side of the bag. *Do not punch your assailant in the face.* The chances of you missing his face and punching the ground are quite good. Practice punching to the body and open hand strikes and elbows to the head. You will want to rise up slightly, tilting your shoulders as you drop the elbows or other strikes straight down.

If you wind up on their side, knee drives to the ribs, head, and legs are effective. So is dropping elbows to the opposite side of the body and head. Just don't stay here too long. It's better to have a full mount position. It's also important to have a solid base. If your knees are too close together, you will be rolled over. Practice your mount position, striking from it and moving from side to side.

Hands (Boxing Drills)

Our boxing coach, Joe Rubino, put together this incredible boxing training sequence for developing muscle memory and conditioning for striking with your hands. If you want to develop more strength and conditioning, use 14- to 16- ounce gloves. For improving the conditioning of your hands, use thin bag gloves.

One overbearing, essential component to working the heavy bag properly is to do so as if you were fighting. This means head movement, moving in and out on the bag, keeping your hands up. Chin to hand or hand to chin after you punch. Practice your bobs, weaves, and slips as you move and strike. Stay on the balls of your feet and perform your herky-jerky[47] movement.

---

[47] Herky-jerky movements involve stomping the floor, feinting in and out of your opponent's range, and throwing off their rhythm with your arrhythmic motion. It's a great strategy to draw another out and get them to commit or to stop their movement, allowing you the opportunity to launch an attack.

Coach Joe Rubino's Heavy Bag Routine

Round 1 – Working the jab around the bag
Round 2 – Working the 1–2 combination around the bag
Round 3 – Slipping, bobbing, and weaving with combinations
Round 4 – Fast combinations around the bag (staying tall)
Round 5 – Fast combinations up and down around the bag
Round 6 – Punching from angles (swing the bag)
Round 7 – Hand speed short, quick punches after working your way inside
Round 8 – Power shots
Round 9 – High/low combinations
Round 10 – Working the inside position (use elbows and forearms to control bag)
3 minute rounds with 30 seconds rest between rounds
OR
2 minute rounds with 1 minute rest between rounds

Kickboxing: Mixing the Strikes of the Hands and Feet

Now we are going to add kicks to the mix. Here's a routine that I have been using for quite a few years. Mind you, there are many other combinations and sequences that work, but this one is a standby and a great place to start with.

Our striking sequences are primarily done in a circle fashion, as opposed to an X. To illustrate this point, we will consider the first combination. Start in your orthodox stance and then throw a right cut kick, followed by a right jab, a left cross, and finish with a left-cut kick. That would be an example of a circle striking configuration. An example of an X would be, starting in the Orthodox stance, a left jab, step across, and throwing a right-cut kick. Another example would be a left jab, right cross, and a left roundhouse kick. When "mirror image" with my opponent, both fighters either in Orthodox or South Paw, it's recommended to use more X style of striking. When you are "chest to chest" with your opponent, both fighters in the same stance, "circle striking" works the best. These are not hard and fast rules, but more like guidelines.

Please do not deliberate on the Circle vs. the X for striking. Practice both and use what works best for you. However, understand that as a general rule, the circle is quicker, and the X has more power. I have discovered that it's easier to put more power into my circle attacks than it is to add more speed to my X.

Additionally, when training the kickboxing sequence, we work both orthodox and southpaw stances. In fighting and kickboxing, it's important to be able to switch your stances on the fly. Switch sides either halfway through the round or every other combination.

Kickboxing Sequence

Round 1 - Right cut kick, right jab, left cross, left-cut kick.
Round 2 - Lead leg roundhouse kick, jab, and cross.
Round 3 - Lead leg side kick, backfist, cross.
Round 4 - Full leg (back one) rapid fire cut kick, round kick, lead hook (hand), cross and lead hook again. After your full cut kick, your rear becomes your lead; you bounce your foot off the ground quickly as you deliver the next two kicks. After the kicks, execute a lead hook punch with the same side.
Round 5 - Piet a te, lead jab, cross, rear leg cut kick
Round 6 - Back kick, spinning backfist, stick punch
Round 7 - Lead jab, spinning backfist, stick punch, double knee
Round 8 - Double jab, body shot (rear hook to the body), cut kick, spinning crescent, hook or wheel kick (vary the kicks)
Round 9 - Fake (feint) the jab, slide lead foot across and throw an overhand right, pivot on the lead foot and throw in a lead hook followed by a rear elbow
Round 10 - Lunging front kick, side step and shin kick, lead hook, rear uppercut
2 minute rounds with 30 seconds rest between rounds
OR
minute rounds with 1 minute rest between rounds

The Four Ranges of Combat

Kicking range. This is the distance where the feet are most effective. Closing the gap and covering distance are best accomplished with your feet. They are your first line of defense.

Punching range. This is a range that you may begin at dependent upon your proximity to your opponent. The clenched fist, open handed strikes, finger jabs, axe hands, chops, and smashes are most effective at this distance. A good guard is essential here, so keep your hands up.

Trapping range. Potentially the most ignored range in the martial arts. This is an intermediary and a "gateway" from striking to grappling. At this distance, you "trap" your opponent's weapon (arm or leg) and deliver your strike—elbow, knee, or head butt. There are a plethora of other weapons you have available to you at this range. They are as follows: hips, shoulders, thigh, forearms, neck, etc... Some styles advocate this range as two distinct distances, but in practice, I have found them to be one in the same. In this range, we also practice the art of "dirty boxing."

Grappling range. If your confrontation lasts more than 3 to 5 seconds, you will be at this range, like it or not. At this distance, leverage, balance and knowledge of the body are most critical. All your takedowns, choke-outs, submission holds, throws and joint manipulation occur at this distance. Please note that striking often occurs at this range as well. There is such complexity to body position and weight shifting that several arts focus solely on this range.

How to Train

When you get in a fight, keep your hands up. When you are in the fracas, get your hands up to protect your head. Keeping your hands up is the soundest advice I've been given.

It is best to start at one range and move into another. Moving to a third and a fourth range is not helpful, because you cannot effectively practice combinations to compensate for the variables, which may occur. We train in this manner.

Round 1: Start at range 1, then go 1 to 2, then 1 to 3, then 1 to 4.
Round 2: Start at range 2, and then go 2 to 3, then 2 to 4, then 2 to 1.
Round 3: Start at range 3, and then go 3 to 4, then 3 to 1, then 3 to 2.
Round 4 - Start at range 4, and then go 4 to 3, then 4 to 2, then to 1.

Please note that you will not always be afforded the luxury of beginning in a range that is comfortable for you. However, through practice, you will be able to enter your most effective distance efficiently and rapidly.

15

DOG ATTACKS

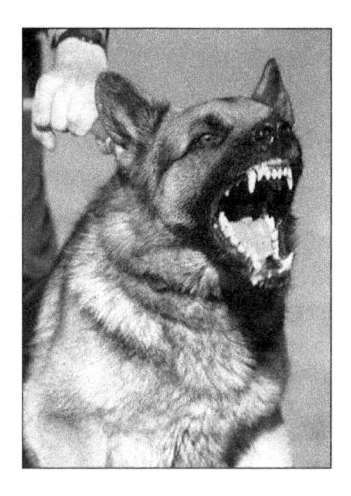

Man's best friend can also be his worst enemy. There are many breeds that are large, powerful, and created for fighting, crowd control, and intimidation. Just imagine 125 pounds of fangs, fur, and fury charging at you! These fierce animals are extremely difficult to deal with, but you are not without recourse.

There are certain considerations to bear in mind. Chances are very good that you will suffer a bite in a confrontation with a dog. Know this going in. The bite pressure, in PSI (pounds per square inch) of some domesticated dogs can be more than that of cougars (350 PSI) and wolves (406 PSI). These wild animals are able to crush the skulls and bones of their prey. Due to their massive heads and powerful neck and jaw muscles, the mastiff has the highest bite force of all domestic dogs, with a PSI of 556. The Rottweiler comes in at second with a PSI of 328, third goes to the German Shepherd at 238 and then fourth is the American pitbull at 235 PSI. The adult human male has a PSI of 150.

Awareness of the psyche of the dog is tantamount to the success of your defense. There are postures and voice commands that can help you avoid the attack. A dog likes to have it's feet planted on the ground. By lifting a dog off the ground, you disrupt his ability use his legs to drive off of the ground and significantly reduce his security. Many types of guard or catch animals have their tails docked to eliminate the tail becoming a handle. If they have a tail, use it to lift them off of the ground, thus rendering them unable to use their back legs to drive from. If they do not have a tail, grab their back legs.

First line of defense is to use your voice command: loud, concise, and pointed. This works very well in a surprisingly high percentage of instances. Next, position yourself to deliver a strong kick, aiming for the snoot, ribs, underbelly, or hind quarters.

If this does not work or you are not positioned to deliver a kick, offer up an arm and when the dog bites, lift the bitten arm up quickly and deliver a downward hammerfist smash the dog's first vertebra where skull meets the spine. Your goal will be to break the attacking canine's neck. If you have a knife, offer the arm and thrust the knife into the dog's throat.

Don't try to pull away from the dog once engaged. Shove your arm or fist deep into their mouth and attempt to knock them over. Stick your thumb in their eyes and deliver knee strikes to their ribs and underbelly. If there are multiple dogs, keep the fight standing delivering knee strikes and elbows as you move and position yourself so you are not engaged with both dogs at once.

If the dog bites your hand, grasp the lower jaw firmly, and pull down. Wrap your other arm around the dog's neck and apply a one-armed choke as you yank down on his jaw. A dog will bite and shake. Pulling down on its jaw makes it less able to bite down and securing a headlock like choke reduces his ability to thrash his head about. The dog may simply just try to get away from you at this point.

Different types of dogs attack in various manners. For example, German shepherds and Dobermans will repeatedly bite and release until they can gain a full mouth bite, and then they will grab and shake. The bully breeds, pit bulls, bulldogs, mastiffs, and the like tend to grab, hold, and shake as opposed to biting and releasing. Your general defense to either type of attack will not vary, but I think that it was worth mentioning. However, if any dog has had Shutzund, or "bite training," their approach will be in accordance with how they were trained. It is comforting to know that most trained dogs will go after the first limb that gets presented and are generally trained to bite their opponent's arm once engaged.

16

UNCONVENTIONAL WEAPONS

PRACTICE IS ESSENTIAL

Practice with your weapon on a regular basis. There are many instances when a person is trying to defend themselves and the weapon gets taken away and used on them. Get used to its weight, size, and how it reacts when you use the weapon.

Unconventional weapons, as with conventional, require practice to become proficient. They are easy to travel with, and you will not get questioned by the TSA while traveling. Some of these weapons are readily available in the environment.

Here is the Unconventional Weapons Real Life Story that I've selected to relay. Always consider all options and keep your wits about you.

***

One of my martial arts students, John Geraghty, was traveling abroad in India for business. The area in India that he was traveling in was an exceptionally impoverished region. He was at a business dinner with a gentleman in his late sixties, and they were taking a cab back to the hotel. There was quite a bit of drinking at the dinner; wisely, John did not partake.

The arrangements for the cab were made by a third party. As they neared the hotel, which had barbed wire and armed guards at the gate, the cab drove past. John was very aware, but his comrade was not. Traveling internationally with conventional weapons is frowned upon, but John did remember that in class, we had learned how to use a rolled-up magazine as a defense weapon. He had one in his hand.

The cab traveled past the secure entrance to the hotel, and John questioned the driver. He told them to "Get out here." John got out of the cab with his slightly inebriated partner in tow and was surrounded by a group of six or so assailants. The cab sped off.

John took his adjusted his makeshift weapon in the back seat of the cab prior to getting out. As the group descended upon them, he had to act quickly. The closest assailant was the recipient of the butt of the rolled-up magazine applied to the occipital region of his head. He dropped to the ground as John grabbed his compatriot by the belt and fled quickly to the hotel gate as the gang was in disarray.

John employed awareness skills, an unconventional weapon, listening to the survival voice, willingness to act and act decisively with conviction and knowing where to place a strike saved his life and that of his business associate. This all happened so quickly that the travel partner was in total shock and 100 percent unaware of what had just transpired until he witnessed the aftermath.

UNCONVENTIONAL

Pen, towel, brush, sock with batteries, magazine, chair, umbrella, garbage can lid, change, brief case, belt with buckle, Chemical deterrents, hornet spray, and air horn.

Various strikes, parries, techniques, and strategies.
Diamond defense with a chair.
Breaking a board with a magazine.
Throwing change into the eyes and face of assailant.

Pen: A pen may be used to slash and stab an opponent with. Both the ice pick and fencing grips may be used. The target areas for the slash are the eyes and throat. Thrusts are directed to the temple, eyes, neck, and groin.

Towel: A towel may be used to wrap your hand in to battle a knife-wielding assailant. You may also use it to ward off blows and offensively as a means to apply a choke or to tie up an assailant.

Brush: A hairbrush may be used in two different applications. Rake the bristles across the eyes of an assailant, or use the butt end of the handle to strike vital and semivital target areas.

Sock with batteries: Take an athletic tube sock or another calf-covering sports sock and place two size D batteries in it. This may be used to swing, hitting vital and semivital target areas.

MagLite: A flashlight is a great emergency tool to have, why not have one that doubles as an effective weapon? I recommend that you get the version that requires four or more size D batteries. If you are defending yourself in a dark setting, hold the MagLite with your knuckles facing upward and the light section by your pinky. The long end is facing backward. Keep the light off until the last second. Turn it on and temporarily blind the assailant, and then smash him over the top of the head with the long end of the light. Immediately turn your palm down and strike the side of their head with a backstroke. If necessary, turn your palm up on the follow-through and hit the other side of the head on the way back.

Magazine: Procure a magazine, preferably a thicker one—*Cosmo, Muscle & Fitness, Glamour,* etc. . . Roll it up very tight and keep it in your hand at the ready. You have just made a club. The primary use will be for hammer strikes downward or across to the neck, jaw, temple, or nose. Thrusting may be used on the solar plexus, throat, or groin.

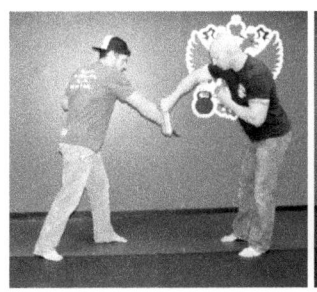

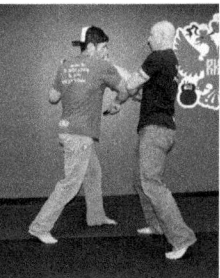

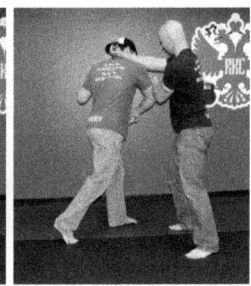

Chair: Chairs are available in most places. Can you use a chair like they do in the WWE? Yes, you can grab a folding chair and hit someone over the head or across the back with it. However, there is a much more effective manner to use a chair. Position the chair in your hands with the four points facing the opponent in a diamond formation. This will position the top and bottom points at your adversary's groin and face. The other two legs are to the outside, making it difficult for your attacker to hit you. The chair defense is good for defending against a knife attack. Be very aggressive with the chair and back the attacker up with jabs and thrusts.

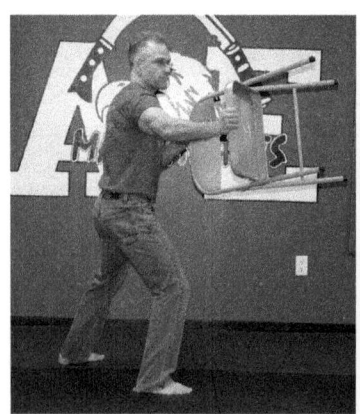

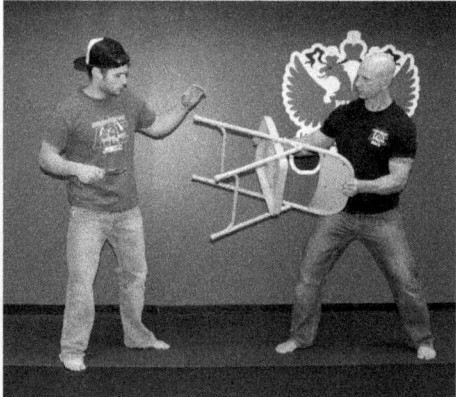

Umbrella: The large gold umbrellas work best. Use the point to jab and thrust into the vital and semi-vital target areas. If the handle is hard plastic, that can be used to add power to your strikes as well.

Garbage can lid: Pick up a garbage can and hit the adversary with it. Grab a lid to block strikes, knife thrusts. Use the edge of the lid to administer strikes as counteroffensives.

Change: Have loose change available in your pocket. When faced with an assailant, throw it in their face as a distraction and follow immediately with your counterattack.

Briefcase: Most of us don't carry a briefcase any longer, but you still should apply the principles here. Use the edge and corners of the case to strike the groin, knees, and up in to the chin of an assailant. You'd be surprised how effective this technique is!

Belt with buckle: Having a good-sized belt buckle has its advantages. Pull your belt off quickly and wrap the strap around your hand, leaving a short length (approximately 3 to 5 inches) unwrapped before the buckle. The leather strap adds protection to your hand for punching, and the buckle can be used to swing and cut the face of your target.

Chemical deterrents: There are a variety of chemical deterrents available on the market. The most well-known, the pepper spray, or OC (oleoresin capsicum) spray, or Mace Phenacyl chloride (CN/tear gas). The two are often referred to as one and the same; however, they are not. Pepper spray is more effective and legal in most states. Mace was proven ineffectual when used in many situations when the assailant is intoxicated or under the influence of certain narcotics. Pepper spray irritates and inflames the mucus membranes, resulting in breathing difficulty, temporary blindness, and confusion. As a side note, Mace brand still carries their Triple Action Defense Spray, which is claimed to be a combination of OC pepper spray, CN tear gas, and UV marking dye. When using pepper spray, it is important not to be downwind, or you will risk the chance of having the spray blown back into your face. Also, employ the sign of the Cross when spraying. By spraying in both the vertical and horizontal planes, your coverage of the assailant will be maximized. This strategy will allow the fumes to travel upward toward their mouth and nose, making the effect more effective. It is easy for one to miss the attacker's face when aiming directly at it.

As an aside, if the assailant is covered with vomit, feces, or urine, it will nullify the effects of any chemical sprays. This tactic has been successfully employed by prison inmates.

Hornet (wasp) spray: Depending on the laws in your jurisdiction, carrying a chemical deterrent may or may not be legal. There are no laws against hornet or wasp spray anywhere, though. The range of the spray is up to 20 feet. This is quite a bit farther than that of the commercial chemical deterrents available on the market.

Air horn: This little device is readily available and 100 percent legal to carry. If you are confronted, literally shove the horn in the face of the assailant and then press the button. There will be a moment of "shock" that will afford you the opportunity to deliver a well-placed kick and escape to safety. Additionally, it's loud and will attract attention.

17
CONVENTIONAL WEAPONS

Practice with your weapon on a regular basis. There are many instances when a person is trying to defend themselves and the weapon gets taken away and used on them. Get used to its weight, size, and how it reacts when you strike or stab something or when you fire it, if it's a gun. We are providing a simple overview of weapons use here. Whole books can and have been dedicated to each of the weapons listed below.

WEAPONS OF CHOICE

There are so many weapons to choice from. There a great deal of laws to consider, but we are not going to address the legality of weapons. I am simply going to list my favorite weapons and how to best use a few of them: expandable baton, baseball bat, short stick, 12 gauge shotgun, Glock 9mm, Special Ops folding knife, KBar, black jack, sap, and sap gloves.

It is essential to practice drawing, shooting, striking, or cutting with your weapon. Become familiar to it in your hand, its weight, shape, and general "feel." You must be very comfortable with the weapon if you want to use it effectively in a stressful situation.

Gun: When using a gun, shoot to kill. Aim for the center mass. Wounding someone will only make them more enraged and increase the chance of them getting to you and causing serious injury or death. There is no such thing as "shooting someone in the leg to wound them." Shoot to kill, period.

I prefer a 12 gauge pump action Remington 870 Express. When you lock and load and the intruder hears the *click, click*, they know they are in trouble, and sometimes it will be enough to scare them off. If not, the intruder knows where you are, so be prepared to shoot.

As far as pistols go, I like the Glock, either a 9mm or .40 caliber. I have put over 10,000 rounds through my Glock 19, and it still fires true. I found the pistol grip a little small for my hand, so I put a rubber grip sleeve over the handle.

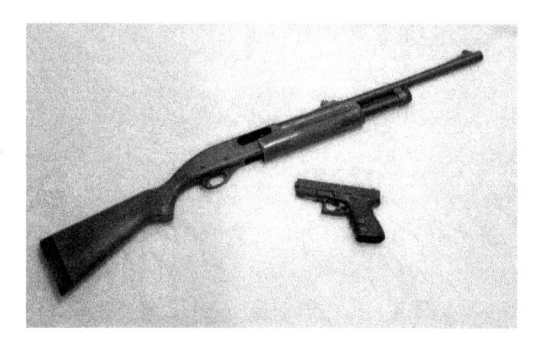

Join a shooting club, get some lessons, and practice until you are comfortable. Make your shooting part of your training routine.

KNIFE

I love knives. I carry one with me at all times. My house also has several knives strategically placed throughout for easy access in an emergency. Once you get used to carrying a knife, you'll feel naked without it. I have to purposely remind myself to take my knife off and leave it home when I go to the airport. Keep your knives sharp and available.

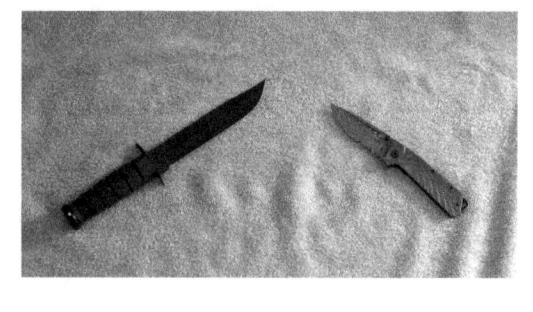

The basic knife movements include the thrust, slash, and flick. The basic defensive maneuvers are parries and blocks. You also must consider how you grip your knife when holding it. I prefer the "fencing" grip, with the blade facing toward my opponent as opposed to the "ice pick" grip. I'd only use the ice pick grip (blade downward), if I did not want to reveal that I was carrying a knife. There are may more options with the fencing grip style, plus I'd rather have my cold steel between me and an assailant. If your knife has a hilt, practice pressing your thumb into the hilt, this will make your grip more stable.

Thrust: This is a straight and powerful attack. Aim for soft target areas—abdomen, low back and side, groin, neck, and throat. To inflict maximum damage, twist the knife upon exit. A thrust is meant to finish an individual off.

Slash: Slash on angles primarily downward, but upward works in some instances. Aim for the neck, wrists, arms, inner thighs, and groin. Slashing is designed to make you bleed and set up the opponent for a finishing thrust.

Flick: This is thrown as you would a backfist. It's very quick and difficult to avoid or block. Flicks are thrown to the face and throat. They are designed as an entry technique to help you administer a more lethal attack.

Parry: Use the flat of the blade to redirect a thrust or a slash. Follow up with another redirect or parry with your free hand and then counterattack with your knife.

Block: The edge of the knife is best suited for blocking. The block can also double as a slice used to cut the attacking limb. When facing an armed foe, it's better to go metal to metal when blocking a blade coming at you.

Baton: There are different types of batons that you may choose to work with. Bando short stick, expandable baton, Police billy club, baseball bat, and I would even include rattan (arnis) in this group. You want focus on what works best for you. Personally, I keep an expandable baton with me and keep both a baseball bat and a bando short stick at the ready in my house.

When you practice, mix your strikes, swings, and thrusts. Set up a station that you can practice on. Take a garbage can and flip it over.

Next, place a piece of wood on top of the can's bottom and strike the split log, knocking it off. Another method is to find a dead tree in the woods or some pole. If the tree is alive, wrap it up with carpet. Practice your strikes. These methods will provide you with feedback of the effectiveness of your strikes, how your grip is, and the best angles for maximum striking power.

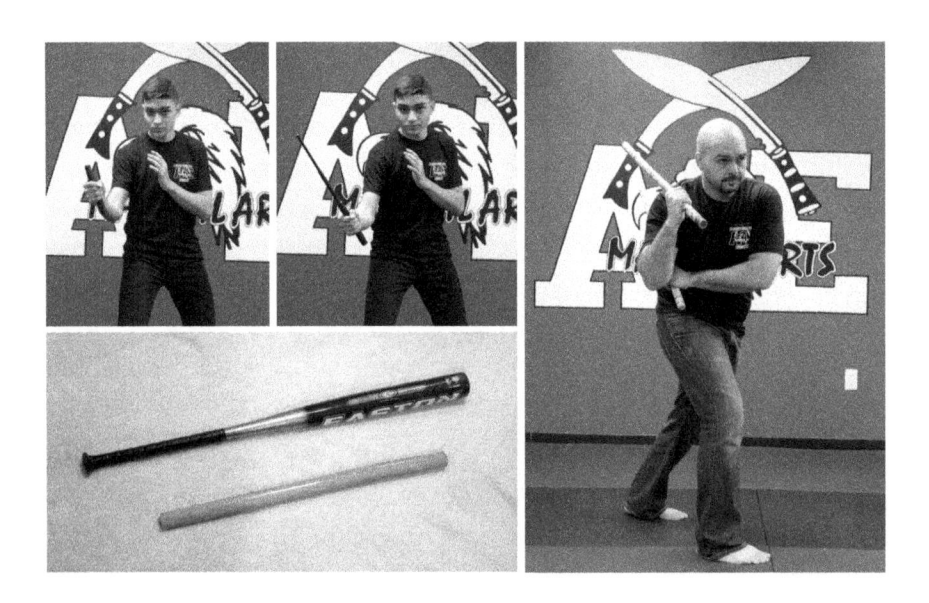

18
HOME PREPAREDNESS

Have some type of alarm or home warning system, or at least a window sticker. Some deterrent is better than none.

A dog is great for home protection. Most criminals will pass up on a house with a large dog and move on to one without a canine. They will travel the path of least resistance.

Have the emergency numbers coded into your phone and written down. Your electronic devices may be compromised.

Secure your windows and doors. Keep them locked and place a pole or dowel in the floor track of your sliding glass door. A sturdy dowel makes for an effective weapon too!

Strategically place weapons in every section of your house. Firearms, clubs, knives, swords, baseball bats, saps, black jacks, expandable batons, etc…should be available to you in an emergency. However, they need to be secured so that no unauthorized family members, especially the very young, can gain access to them. Also, be sure that you know who comes in and out of your house. More often than not, the friends of your children are very curious and coax your young ones into "showing" them a weapon. That's how accidents happen. Use your better judgment when it comes to the accessibility of weapons and "who" knows "where" "what" is. Nothing works better than common sense in action.

Have a plan *and* a backup plan. Murphy's law usually doesn't apply to backup plans. Make certain that everyone in the house knows the plan. "Man plans and God laughs. Man has a backup plan, and he smiles." Or so the saying goes.

Have a survival kit for natural disasters in addition to your weapons. Water, batteries, generator(s), canned goods, emergency food packs, etc.

Fire safety: Window ladders, smoke detectors, and fire extinguishers. Every floor should have a fire extinguisher, and all upper floors a window ladder. Make sure that your smoke and carbon monoxide detectors are fully operational, strategically placed, and have fresh batteries. A fire extinguisher is also a great weapon, both for spraying and to strike with.

The door: Do not open the door for uninvited, unscheduled guests. Period. Have them make an appointment—*then* show identification and clearly state why they are there before you even entertain letting them in. Many home invasions occur without forced entry. People are often duped to letting unidentified strangers into their homes.

Get a firearm and learn how to use it. The best home protection weapon is a pump-shot gun, preferably a 12 gauge. The ammunition should be shells loaded with buckshot. Consult the NRA and/or your local gun shop for firearms safety courses and lessons. Know your weapon and how to handle it. Avoid accidental shootings and keep your weapon in a safe but accessible place.

Practice moving about your home in darkness. Count the steps of your staircases; this will enable you to move more easily in the darkness without having to think. The assailant does not know your home like you do. Use your "home field" to your advantage.

19
Everyday Public Places

No matter how much you fortify your home, you will need to venture out. Now don't be mistaken, I'm not advocating you become a hermit living on some mountain top with an electric fence, a pack of pitbulls in the yard, and an M60 mounted to your roof on a turret; but you will have to take precautions when you go out in public. Bring with you weapons, either standard or unconventional, that you are adept at using and are legal in your jurisdiction. Be alert and watchful. Forget walking around with your headphones on and your eyes glued to your smart phone.

Mall Safety

The malls are a haven for criminals. The mall ownership sequesters the crime statistics, and many crimes go unreported and/or unrecorded. If the general population knew how much crime occurs at the mall, they would sit at home and do their shopping via Amazon! The mall is laden with predators. Look at the bounty they have to choose from! People have money on them, or at least credit cards. They are preoccupied with their task of shopping. The solitary targets generally don't travel in groups of more than two. There are mothers with children in strollers, older folks looking to get out of the house, others in a rush to get in and out. What a cornucopia of potential victims!

First, you must consider the mall parking lot. Shoppers laden with too many bags as they fruitlessly search for their car because they were too busy "updating their status" on Facebook and forgot to check where they parked. Huge mistake. You are a crime statistic waiting to happen.

Most crimes don't happen per chance. You have been targeted. Just like the lion looks for the slow, old, or weak zebra, you have been chosen as easy prey. Criminals, thugs, skells, hoodlums, and dirtbags, whatever you choose to refer to them as are purely predatory creatures. Know this and be aware of this at all times.

Do not be afraid to ask a salesperson to walk you to your vehicle. The retailers and the Mall do not want to be responsible for a theft, injury, or death of a customer, especially if they have asked for help. It's bad for business.

Look under and around your vehicle. Are there "unsavory characters" watching you? Is there someone under your vehicle waiting to slash your Achilles's tendon as you open your car door?

ELEVATOR

There are so many times that our "civilized" upbringing makes us vulnerable. If you are alone on an elevator and a group of rowdy youths enter, leave. When you are getting into the elevator, look at who is in there. If you feel strange passing it up and feel like saying something, say, "Oops, wrong direction!" And then move on. We are so preoccupied about insulting perfect strangers that we compromise our own safety. It is always better to avoid a situation than it is to defend yourself physically; so many things can go awry.

Let us suppose that you are alone on an elevator and you become surrounded by a rambunctious group of individuals. They begin to harass you and close in around you. Let us hope that you have a self-protection weapon at the ready. Most people do not have a concealed firearm carry permit. If you are one of those lucky few, now it's time to have your hand on the weapon. Don't brandish it until it's necessary and don't ever point a gun at something that you don't intend to shoot.

So you don't have a gun and you're faced with four hostile individuals, what's to happen to you? Hopefully, you have prepared yourself with some good training and have one of your weapons of choice with you. If you don't have any weapons, you will need to make the first strike. Go for the vital and semivital target areas—throat, eyes, groins, etc. Hit and move! Strike and spin, like an NFL running back spinning and turning as he cuts through the line. Keep moving. Do not allow yourself to be grabbed. You will have to hope for some good luck as well. As soon as the elevator door becomes open, get out!

Public Bathrooms

As always, look around and see who is sharing the room with you. If you are a female and there's a man in the restroom with you, turn around and get out! Be astute when you are entering the restroom. Was anyone watching you when you went in? Did someone follow you in? Keep your eyes peeled.

Guys, look out for groups of people. Also, you are very vulnerable when you are at the urinal. Once you are urinating, place your other hand against the wall. This will make it more difficult for a perpetrator to sneak up on you and slam you into the wall.

Restaurants

Once you arrive, scan the area. Look at the patrons and general layout. Locate the restrooms and the exits. Have a plan in mind in the event that a robbery or assault occurs. Take a walk through the restaurant and scout it out. Even if you don't have to go to the bathroom, do so. Always sit so that the door is in plain view. While you are out to dinner or in a restaurant, it is also important to recognize that you should never get too inebriated. You will not think clearly, and no matter what you think, your reactions are slower and less precise. Don't get drunk and leave yourself and those you are responsible for exposed.

Parties and Bars

This advice is primarily geared toward the younger set. The dangers that you may encounter when you are simply out trying to have a good time are many. Women are more often the target of drugging, but it may happen to guys well. Follow these rules, as well as all of the other safety rules and be alert. If something feels wrong, extradite yourself from the situation. Have a back-up plan and a means to leave.

1. Never take an open drink. Even if it's from someone you know. Do you trust that they had their eyes on the drink the whole time? No open drinks, even water. Only accept a closed beverage.
2. Keep your hand over the top of your glass and never set your drink down anywhere.
3. Know the people that you are attending the party with and have a meeting place designated.
4. *Do not* get uncontrollably drunk. There are far too many bad things that can happen to you if you are intoxicated or pass out.
5. Go in groups, especially if you are going to an unfamiliar location. There is safety in numbers.

20
Mass Hysteria

The year was 2004, and I was part of a crew working a security detail for an event hall. There were eleven of us working security, and we were equipped with metal detectors and wands to check the attendees for weapons prior to entrance to the party. The establishment was located in Little Ferry, New Jersey on Route 46 West and directly across the river from Paterson. This party was the last event to be held there. The hall was shut down after what transpired that night.

Steve Cirone (in this book) and I were on the detail. Things started to go awry from the beginning. We found out that the party was a jeans-and-boots party. This is not a good thing. The people showing up would not be dressed well, and generally people will act in accordance to their attire. Meaning that if one is dressed up and presentable, they will behave better. If they are wearing boots, jeans, and sweatshirts, they don't care if their clothes get messed up. Call it profiling, call it stereotyping, call it what you want. I'll call it what it is, a fact.

As the night went on, the patrons became more intoxicated. The owner was selling full champagne bottles, even though we advised him not to. There were factions from two rival gangs in attendance as well. That's when things really started to heat up.

Skirmishes were breaking out on and around the dance floor; the DJ was calling for security to intervene. In one skirmish, one of the partiers raised up his champagne bottle to strike someone. I grabbed his hand. I directed him to relax and put the bottle down. His response was not one of compliance. He then came at me, which elicited my survival reaction. I punched him square in the face. All hell broke loose. Steve Cirone planted a boot on the back of a rioter and sent them to the ground. The three of us—Steve, Tony (Blandino), and I—then went back to back to back. We fought our way to the kitchen; people were screaming, running, fighting. The place was in total chaos. I have no idea how we did not get hurt or even hit (that I can remember). We were shoving, kicking punching, bobbing, and weaving as we extracted ourselves from the immediate melee. Normally, I don't remember exactly what happens 100 percent in an altercation, until a witness fills me in. In this case, the witnesses that would have conveyed my actions to me (Steve and Tony) were all involved reacting to the impending situation.

There were cops from fifteen towns there, but none dared to come in. They waited outside in the parking lot. Police would not enter into a situation like this. The chance of them getting their weapons compromised was far too high. They generally wait until it dissipates or, in extreme cases, administer tear gas to move people out. They didn't have to in this case; people came out on their own accord. Someone threw a chair through a wall mirror and a woman screamed, "He has a *GUN!*" Now the brouhaha escalated to an even higher level! People started rushing for the door. We made certain that there was no gun and began to push and shove the crowd, "helping" them to get out of the door and into the parking lot.

Many of the rabble rousers began to fight with the police. It was quite a scene! Police cars, ambulances, blood, fights, rock throwing, bottles being broken, and throngs of people in conflict. The police wound up arresting a bunch, but most of them were simply "pushed" out of the area and toward the bridge heading to Paterson. As security personnel, we had succeeded in getting everyone out of the establishment. However, there were a great deal of mistakes made. Had I been in charge, I would have prompted everyone who was on staff prior to the evening so they were aware of the potential element. With that type of crowd, there should have been a plan in place or some mechanism to keep certain people out to have avoided the situation entirely. Again, I was not in charge. When the fights began, the other eight bouncers were nowhere to be found. They scattered, and the three of us were left to deal with the situation. Also, a staff of 11 bouncers for over 600 people is far too small. There should have been at least double what we had.

The important thing to note is that we kept our heads, knew when to act, when to exit, and where to go when push came to shove. There was a great deal of confusion, and people could have easily been killed, but no one was. However, the situation was a total cluster***k and wound up on the news for a couple of days afterwards. The establishment was shut down by the town after this debacle.

How does this story relate to you? You may never become a bouncer or a protection agent. However, you may find yourself in a situation where a crowd is in panic or is engaged in a riot. In this era of terrorist threats, unruly protesters and out of control mobs, what can you do? It's obvious to state that if you find yourself three feet away from an exploding back pack, then you were simply unlucky. No method, thought process, or training will help you then. The stars were not aligned in your favor. If that's not the case, you will have time to react to protect you and your loved ones.

Where we can help you is in the event of a terrorist attack, an uncontrolled mob, or whether it's a lone assailant, a group of shooters to explosive devices detonated from a distance or some type of chemical attack. The number one thing to remember is that *cooler heads prevail.* So keep your cool. You don't want to panic and run from the frying pan straight into the fire.

In all of these scenarios, *mass hysteria* will set in. People will be screaming and running wildly. I've been involved in a few of these incidents, and it's not a pretty sight. You have to be cognizant of not being trampled and not getting pushed in the wrong direction. Things get more complicated when you have a small child or otherwise "less self-sufficient" companion with you. Protect who you are with and try to have a wall to your back. Avoid getting knocked down and keep a visual on an exit.

We will consider several scenarios. Let us ponder the incident of a lone shooter. This may occur *anywhere.* In a mall, a school, a movie theater a parking lot, you name it. So you must maintain vigilance at all times.

Look, you don't have to run around in a complete paranoid state like John Belushi sneaking into Dean Wormer's office in Animal House,[48] but you do have to be aware. If you are walking around with your ear buds or your headphones blaring the latest Jay Z rap, how can you be in tune with your surroundings? Lose the headsets and anything else that will divert your attention. Be alert.

The first thing you do is to hit the deck and bring your loved ones down the floor with you. Don't stay on the ground long, though; people will begin to run amuck. The thing is, people will panic and will be running wildly. It's frightening to see the look of abject fear on their faces and in their eyes as they scramble aimlessly trying to flee. However, since you have been vigilant, you know where the closest exit is. Stay low and look for cover as you make your way to the nearest, most secure exit.

When considering these next scenarios, your course of action will not much different, just more difficult. If there are several shooters or explosive devices being detonated, please realize that you are most likely in the middle of an organized attack. You are living on borrowed time, so every second that you are alive is bonus time. Use it wisely. Immediately hit the deck and seek cover. Stay low.

Try to determine where the shooters are. In an organized attack, there may be diversions set up that will "funnel" the crowd into an even worse situation, so be cognizant of the options and don't rush toward the most obvious without being certain it's not a setup.

This is typical of terrorist attacks. They are counting on hysteria to maximize their death totals. Hopefully, Lady Luck will be on your side.

There are other situations to consider, albeit not a terrorist situation, but a safety issue. If you are in a public place and a fight breaks out, *move*! Exit the area posthaste. There are far too many incidents of innocent

---

[48] Animal House, released in 1978 by Warner Bros. If you have never seen it, I'd highly recommend this movie as a Comedy Classic.

bystanders getting injured or killed when a fight breaks out. Picture the scene: two or more guys get into a scuffle. Tempers flare, and one of the boneheads pulls out a gun and begins to fire. You have no control of where the bullets go.

You only have control over how you react to a situation. So react by removing yourself from harms way. As we have discussed before, you can avoid over 95% of situations simply by not being there. Exit the area Post Haste. Don't let curiosity do to you what it did to that cat.

21
CAR SAFETY

Make it a habit of being able to see the rear tires of the car in front of you when at a stop light. If you are able to see the rear tires of the vehicle in front of you, you will be able to pull around them.

This will prevent someone from boxing you in. Typically, if you are being set up, criminals will box you in by having a car in front and in back of you. Once you are boxed in, they will converge on your vehicle from both sides. If there is a car in front of you and one behind you and you notice the taillights of the car ahead of you illuminating, *move*! You are most likely being set up and had best remove yourself from the area.

Criminals will stoop to the lowest levels imaginable in order to relieve you of your money and property. There have been incidents of these deviants feigning distress by posing with a "baby" next to a "disabled" vehicle. There have been other occurrences of an attractive woman standing by a car looking helpless and forlorn. In both of these cases, their accomplice was in hiding nearby waiting for their opportunity to pounce on the hapless, Good Samaritan. Do not stop. Keep driving and call 911 to alert them of the person in need of roadside assistance. If you don't have a cell phone or service, wait until you come to a location that has a phone and then call.

You should have at your immediate disposal an expandable baton, club, or some other type of blunt instrument, a knife with a serrated edge and a chemical spray. Not only are these great defensive tactics weapons, but the blunt instrument and the knife can be used to help you extract yourself from a compromised vehicle in the case of an accident. The blunt club or baton may be used to break a window. The serrated knife can serve as a means to cut you loose from a malfunctioning seat belt.

Make certain that you have an emergency kit in your car. Mine includes a compass, pocket fishing pole, fishing lures, water purifying kit, handheld chain saw, fire starters, matches, flint, lightweight thermal blankets, MREs, a Leatherman, sharpening stone, collapsible eating utensil kit and a survival knife. You never know how long you are going to be stuck and who you might run into. There are several very good disaster survival books and courses to read or take. These are written by or conducted by others more qualified than me in these matters. I will defer the details of disaster preparation to these experts. I just felt the subject was worth mentioning.

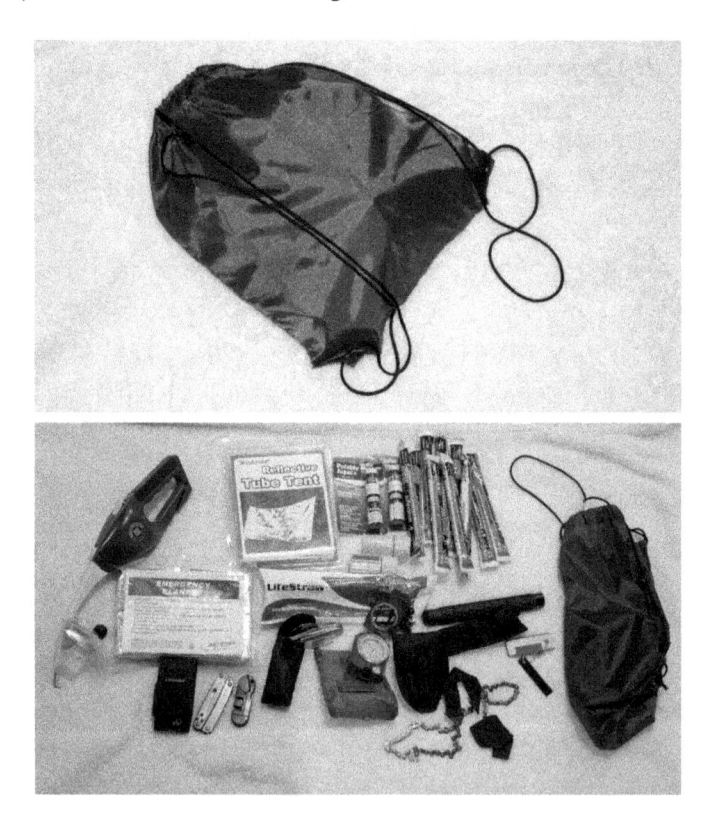

Unmarked police cars. Do not pull over if an unmarked police car tries to pull you over. Immediately call 911, especially if you were not speeding. Just because you are a guy, don't be all "macho" and think that nothing can happen to you. It can and it will. Call 911 and if you do get pulled over, don't open the car door or window until you have positive ID of the officer.

Road rage. As stated before, *cooler heads prevail.* Always keep this in mind. Yes, there are a great deal of bad drivers and complete fools out on the road, but are any of them worth more than your life? Don't ever pull over and get out of your car to "teach this guy a lesson." To many times people have been hurt or killed in this fashion. You may even get run over by an on coming car. There could be more than one person in the vehicle. He or she could have a weapon. Yes, I said she. There are prisons full of women, and the rate is rising. Maybe they want you to pull over so they can rob you. Whatever the case is, stay in your car.

At a stop light, always leave enough room in front of you to be able to see the back tires of the car in front. This ensures that you will be able to pull around the vehicle. If they begin to back up, move quickly!

Obstacles. If there are obstacles in the road, move around them. Do not stop. Flaming tires, road blocks, or crowds out and about on a street in a rough neighborhood late at night. Keep your windows up and keep moving.

Know where you are going. Knowing where you are going avoids a great deal of issues. Use your GPS, but also have printed directions and a map. Remember that a backup plan is essential. Familiarize yourself with you route prior to embarking on your journey.

Have weapons available. Keep some type of weapon in your car. You should have at your immediate disposal an expandable baton, club, or some other type of blunt instrument, a knife with a serrated edge and a chemical spray. If you carry a baseball bat with you, be sure to have a glove and ball in the car as well. You could simply state that you use it in the park to shag fly balls with your friends, if questioned. Not only are these great defensive tactics weapons, but the blunt instrument and the knife can be used to help you extract yourself from a compromised vehicle in the case of an accident. An expandable baton or metal pipe/club may be used to break a window in case of a crash either underwater or if the doors malfunction. Please make sure that it has another "use." A knife with a serrated edge may be used to cut you out of a jammed safety belt in case of a malfunction after an accident. Have your chemical deterrent in the car at the ready as well.

Always abide by this axiom: *It's better to have it and not need it than it is to need it and not have it.* Words to live by.

22

THE IMPORTANCE OF TRAINING: PRACTICE CYCLE

The saying goes: Victory does not favor the righteous or the wicked, *Victory Favors the Prepared.* The benefits and the transformation of your mind and body as a result of regular training are most likely more than you have ever imagined. Do not set limits on yourself and do not think that you are unable to develop the reflexes necessary to defend yourself adequately.

Consider the sport of baseball. It takes 400 milliseconds for the pitcher to deliver a baseball across home plate. The minimum human reaction time is 200 milliseconds. So a hitter must make his decision to swing at a ball by the time it's less than half way from the pitcher's hand to crossing home plate.

You may be asking yourself why this is important. What does it have to do with self defense training? It has everything to do with it. Please note that I stated "minimum human reaction time," Not an "Elite level athlete's reaction time."

Scientists have been studying human reaction times for over 40 years and attempting to link their reaction times to having some type of superior genetics common to elite athletes. Not the case. After many years of administering many tests it was determined that there was Zero difference between an Elite Athlete's reaction and the reaction time of your accountant. You may still be asking why this is important.

The point of this passage is to make apparent that you have the ability to develop quick reactions by training and training often. The only way a professional baseball player is able to hit a ball traveling 95 mph is due to his ability to predict where the ball will cross the plate. He is able to predict this because he has seen thousands upon thousands of pitches over many hours through many years of training. You can do the same thing.

You have the ability to develop IT, Instinctive Technique. Once you have trained yourself and you remove thought from the process.

You have the equipment and now you have the knowledge. It's all up to you to practice and practice properly. In order to give yourself the best chance of victory, you must be PREPARED!

Excuses for not training are far too common. Find a manner to succeed.

There is no way on earth that you will be able to practice all of the techniques, defensive tactics, strength and conditioning movements in this book on a daily basis. There is far too much volume and variations.

While training, you will need to warm-up sufficiently with your jump rope, mobility and flexibility routines for 5 to 7 minutes. Spend 20 to 25 minutes on the strength and conditioning and use the remainder of your session on your defensive tactics. A lot of how much time you spend on the different aspects of the training will depend upon what else you do. For example, if you train at a BJJ (Brazilian Jiu Jitsu) Academy, you will not want to spend too much time with your grappling. If you are a kickboxer, you'll want to spend less time on your striking combinations. If you are extremely fit and work out at a gym a great deal, spend more time working on your strikes, self defense and grappling and less time on the fitness aspects provided in this book.

If you'd like to train in the program 5 or 6 days a week, split it up. Spend an hour ever other day on the fitness and do your bag work, body conditioning, striking and grappling on the alternate days. You also have to consider when a training partner is available or not. If you are training solo, focus on your strength and conditioning, body conditioning (toughening) and your bag work. When you do have a partner, work on the defensive tactics, grappling and partner drills.

Below we have listed a guide to aid you in your training rotation.

SURVIVAL STRONG TRAINING ROTATION

1. Push-ups, Abs & Bridges. Pad Work: Station Rotation.
2. Handstands, Pull-ups & Squats. 4 Ranges of Combat.
3. Walk the Plank, Ab Crawls & Lunges. Ground up Fighting.
4. Dips, Cossacks & Planks. Zones and Herky Jerky.
5. Plyometric (Leap up, Thrusters, Push-ups). Body Conditioning.
6. Push-up, Squats & Bridges. Power Strikes.
7. Walk the Plank, Ab Crawls. Unconventional Weapons
8. Handstands, Bridges, Lunges. Get up from ground with attacker on you; prone and supine. Body Conditioning
9. Push-ups, Pull-ups, Abs, Squats. Multiple Attackers
10. Push-ups, Abs & Jump Rope, Handstands. Knife Attacks.
11. Pull-ups, Hanging Abs, Squats & Lunges. Power Strikes, Slaps & Punch Defense.
12. Handstands, Pull-ups, Bridges. Break Falls, Roll-outs, Upkicks
13. Push-ups, Dips, Abs. Power Strikes, Quick Strike Defense.
14. Push-ups, Squats, Bridges. Movement, Punch Defense and Baseball Bat Defense.
15. Handstands, Lunges, Back Pressure Abs. Cut Kicks, Slaps and Knife Defense.
16. Push-ups, Squats, Bridges, Dips. Knee Drives, Elbows and Bear Hugs.
17. Pull-ups, Dips, Abs, Bridges. Side & Front Kicks, Axehands & Wrist Locks.
18. Push-ups, Squats, Planks. Four Ranges of Combat.
19. Handstands, Bridges, Lunges. Throws and Sweeps.
20. Dips, Hanging Abs, Squats. Ground Fighting & Knife Defense, menacing.
21. Handstands, Bridges, Push-ups. Takedowns, Gun Defense.
22. Squats, Pull-ups, Planks. Dog Attacks, Knife at the throat.
23. Handstands, Dips, Lunges. Chokes: 3 & 4 Point, Front, with entries.

24. Bridges, Handstands, Ab Crawls. Power Strikes: Hands and Elbow with entries.
25. Pull-ups, Push-ups, Hanging Abs. Knife & Knife Vs Gun
26. Partner Bodyweight: Push-ups (hold ankles or on back), Abs (Standing or Dog Stance), Bridge Back (Greco Drill) & Squats (on back). Wrist Locks.
27. Dips, Plyo Squats/Box Jumps, Levers & "Phil-Ups". Club attacks.
28. Push-ups, Bridges, Lunges. 4 Ranges of Combat.
29. Handstands, Abs & Squats. Open hand strikes.
30. Pull-ups, Dips (rings too), Bridges. Kick Defense
31. Push-ups, Lunges, Abs. Choke and Guillotine Defense
32. Pull-ups, Bridges, Squats. Ground Attacks
33. Handstands, Hanging Abs, Plyo Squats. Wrist Locks.
34. Push-ups, Bridges, Squats. Knife Attacks, held to the neck.
35. Plyometrics – Push-ups & Squats. Kicks
36. Handstands, Abs. Elbows & Bear Hugs.
37. Bridges & Squats. Body Conditioning, Quick Strike Defense.
38. Push-ups & Abs. Ground up defense and Arm Drags to take down.
39. Pull-ups, Lunges, Dips. Kicks, Combos, Choke from behind
40. Dips, Plyometric Squats, Lying Abs. 1-6 Punches and Combinations.
41. Bridges, Handstands, Lunges. Power Strikes, Elbows and Knees
42. Terrorist Attacks: 1) Holstered, 2) Reloading, 3) From behind & 4) From the Front, you will need to drop and bear crawl or forward roll.
43. Dynamic Tension with Push-ups, Squats and Bridge and Hold. Ground Defense with arms pinned. Takedown and mount.
44. Plyo Push-ups, Spilt Squats and Table Top Bridge. Defense from the ground while being choked. Ground and pound from the top, once you reverse.
45. Handstands, Pull-ups. Knife Basics.
46. Push-ups, Abdominals. Throws: Hip Toss, Body Lock and Head Locks.
47. Squats (One and/or two legs), Bridges. Body Conditioning and Pad Work.

48. Lunges, Dips and Plyo Push-ups. Choke defense, standing and on the ground.
49. Bridges, Plyo Squats or Box Jumps. Four Ranges of Combat.
50. Handstands, Hanging Abs (or Abs), Push-ups. Car scenarios, Multiple Attackers.

The beauty of this information is that you are able to cater it to fit your needs, ability and time constraints. The most important aspect to bear in mind though is to train on a consistent basis. Once a month or once a week is not enough, three times is a *minimum*, but four or five times a week is recommended.

23
Breathing and Meditation

Breathing will help calm you and reduce anxiety during a stressful situation. When we experience adrenaline dumps, our breathing becomes shallow. If you are "chest breathing", you will run out of air quickly and become exhausted. This is *not* conducive to effectively defending yourself.

Get into the habit of breathing exercises and meditation. There are many effective methods to employ. I developed a Meditation CD, Powerful Spirit; it is twenty-three minutes long and based on self-hypnosis and the positive imagery as instructed at the West Point Military Academy. I've had significant success with my fighters and wrestlers using the CD. Even my mother's friends use it to fall asleep to!

I would recommend that you read some books on the powers of Zen and meditation. The knowledge will prove helpful for your training and overall mental health.

Epilogue

There are no short cuts to self defense, strength development and honing your survival skills. You must make your training a lifestyle and adapt the mindset of vigilance and preparedness. When I first embarked on this book, the dangers of terrorism and social unrest were already on the rise and I observed the ever growing constraints placed upon law enforcement and the general population. People, on a whole are good hearted and just simply want the live their lives. Unfortunately, there are factions whether they be radical religious fanatics, sociopaths or hardened criminals, that we may have to deal with. No one is immune. We must realize that the police and the government will not be there to provide protection at all times and that protecting ourselves is ultimately our responsibility.

This information contained in this book has an incredible amount of material, advice and techniques. However, the movements and strategies must be practiced on a regular basis and there is no substitute for hands on instruction by a qualified instructor. If you cannot find a suitable instructor in your area, we conduct Survival Strong Seminars and Workshops and can come to your facility.

The movements and exercises in this book are relatively basic and can be learned and executed by virtually anyone. More advanced movements, more difficult strength exercises and in depth weapons, blunt and edged as well as grappling and striking will be covered in future publications.

Good luck in your training and other than the strength and conditioning in this book, I hope that you never have to use any of the techniques in a real life situation. If you do, let's hope that the avoidance strategies have enabled you to avoid the conflicts. If not, I'm confident that if you have practiced hard and often, developed your

"IT", you will react properly. Remember to act concisely, decisively and with great fervor.

Strength and Honor,

Coach Phil

Recommended Training Aids

There are a certain minimum amount of items that you will need to maximize your training efforts. Listed below are some equipment, books and videos that I have found extremely beneficial to my mindset and physical conditioning.

Equipment

Focus mitts
Rubber knife and gun
Clubs or baseball bats (wiffleball bats acceptable for training)
Jump rope
Kicking shields
Various unconventional weapons as previously listed
Body conditioning (hardening) tools
Staff or dowel, 6 feet
Martial arts belts
Towel
Abdominal wheel (wheel of death)

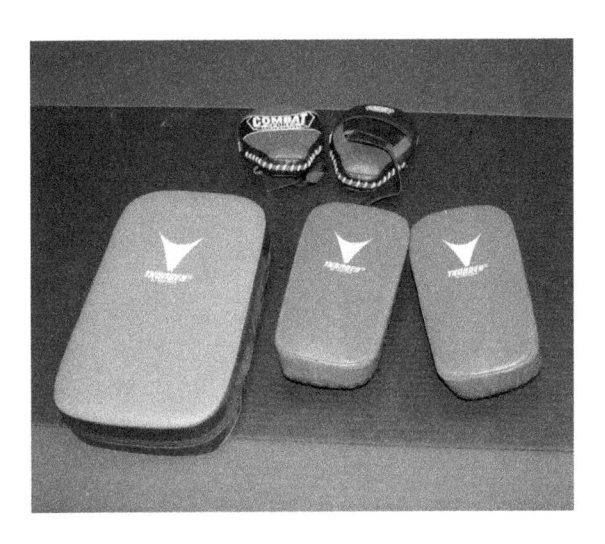

RECOMMENDED TRAINING MATERIAL:

The Convict Conditioning Series (1, 2, and 3)
By Coach Paul Wade

Ferocious Fitness (available Fall 2016)
By Phil Ross
These books are available from Dragon Door
http://www.dragondoor.com/?apid=4640

Main Site: www.philross.com and/or
http://www.survivalstrongofficial.com/

Phil Ross' *S.A.V.E. Video Training Series*
Complete Set, 4 videos & Audio CD Mental Preparation CD

To increase your strength and conditioning, delve into kettlebell training. The Kettlebell Workout Library has Bodyweight, Plyometrics and Flexibility as well as 104 Kettlebell Based Workouts on 20 hours of Video Footage, and a 144 page full color manual depicting every workout.

www.kettlebellking.com or Call: **877-382-8010, 201-612-1429**

OTHER SOURCES

www.juijitsustrength.com

SUGGESTED READING MATERIALS

I have read a multitude of books over the years, and several of them have had a profound impact on my thinking and training. Either by reaffirming what I had already experienced or by enhancing my training in a positive direction.

The Way and the Power: Secrets of Japanese Strategy
Frederick J. Lovret

Kill or Get Killed
Col. Rex Applegate
MMA for Dummies
Frank Shamrock

Infinite Insights into Kenpo
Ed Parker

A Book of Five Rings
Miyamoto Musashi

Ultimate Athleticism
Max Shank
http://ultimateathleticism.com/

A Guide to Martial Arts Training with Equipment
Dan Inosanto

Appendix:

Accomplishments and Credentials
2014:   Chief Instructor for Survival Strong
2014:   Kettlebell and Bodyweight Consultant for Parisi's
2013:   Progressive Calisthenics Certified
2012:   Promoted to Master RKC Kettlebell Instructor
2012:   Team Alliance Brazilian Jiu Jitsu Instructor
2011:   East-West Martial Alliance: Appointed as System Head (Naban)
2010:   NAGA Battle of the Beach: Expert Submission Fighting Champion
2010:   RKC Team Leader and CK-FMS Certified Movement Specialist
2009:   Region 2 Wrestling Team of the Year, Head Coach, Mahwah
2009:   NBIAL Wrestling Champs, Head Coach, Mahwah
2008-2012: UFC Fight Trainer, Corner and Coach
2008:   County Wrestling Champs, Head Coach, Mahwah
2008:   RKC Certified Level 2 Instructor
2008:   Asst. Wrestling Coach of the Year, District 5 NJSAAI
2007:   RKC Certified Kettlebell Instructor
2007:   Head of Security, NJ All-Star Girls Soccer Team to Brazil
2007:   NJ Licensed Mixed Martial Arts Trainer and Manager

2006: Mahwah HS Wrestling Coach, League Champs, State Sectionals
2005: Certified Shamrock Submission Fighting Level II Instructor
2005: Inducted to the Action Martial Arts Hall of Fame
2004: Certified Shamrock Submission Fighting Level I Instructor
2003: AFPA Certified Personal Trainer
2000: Garden State Games Black Belt Heavyweight Sparring Champion
2000: Garden State Games Karate Masters' Kata Champion
1999: Certified CDT Master Tactical Instructor
1998: Medalist in Weapons, Kata & Free-Fighting, Bando Nationals
1997: President Elect of the International Federation of Fighting Arts
1997: NRA Certified in Use of Handguns for Protection Purposes
1997: Featured in the CDT Police and Bodyguard Manual
1996: MVP Award in the New York vs. New Jersey Team Challenge
1996: United Kung Fu Federation - Competitor of the Year Award
1995: Amateur National Heavyweight Freestyle Fighting Champion
1995: Garden State Games Empty hand and Weapons Dual Medalist
1994: World Martial Arts Hall of Fame – "Man of the Year"
1994: Instructor, NJ Department of Criminal Justice, Defensive Tactics
1994: Captain of Garden State Games – Black Belt Championship Team
1994: Captain of World Karate Union – Team New Jersey
1993: Instructor for the State of the Art Security Training Commission
1993: NJ State AAU Tae Kwon Do Chairman
1992: Bronze Medalist – AAU Tae Kwon Do Nationals
1989: Featured Performer ABC WWS "Oriental World of Self Defense"
1989: Garden State Games, Black Belt Heavyweight Gold Medalist
1988: Big Apple Challenge Heavyweight Karate Champion
1987: Reebok Classic Powerlifting Champion – 181 lbs.
1983: Mr. DC – Middleweight Bodybuilding, 3rd Place
1982: University of Maryland Olympic lifting Champion – 181 lbs.
1981: Empire State Games Karate Champion
1981: Mr. Wilkes Bodybuilding Champion
1979: AAU Junior Olympic Eastern National Greco-Roman Runner-Up

CPSIA information can be obtained
at www.ICGtesting.com
Printed in the USA
FFHW020801010219
50389209-55525FF

9 781514 455135